Building Better Caregivers

A Caregiver's Guide to Reducing Stress and Staying Healthy

Kate Lorig, DrPH • **Diana Laurent**, MPH
Robert Schreiber, MD • **Maureen Gecht-Silver**, OTD, MPH, OTR/L
Dolores Gallagher Thompson, PhD, ABPP
Marian Minor, RPT, PhD • **Virginia González**, MPH
David Sobel, MD, MPH • **Danbi Lee**, PhD, OTD, OTR/L

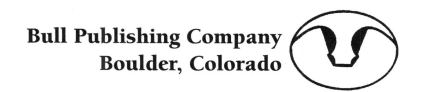

Copyright © 2018 Bull Publishing Company and the Self-Management Resource Center

All rights reserved. No part of this publication may be reproduced, distributed, or transmitted in any form or by any means, including photocopying, recording, or other electronic or mechanical methods, without the prior written permission of the publisher, except in the case of brief quotations embodied in critical reviews and certain other noncommercial uses permitted by copyright law.

Published by Bull Publishing Company
P.O. Box 1377
Boulder, CO, USA 80306
www.bullpub.com

Library of Congress Cataloging-in-Publication Data

Lorig, Kate

Building better caregivers / Kate Lorig, DrPH, Diana Laurent, MPH, Robert Schreiber, MD, Maureen Gecht-Silver, OTD, MPH, OTR/L, Dolores Gallagher Thompson, PhD, ABPP, Marian Minor, RPT, PhD, Virginia González, MPH, David Sobel, MD, MPH, Danbi Lee, PhD, OTD, OTR/L

pages cm

Includes bibliographical references and index.

Cataloging-in-Publication Data is available at the Library of Congress.

ISBN 978-1-945188-16-9 (paperback)

Printed in U.S.A.

23 22 21 20 19 18 10 9 8 7 6 5 4 3 2 1

Interior design and project management: Dovetail Publishing Services

Cover design and production: Shannon Bodie, BookwiseDesign.com

To David Bull, who made this book possible

The Authors

Kate Lorig, DrPH, is professor emerita at Stanford University School of Medicine and a partner in the Self-Management Resource Center (SMRC). As director of the Stanford Patient Education Research Center she was a co-developer of the Building Better Caregivers educational program. For 20 years, Kate watched her mother care for her father, who was severely disabled by a stroke.

Diana Laurent, MPH, is a health educator and partner in the Self-Management Resource Center. During her over 30 years at Stanford School of Medicine, she co-developed the Building Better Caregivers program, as well as several other educational programs. Diana was and is a caregiver of her parents and in-laws; she also has experience in participating in the care of relatives who have dementia.

Rob Schreiber, MD, is a board-certified geriatrician/internist and the vice president/medical director of Summit ElderCare, the largest PACE (Program of All inclusive Care for the Elderly) program in Massachusetts. Previously, he was the physician-in-chief at Hebrew SeniorLife in Boston, Massachusetts, and on the faculty of Harvard Medical School for over 20 years. Rob has been a caregiver for his parents, as well as multiple other elderly family members and actively works with caregivers in his role at Summit ElderCare.

Maureen Gecht-Silver, OTD, MPH, OTR/L, is an assistant professor of clinical family medicine and occupational therapy at University of Illinois at Chicago. In her clinical and academic roles, she has worked towards improving self-management skills and quality of life for people with chronic conditions and disabilities as well as their caregivers. Maureen, along with her sisters, was a caregiver for her father, who lived to age 98.

Dolores Gallagher Thompson, PhD, ABPP, is board-certified in clinical psychology and geropsychology and is professor emerita at Stanford University School of Medicine and co-director of the Optimal Aging Center in Los Altos, California. She has 30 years of experience in conducting funded intervention research with family caregivers and worked directly with caregivers in her clinical practice at Stanford. Dolores entered this field after being a long-distance caregiver for her mother who suffered multiple strokes before her death; at that time few resources for caregiving families were available and her experience shaped her subsequent career choices.

Marian Minor, PT, MSPH, PhD, is a professor emerita at the University of Missouri School of Health Professions where she taught and did research on exercise. She has contributed exercise information for self-management education for a variety of populations. Marian has been a caregiver herself and has supported other caregivers for many years.

Virginia González, MPH, is a health educator and partner in the Self-Management Resource Center (SMRC). She has over 15 years of experience working at the Stanford School of Medicine, where she was a co-developer of various self-management programs and was instrumental in the cultural adaptation and Spanish translation of these programs for Latino/Hispanic communities. After leaving Stanford and before becoming a partner in SMRC, Virginia was raising her children, while caring for her aging, chronically ill parents and in-laws. She also has personal experience with caring for extended family members with dementia and mental illness.

David Sobel, MD, MPH, is adjunct lecturer in the Department of Medicine, Stanford University School of Medicine. As the medical director of Patient Education and Health Promotion for Kaiser Permanente Northern California, he has developed and evaluated programs to serve over five million Kaiser members. In addition to assisting in the care of both his parents during their nineties, David is currently helping to manage the care for a family member with advanced dementia.

Danbi Lee, PhD, OTD, OTR/L, is an assistant professor in the Department of Rehabilitation Medicine at University of Washington in Seattle, Washington. Her work is focused on improving the experiences of people with disabilities and their caregivers as they transition into meaningful community activities and roles after rehabilitation. Danbi has personal experience supporting family members with dementia and stroke.

Acknowledgments

Many people have helped us write this book. Among the most important are the first 200 participants of the Stanford University Building Better Caregiver studies. These have been followed by thousands of other online and small group workshop participants. These caregivers, along with our wonderful workshop leaders, have told us what information they needed and helped us make adjustments as we went along.

There are also many professionals who have assisted us: We are especially thankful to the guidance and insights of Laural Traylor, MSW, and Theodore J. Hahn, MD, from the Veterans Administration, Bonnie Bruce, RD, DrPH, Cindy Tan, MPH, Chaplain Bruce Feldstein, MD, Catherine Regan, PhD, and Richard Seidel, PhD. To all of you, your help has been gratefully received.

There are also many friends, leaders, and trainers who have given us wonderful advice and added richness to our thinking: Fran Rice and Jean Thompson.

We would also like to thank the publishers for permission to adapt sections from *The Healthy Mind, Healthy Body Handbook* (also published as *The Mind & Body Health Handbook*) by David Sobel, MD, and Robert Ornstein, PhD (published by DRx).

Finally, thanks to David Bull to whom this book is dedicated. David was our first publisher and had faith in this project that allowed us to proceed. Without him, there may never have been a book. His son Jim has continued the family tradition with support and encouragement.

If you would like to learn more about our continuing work, online internet programs, trainings, and materials see our website:

https://www.selfmanagementresource.com

If you would like to find workshops near you see:

http://www.eblcprograms.org/evidence-based/map-of-programs/

We are continually revising and improving this book. If you have any suggestions or comments, please send them to:

smrc@selfmanagementresource.com

Contents

1 Introduction: A Blueprint for Better Caregiving 1

2 Becoming a Better Caregiver: The Basics 9

3 Dealing with Stress and Difficult Care Partner Behavior 25

4 Dealing with Difficult Emotions 35

5 Using Your Mind to Manage Stress 49

6 Communicating Effectively 71

7 Getting Help 93

8 Preventing Injuries 109

9 Exercising for Health and Wellness 145

10 Healthy Eating 169

11 Understanding Your Care Partner's Brain 195

12 Managing Medications 215

13 Making Treatment Decisions 231

14 Planning for the Future: Fears and Reality 237

Index 259

Disclaimer

This book is not intended to replace common sense, or professional medical or psychological advice. You should seek and get appropriate professional evaluation and treatment for problems—especially unusual, unexplained, severe, or persistent symptoms. Many symptoms and diseases require and benefit from specific medical or psychological evaluation and treatment. Don't deny yourself or your care partner proper professional care.

- If your or your care partner's symptoms or problems persist beyond a reasonable period despite using self-care recommendations, you should consult a health professional. What is a reasonable period will vary; if you're not sure and you're feeling anxious, consult a health care professional.
- If you receive professional advice in conflict with this book, you should rely upon the guidance provided by your or your care partner's health care professional. They are likely to be able to take your specific situation, history, and needs into consideration. If you are experiencing violence in your home, get out and seek help from health care professionals and/or law enforcement.
- If you are having thoughts of harming yourself in any way, please seek professional care immediately.

Medical treatment and knowledge are continually evolving. This book is as accurate as its publisher and authors can make it at the time of publication, but we cannot guarantee that it will work for you or your care partner in every case. The authors and publisher disclaim any and all liability for any claims or injuries that you may believe arose from following the recommendations set forth in this book. This book is only a guide; your common sense, good judgment, and partnership with health professionals are also needed.

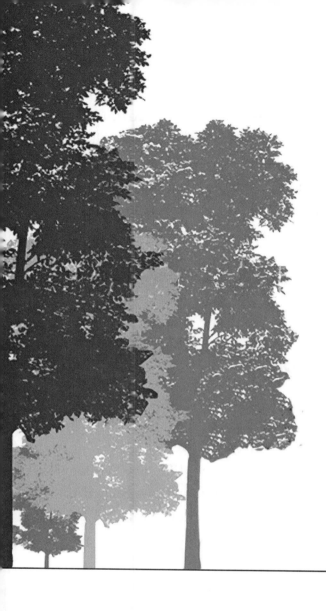

CHAPTER 1

Introduction: A Blueprint for Better Caregiving

As we plan for our lives, there are many things we prepare for and expect. Many of us go to school, get married, have children, lose love ones, become empty nesters, go to work, etc. Caregiving is not usually part of our expected life plan. Most people do not ask to be caregivers, prepare to be caregivers, and sometimes do not want to be caregivers. Nevertheless, we are caregivers and, more importantly, we have chosen to be caregivers.

The last statement may seem a little strange. We did not choose to have our relative, spouse, or friend become ill or injured and need care. What we did choose, however, was to care for them. Many people for one reason or another do not make this choice and do not provide care to others. So, congratulations for making that choice and being a caregiver! You are a very special person! As the authors of this book, we are here to share our expertise and the best in caregiving research. We also share what we have learned from thousands of people like you as well as our own experiences as caregivers. Together, we hope to help you gain skills you need to take care of yourself and your care partner. Probably the most important thing that these skills will give you, though, is confidence to manage your life and reduce your stress. Our goal is to improve the quality of life for both you and your care partner.

Right now, you may be wondering just what a care partner is. Your care partner is the person for whom you are caring. Your care partner may be Sally, or Jose, your "Sweetie," your "Dad," or your "Old Man." No matter what you call the person, in this book, we use the term *care partner* to refer to this person. We do this primarily because it is awkward to always say "the person you are caring for." A wonderful group of caregivers suggested this name and it works well for our purposes in this book.

How to Use This Book

Before we go any further, let's talk about this book and how to use it. Throughout, you will find information to help you learn and practice your caregiving skills. Some of these skills will help your care partner, but most of the skills are aimed at helping you to both care for someone else and to care for yourself. This is not a textbook. You do not need to read every word in every chapter. Instead, we suggest that you read the first four chapters and then use the table of contents or the index to seek the information you need. Feel free to skip around. In this way, you will learn the skills you need to negotiate your individual path.

So, what is in this book? You will not find any miracles or cures in these pages. Rather, you will find hundreds of tips and ideas to make your life easier. This is your "Caregiver's Toolbox." This advice comes from physicians and other health professionals, as well as caregivers like you. The content is supported by research and studies and it is as up-to-date as possible.

Caregiving is a great leveler. It does not matter if you went to school for five years or 20 years. Nor are caregiving skills related to race, age, gender, or genetics. Everyone can learn them. The good news is that there is no test, not even pass or fail.

Our assumption is that most caregivers are doing a terrific job under conditions that are often difficult. In addition to being a challenging job, caregiving can also be isolating. You may be cut off from friends and even family. This makes learning from others difficult. To help you overcome this isolation, we have talked to hundreds of caregivers as well as people who study caregiving. What we have learned, we have put into this book. Our hope is that sharing by this wisdom and knowledge from others, we can help you and others like you become better caregivers.

Stress and Caregiving

Caregiving is stressful. This is one of the things that we have been told by everyone who has experience with caregiving and caregivers. It is almost impossible to be a caregiver without experiencing increased stress. For some, this may be a little stress and for others, lots of stress. The figure shown here illustrates stressors—the things that can cause caregiver stress. In this book, we will discuss each of these stressors in detail and give you some information on how to develop the skills needed to deal with these stressors. As you gain more confidence in your skills, our hope is that your stress decreases.

But what is stress? In the 1950s, the physiologist Hans Selye described stress as "the nonspecific response of the body to any demand made upon it." Others have expanded this definition to explain that the body adapts to demands, whether pleasant or unpleasant. In short, stress is how we react emotionally to a stressor. The stressor can be a dog barking, receiving bad or even good news, someone saying unkind words, or fear of the future. For caregivers, it is often the frustrating or difficult behaviors of our care partners (more about this later). When we are exposed to stressors, not only do we have an *emotional* reaction, such as anger, sadness, or crying, but our bodies also react *physically* with muscle tension, headaches, fatigue, or pain. Our hearts may beat faster and we might have problems breathing. Stress can cause us to shout, weep, go quiet, flee, or smile nervously.

If all this seems complex, you are right. Stress is complex. Thankfully, you do not have to understand how stress works to do something about it. Consider the following two people and their stories:

- John has been a caregiver for Julianna for many months. He has lost contact with most of their friends. Julianna has Alzheimer's disease, and it seems like every day she remembers less and less. John is worried about his ability to cope and one day when Julianna cannot remember his name. John becomes

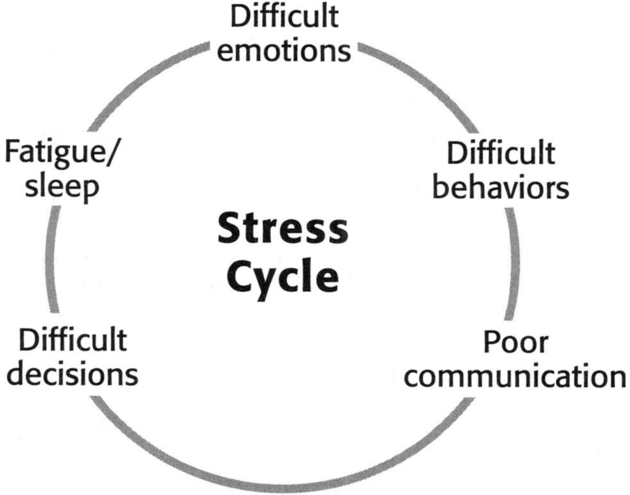

angry, sits down, and cries. Julianna looks confused and frightened.

- Ellen has been the caregiver for Jose for many months. He has Alzheimer's disease and it seems like every day his memory gets worse. Ellen is worried about her ability to cope, but she has found an online support group and she also talks to her friends about her concerns. One day, Jose cannot remember her name. Ellen is sad and mourns for all they both have lost. She takes a few minutes for herself and then gives Jose a dish of his favorite ice cream. He smiles.

These two examples are similar. The stressor—a care partner not remembering a spouse's name—is the same. The immediate emotional reaction of the two caregivers is also similar; they both feel sadness. There are also differences. Ellen has some support. She has both maintained contact with friends and joined an online support group. John does not seem to have any support. John's sadness is accompanied with anger that frightens his care partner. Ellen's sadness prompts her to try to show her love to her care partner. Her reward is a smile.

In the chapters to follow, you will find many tools for dealing with stress. Chapter 2, Becoming a Better Caregiver: The Basics, gives you the basic tools discussed in this book and Chapter 3, Dealing with Stress and Difficult Care Partner Behavior, is a thorough introduction to the basics of stress.

Thinking about Caregiving

By itself, changing the way you think cannot cure stress. However, positive thinking and certain caregiver skills can make caregiving easier. What you do about something is largely determined by how you think about it. For example, if you think that being a caregiver is like falling into a deep pit, you may have a hard time motivating yourself to crawl out, or you may think the task is impossible. The thoughts you have can greatly determine what happens to both you and your care partner.

The following are some of the thoughts that caregivers have shared with us and some suggestions for ways to address the problems that these thoughts present:

"When things do not go right or my care partner behaves badly, it is my fault."

You are not to blame. You did not cause your care partner's condition. Your care partner's behavior is the result of trauma or genetic, biological, environmental, and/or psychological factors. We do not feel guilty when a young child has a tantrum or wets his pants. These behaviors are part of a developmental process. Similarly, your care partner's behaviors are caused by a disease, not by you. However, in both cases you are responsible for helping to manage these behaviors. We talk more about strategies to manage care partner behavior in Chapter 3, Dealing with Stress and Difficult Care Partner Behavior.

"I feel so guilty."

Guilt is a common caregiver feeling. You are probably doing the very best you can. You may also feel guilty because you want your old life back. Believe us when we say that almost every caregiver feels this way.

"I should have done that when I had the chance."

There are lots of "if only I had (fill in the blank with anything you wish you had done) when I had the chance." Well, you have a chance now. We cannot remake the past, but we can to some extent determine the present and the future.

"I am so isolated; I feel so alone. No one offers any help."

You don't have to do it alone. One of the common side effects of caregiving is a feeling of isolation. As supportive as friends and family members may be, they often cannot understand what you are experiencing as you struggle to cope and survive daily. They do not know how to help and they stay away. You may have told them that there is nothing they can do.

Connecting with other people with similar situations can reduce your sense of isolation and help you understand what to expect based on a fellow caregiver's perspective. Other people can offer practical tips on how to manage on a day-to-day basis, give you the opportunity to help others cope with their caregiving, help you appreciate your strengths, and realize that things could be worse. They can inspire you to become a better caregiver. Support can come from reading a book or a newsletter about the experiences of other caregivers. Or it may come from regularly scheduled family meetings or from talking with others on the telephone, in support groups, or connecting online through computer and electronic support groups. Invite people to bring in a meal, use social media such as Facebook or Instagram, use FaceTime or Skype to video chat with distant friends and relatives. You will find more about getting support in Chapter 3, Dealing with Stress and Difficult Care Partner Behavior, and Chapter 7, Getting Help.

We know that caregivers do not have much time, but we also know that good caregivers do not do it alone. You need consultants such as other caregivers, family, friends, health professionals, and social service agencies. Your job is to learn from and to manage these consultants. As a caregiving manager, you gather information, make decisions, and perhaps hire a consultant or team of consultants, such as a health care professional or caregiving help. Then you must follow through.

Succeeding as a Caregiver

In this book, we describe many skills and tools to help you succeed as a caregiver and address real problems such as how to relieve caregiving stress. You may find that some are more helpful than others. Some may not be helpful at all. What we ask is that you try something before you reject it. You might be surprised and have a new caregiving tool. We do not expect you to use them all. Pick and choose. Experiment. Set your own goals. *What you do may not be as important as the sense of confidence and control that comes from successfully doing something you want to do.*

We have all noticed that some caregivers get on well and seem content with their task, while others have daily problems and are miserable. The difference often lies in their caregiver skills and management style.

The keys to success in any undertaking are, first, to define the problem and explore possible solutions; second, you must decide what you want to do and how you are going to do it; and third, you must learn a set of skills and practice them until they have been mastered. But we have learned that knowing the skills is not enough. To succeed, we need a way of incorporating these skills into our daily lives. Whenever we try a new skill, the first attempts may be clumsy, slow, and might not work. It is easier to return to old ways than to continue trying to master new and sometimes difficult tasks. The best way to master new skills is through practice and evaluation of the results. In Chapter 2, Becoming a Better Caregiver: The Basics, we introduce and discuss three core caregiving skills: problem-solving, decision-making, and action-planning.

You Are More than a Caregiver

When you are a caregiver, too often there seems to be nothing more to life than caregiving. But you are more than a carer for your care partner. It is essential to grow areas of your life that you enjoy. Small daily pleasures can help balance the other parts in which you must manage uncomfortable and demanding tasks or emotions. Find ways to enjoy nature by growing a plant or watching a sunset, or indulge in the pleasure of human touch or a tasty meal, or celebrate companionship with family or friends. Finding ways to introduce moments of pleasure is vital.

Focus on your abilities and assets rather than disabilities and deficits. Celebrate small improvements—improvement in your caregiving, in your stress level, and in your care partner's emotions and behaviors. If caregiving teaches anything, it is to live each moment more fully. Within the true limits of whatever problems you and your care partner have, there are ways to enhance your sense of control and enjoyment of life.

Some of the most successful caregivers are people who think of caregiving as a path. This path, like any path, goes up and down. Sometimes it is flat and smooth. At other times, the way is rough. To negotiate this path, one has to use many strategies. Sometimes you can go fast; other times you must slow down. There are obstacles to negotiate.

As we build better caregivers, we first must prepare to create an overall plan. In this chapter, we outlined some of the many challenges caregivers face and some basic ways you can approach those challenges. In the next chapter, we build the foundation and structure and walk you through building a personal action plan of your own. After that, you can read the chapters in whichever order you prefer and pick and choose the skills that will be most helpful to you. At the end of most of the other chapters, we list suggested readings and other resources. You will see some of these more than once, as certain resources cover several topics. Just remember, this is your Caregiver's Toolbox. You are the builder and we are here to help.

Suggested Further Reading

Blum, Alan, and Stuart Murray. *The Ethics of Care: Moral Knowledge, Communication, and the Art of Caregiving*. New York: Routledge, 2017. Offers discussions from a variety of disciplinary approaches, including sociology, communication, and social theory. http://amzn.to/2Cq1YRG

Bucher, Julia A. *American Cancer Society Complete Guide to Family Caregiving*. Atlanta: American Cancer Society, 2011. Offers information, techniques, resources, and insights into caregiving. Includes checklists, questions to ask the doctor, signs and symptoms, and a glossary of terms. http://amzn.to/2BuRRxU

Burgio, Louis D., Joseph E. Gaugler, and Michelle M. Hilgeman. *Spectrum of Family Caregiving for Adults and Elders with Chronic Illness*. Oxford: Oxford University Press, 2016. Written for individuals who serve family caregivers who are supporting an adult or elder with a chronic condition. It includes eight disease-specific chapters written by experts from various disciplines. http://amzn.to/2o1QqPY

Casey, Nell. *An Uncertain Inheritance: Writers on Caring for Family*. New York: Harper Perennial, 2008. A collection of essays from accomplished writers examining caregiving from every angle. http://amzn.to/2EJKTHw

Gaugler, Joseph. *Family Caregiving in the New Normal*. Cambridge, MA: Academic Press, 2015. Discusses how sociodemographic trends like divorce, increased participation of women in the workforce, geographic mobility, fewer children in post-baby boom families, chronic illness trends, economic stressors, and the current policy environment have started a new conversation on how family care for older adults will evolve. http://amzn.to/2sxok3F

Hewitt-Taylor, Jaqui. *Children with Complex and Continuing Health Needs: The Experiences of Children, Families and Care Staff*. London: Jessica Kingsley Publishers, 2008. A book of case studies that illustrate the experiences of children, parents, siblings, and extended families, as well as professionals in health and social care. http://amzn.to/2C0Cz5d

Mace, Nancy L., and Peter V. Rabins. *The 36-Hour Day: A Family Guide for People Who Have Alzheimer Disease, Other Dementias, and Memory Loss*. 6th ed. Baltimore: Johns Hopkins Press Health Book, 2017.

Marriott, Hugh. *The Selfish Pig's Guide to Caring*. London: Hachette, 2012.

Other Resources

AARP has a section of various resources for family caregivers, including information about where to find local resources. https://www.aarp.org/caregiving/

Caring.com supports caregivers as they care for aging parents, spouses, and other loved ones 50+ by providing articles, helpful tools, a comprehensive local directory of caregiving services, and the collective wisdom of an involved community. https://www.caring.com

CaringInfo by the National Hospice and Palliative Care Organization offers free resources and information (online and over the phone) about end-of-life care and services including information about advance care planning, financial assistance, hospice care, and grief. http://www.caringinfo.org

Family Caregiver Alliance is the first community-based non-profit organization in the country to address the needs of families and friends providing long-term care for loved ones at home. The services, education programs, and resources FCA provides offer support, tailored information, and tools to manage the complex demands of caregiving. https://www.caregiver.org. Refer to Fact and Tip Sheets for specific information. https://www.caregiver.org/fact-sheets

The National Volunteer Caregiving Network (NVCN) provides technical assistance, educational webinars, national conferences, information, referrals, and mentorship, among other benefits for members. http://www.nvcnetwork.org

The Senior List is a lifestyle brand focused on the needs of boomers and older adults across the United States that engages in discussions about caregiving. https://www.theseniorlist.com/category/caregiving

Today's Caregiver provides online information and support to family caregivers, including a resource that helps to identify and locate caregiver support groups and other caregiver resources in specific counties, including non-profit organizations, rural caregiver resources, and products and services. https://caregiver.com

Well Spouse Association is a national, non-profit membership organization that provides support to wives, husbands, and partners of the chronically ill and/or disabled. http://www.wellspouse.org

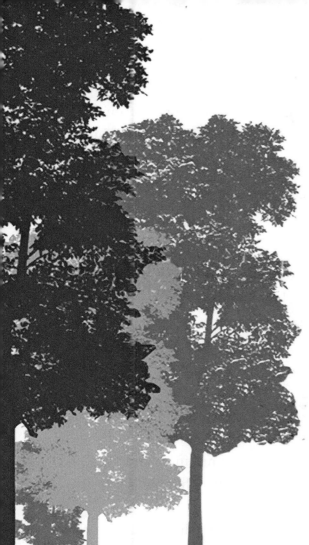

Chapter 2

Becoming a Better Caregiver: The Basics

You know better than anyone that becoming a caregiver means making many changes—changes in what you do and how you do it, and changes in how you socialize. It may mean giving up a paid job or working less. It also changes the dynamics of families and friendships. For some people, caregiving is full time, 24 hours a day every day. For other people, it takes up a few hours a week.

No matter how much time it takes or how complex the caregiving, as a caregiver you have a major decision to make. Are you going to take it one day at a time and cope the best you can, or are you going to become a better caregiver by learning skills, problem-solving, and planning? Please note the word *decision*. There is no way to avoid deciding. If you choose to do nothing, that is one way of deciding. If your decision is to become a better caregiver, then let's get started.

Like any skill, active caregiving must be learned and practiced. This chapter will start you on your way by presenting the three most important caregiving tools: problem-solving, decision-making, and action-planning. Remember, you are the manager. Both at home and in the business world, managers direct the show. They don't do everything themselves; they work with others, including consultants, to get the job done. What makes them managers is that they are responsible for making decisions and making sure that their decisions are carried out.

Like the manager of an organization or a household, you must do all the following things:

1. Identify problems and seek solutions.
2. Make decisions for both you and your care partner.
3. Take action.

In the rest of this chapter, we will explore each of these skills and discuss ways you can be a better manager.

Solving Problems

Problems sometimes start with a general uneasiness. In order to think more about problem-solving, imagine yourself as the caregiver in the following story. You may feel unhappy but are not sure why. Upon closer examination, you find that you want some caregiving help from your family. Some of them live quite close, but except for an occasional phone call, they have all but disappeared from your life.

Your first thought is that they just don't want to be bothered and so you must do it all yourself. The more you think about this, the more you realize that this is not a solution. A solution would fix the problem, but you still have the problem. You also realize that you are not sure exactly why they are staying away or exactly what help you need. You consider calling and telling them what you're are thinking, but you are afraid your concerns will be made light of or you will be blown off. You think about getting help elsewhere but do not know how to start, and besides it may be too expensive. You talk about this with a good friend who suggests a family meeting. (We discuss more about family meetings in Chapter 7, Getting Help). You had never thought about this but decide to learn more.

The problem of getting help still seems overwhelming, as this idea of gathering the family for a meeting is all so new and you are not sure you have the time or strength to face all that you must do. However, you decide to take the first step by finding out more about family meetings. You make this an action plan.

To start your action plan (more about this later in the chapter), you promise yourself that this week you will gather more information about family meetings. You begin by looking at the content in this book about family meetings. You find this information helpful but you need more. So, you search the topic on the internet. A search of the internet for family meetings leads to lots of stuff for families with young children, but that is not what you need. You decide to add the word *caregiver* and find lots of information. Now you know more than you did, but you think that you may need more help. You decide to call the local Alzheimer's Association to see if they can help. You have just used the problem-solving tool in your Caregiver's Toolbox to achieve your goal of getting your family to help.

Let's review the specific steps you, as the caregiver in this situation, took to solve your problem:

1. **Identify the problem.** This is the first and biggest step in problem-solving—and usually the most difficult step as well. You may know that you are unhappy or stressed, but you may not know why until you think it over. With a little thought, you realize that you could use help and that your family has not been very helpful. In this scenario, the problem is needing help and feeling unhappy that family has not helped.
2. **List ideas to solve the problem**. You may be able to come up with a good list yourself. You may sometimes want to call on "consultants" to help you make that list. These can be friends, family, members of a health care team, or community resources. One note about using consultants: These folks cannot help you if you do not describe the problem well. For example, there is a big difference between saying you are unhappy and saying that you need help and are disappointed that your family is not helping more.
3. **Choose an idea to try**. As you consider trying something new, remember that new activities are usually difficult and that feeling nervous or discouraged may be part of the process. Be sure to give your potential solution or problem-solving method a fair chance before deciding it won't work. Sometimes, you have to try a couple of things. In our example, the first internet search was unsuccessful, but adding an extra search term helped uncover more helpful information. The thing to remember is to keep trying.
4. **Check the results** after you've given your idea a fair trial. If all goes well, your problem will be solved. In the example, you still may not have help, but two things have happened. First, you are working on a way of approaching your family for help. Second, you have reached out to a consultant, the Alzheimer's Association.
5. If you still have the problem, **pick another idea from your list and try again**. In our example, maybe the caregiver will decide not to have a family meeting or the family meeting fails. You go to the list for another idea.
6. If your original list of ideas is not proving useful, **use other resources** (for example, your consultants) for more ideas if you still do not have a solution. Then go back to step 3 with your new list.
7. Finally, if you have gone through all the steps until all ideas have been exhausted and the problem is still unsolved, you may have to **accept that your problem might not be solvable right now**. This is sometimes hard to do. However, living with uncertainty is something we must all learn to do, and a caregiver's life contains more uncertainty than most. The fact that a problem can't be solved right now doesn't mean that it won't be solvable later or that other problems cannot be solved. Even if your path is blocked, there are probably alternative paths. Don't give up. Keep going.

Problem-Solving Steps

1. Identify the problem.
2. List ideas to solve the problem.
3. Choose one solution or method to try.
4. Check the results.
5. Pick another idea if the first didn't work.
6. Use other resources for a new list.
7. Accept that the problem might not be solvable now.

Living with Uncertainty

Living with uncertainty is one of the hardest caregiving tasks. It is something that most of us cannot avoid. Uncertainty can be a stressor and one of the causes of emotional ups and downs. Facing the decline of someone important to us and becoming a caregiver takes away some of our sense of security and control. These processes can be frightening and introduce uncertainty into our lives in a whole new way. We are following our life path, and suddenly we are forced to detour to a different, unwanted path. If you have been a caregiver for many months or even years, this uncertainty continues. Of course, we all have an uncertain future, but most people are able to avoid thinking about it. When we become a caregiver, however, this becomes an unavoidable part of our lives. We are uncertain about our care partner's health and function, and perhaps about our ability to continue as a caregiver. Often this uncertainty is the reason given for avoiding making decisions. Remember, no matter what you do, you are making a decision.

Making Decisions: Weighing the Pros and Cons

Decision-making is another important skill in your Caregiver's Toolbox. There are some decision-making steps that are a little like problem-solving. Each of these steps can be a tool in your Caregiver's "Tool Box."

1. **Identify the options.** For example, you may be feeling overwhelmed with housework and yard work. You have to make a decision. Your options include getting help in the house or continuing to do all the work yourself. Sometimes, the options are to change something or to not change something.
2. **Identify what you want.** What is important to you? Do you want to spend more time with your care partner or to take time to have a break from your care partner? Maybe what you really want to do is spend that

time shoveling the walkway, cutting the grass, or cleaning the house. Sometimes, identifying your deepest values helps you set priorities and increases your motivation to change.

3. **Write down pros and cons for each option.** List as many items as you can in two columns, one column for the pros and the other for the cons. Don't forget the emotional and social costs of your options.
4. **Rate each item on the pros and cons list** on a 5-point scale with 0 indicating "not at all important" and 5 indicating "extremely important."
5. **Add up the ratings for each column** and compare them. The column with the higher total should help you identify the best decision for you. If the totals are close or you are still not sure, skip to the next step.
6. **Apply the "gut test."** For example, does hiring someone to help you around the house feel right to you even if it means you might have to work more hours or make some financial sacrifices? If so, you have probably reached a decision. If not, the way you feel should probably win out over the math.

You may wonder, "If I am going to go with my gut, why do I have to do all the math?" This is a good question. The reason is that the thinking that goes on in steps 1–3 help you to understand your gut decision and clarify issues.

Decision-Making Example

Should I get help in the house?

Pro	Rating	Con	Rating
I'll have more time	4	It's expensive	3
I'll be less tired	4	It's hard to find good help	1
I'll have a clean house	3	They won't do things my way	2
		I don't want a stranger in the house	1
Total	11		7

Add up the points for the pro and con lists. The decision in this example would be to get help because the pro score (11) is significantly higher than the con score (7). If this feels right in your gut, you have the answer.

Now it's your turn! Try making a decision using the following chart. It's OK to write in your book.

Decision to be made ______________________________

Pro	Rating	Con	Rating
Total			

This is a special note for caregivers: The intent of this exercise is to help *you* make a decision. It is not for your care partner. Many caregiving problems come from asking care partners to make choices that they may not be able to make. For example, you are going for a ride and ask your Maria where she would like to go. She says she'd like to see her sister in St. Louis (this is 500 miles away). You say that this is not possible and your care partner is very unhappy. The problem is that the question was open-ended. It's better to ask, "Would you like to go to the grocery store or to the park?" We will talk much more about frustrating or problem care partner behaviors in the next chapter.

The key to successful problem-solving and decision-making is taking action. We talk about this next.

Taking Action

Simply knowing you want to do something is not enough. Once you have looked at a problem and made the difficult decision to take action, how can you begin? We suggest that you start by doing one thing at a time.

Setting Goals

Before you can take action, you must decide what you want to do first. Be realistic and specific when stating your goals. Think of all the things you would like to do. One caregiver wanted to have a few hours a week away from home. Another wanted to overcome anxiety and sleep better. Still another wanted to continue to ride her motorcycle but could no longer lift the 1,000-pound bike when it was lying on the ground. (Note that the tools in this chapter are not just for caregiving but can be used for solving most problems, making decisions, and taking action.)

One of the problems with goals is that they often seem like dreams. They are so far off, big, or difficult that we are overwhelmed and don't even try to accomplish them. We'll tackle this problem next. For now, take a few minutes and write your goals below (use an additional sheet of paper if you need to).

Goals

____

____

____

____

____

Put a star (☆) next to the goal you would like to work on first.

Don't reject a goal as unreachable until you have thought about all the possible alternatives. Sometimes, we reject options without knowing much about them. In the earlier example, the caregiver looked for some ways to get the family to help and chose to learn more about family meetings. Although this was not a familiar option, it was not rejected out of hand.

Exploring Options

There are many ways to reach any specific goal. For example, a caregiver who wants a few hours away each week could ask a friend to stay with their care partner or might employ someone for a few hours. Maybe there is a high school student that could come in as part of a community service requirement. Or maybe ask for help in a church bulletin or email list. The caregiver who wants to be less anxious and get more sleep might look into relaxation exercises or yoga videos. They may make a list of the things interfering with sleep so they could start problem-solving how to change them. They might decide to talk to her health care provider about options. Our motorcycle rider could buy a lighter motorcycle, use a sidecar, put "training wheels" on the bike, buy a three-wheeled motorcycle, or give up riding.

As you can see, there are many options for reaching each goal. The idea here is to list all the options you can think of and then choose one or two to try out.

Sometimes, it is hard to think of all the options yourself. If you are having problems, it is time to use a consultant, just as you would in problem-solving. Share your goal with family, friends, and health professionals. You can call community organizations such as Catholic or Jewish Family Services, a senior center or the Area Agency on Aging. You can use the internet.

Don't ask what you should do. Rather, ask for suggestions. It is always good to add to your list of options and to get a fresh perspective from a person who is new to the problem.

A note of caution: Many options are never seriously considered because people assume they don't exist or are unworkable. Never make this assumption until you have thoroughly investigated the option. One woman we know had lived in the same town all her life and felt that she knew all about the community resources. When she was having problems with her health insurance, a friend from another city suggested contacting an insurance counselor. The woman dismissed this suggestion because she was certain that this service did not exist in her town. It was only when, months later, the friend came to visit and called the Area Agency on Aging (which exists in most counties in the United States) that the woman learned that there were three insurance counseling services nearby. Our motorcycle rider thought that training wheels on a Harley was a crazy idea, but then explored the idea at a motorcycle shop owners' suggestion. This extended riding life 15 years by using training wheels. In short, never assume anything. Assumptions are major problem-solving and decision-making enemies.

Write the list of options for your main goal here. Then put a star (☆) next to the two or three options you want to research further.

Options

____

____

____

____

____

Making Short-Term Plans: Action Planning

For most of us, once we make a decision, we have a good idea of where we are going. However, some goals may seem overwhelming. How will we ever be able to move, how will I ever be able to make a life for myself again, how will I ever by able to ____________ (you fill in the blank)? The secret to success is to *not* try to do everything at once. Instead, look at one thing that you can realistically expect to accomplish within *the next week*.

We call this approach to moving forward an *action plan*. An action plan is something that is short-term, is doable, and sets you on the road toward your goal. Your action plan should be about something you want to do or accomplish. It should help you solve your problem and reach your goal. It is a tool to help you do what *you* wish. Do not make action plans to please your care partner, friends, family, or doctor.

Action plans are probably your most used tool for success as a caregiver. Most of us can do things to make caregiving easier, but we fail to do them. Often, failing has more to do with not knowing how to make these new skills part of our daily routine than a lack of will or ability to master the skills. For example, most caregivers have the ability to practice the skills that will lessen their care partners difficult or frustrating behaviors. However, few caregivers have a systematic plan for doing this. Think about your and your partner's activities of daily living (ADLs). ADLs are everyday things such as getting out of bed, bathing, dressing, preparing and eating meals, cleaning house, shopping, and paying bills. Can an action plan help you accomplish any of these tasks more efficiently? Can it help you find the energy to accomplish these and be less stressed out?

An action plan helps us do the things we know we *should* do, but to create a successful action plan, it is best to start with something that we *want* to do. You can start with *anything*. In the following material, we go through the steps for making a realistic action plan.

Creating a Realistic Action Plan

First, decide what you will do this week. For someone seeking information this might mean setting aside 15 minutes on each of three days this week to read, call community agencies, or look things up online. For the caregiver who wants to be less anxious and to sleep better, it may mean practicing a relaxation exercise at bedtime for four nights. The caregiver who wants to continue riding a motorcycle might spend half an hour over two days researching lighter motorcycles and motorcycle training wheels.

Make very sure that your plans are "action-specific"; that is, rather than just deciding "to lose weight" (which is not an action but the result of an action), you will "replace soda with tea" (which is an action).

Next, make a specific plan. Deciding what you want to do is worthless without a plan to do it. The plan should answer all of the following questions:

- Exactly *what* are you going to do? Are you going to take a walk when you get stressed out, or try to avoid overeating when you feel anxious? Will you call someone? What relaxation technique will you practice?
- *How much* will you do? This question is answered with something like time, distance, portions, or repetitions. Will you walk one block, walk for 15 minutes, eat half portions at lunch and dinner, practice relaxation exercises for 15 minutes?
- *When* will you do this? Again, this must be specific: in the late afternoon (when you know you are likely to be tired and more susceptible to stress and losing your temper), before lunch, at the evening meal, before going to bed. Connecting a new activity with an old habit is a good way to make sure it gets done. Consider what comes right before your action plan that could trigger the new behavior. For example, you will do five minutes of relaxation breathing each afternoon right after you do the lunch dishes. Another trick is to incorporate your new activity into your routine right before an old favorite activity such as walking around the block before reading the paper or watching a favorite TV program.

Success Improves Health

The benefits of change go beyond the payoffs of adopting healthier habits. Obviously, you will feel better and be a better caregiver when you are less stressed, communicate positively with your care partner, exercise, eat well, keep regular sleeping hours, stop smoking, and take time to relax. But regardless of the behavior that's altered, there's evidence that the feelings of self-confidence and control over your life that come from making any successful change improve your health.

Being a caregiver is sometimes not good for our self-image. For many people, it is discouraging to be faced by many new problems and stressors each day and to find they do not possess all the coping skills they wish they did. By changing and improving one area of your life, whether it is approaching care partner problems differently, boosting your physical fitness, or learning a new skill, you regain a sense of optimism and vitality. By focusing on what you can do rather than what you wish you could do, you're more likely to lead a more positive and happier life. Taking steps to improve your self-confidence can make you feel better inside and out.

- *How often* will you do the activity? This is a bit tricky. We would all like to engage in positive habits every day, but that is not always possible. It is usually best to decide to do an activity three or four times a week to give yourself "wiggle room" if something comes up. If you do more, so much the better. However, if you are like most people, you will feel less pressure if you can do your activity three or four times a week and still feel successful.

Here are some general guidelines for writing your action plan that may help. First, *start where you are*, start small, or start slowly. If you can walk for only one minute, start your walking program by walking one minute once every hour or two, not by trying to walk a block. If you have never done any exercise, start with a few minutes of warm-up. A total of 5 or 10 minutes is enough. If you want to avoid stress overeating, set a goal based on your existing eating behaviors, such as having half portions. For example, "losing a pound this week" is not an action plan because it does not involve a specific action; "not eating after dinner for four days this week," by contrast, is a fine action plan.

Second, *give yourself some time off*. All people have days when they don't feel like doing anything. That is a good reason for saying that you will do something three times a week instead of every day.

Third, once you've made your action plan, *ask yourself* the following question: "On a scale of 0 to 10, with 0 being totally unsure and 10 being totally certain, how sure am I that I can complete this entire plan?"

If your answer is 7 or above, this is probably a realistic action plan. If your answer is below 7, you should look at your action plan again. Ask yourself why you are unsure. What problems do you foresee? Then, see if you can either solve the problems or change your plan to make yourself more confident of success.

Elements of a Successful Action Plan

- The plan is something ***you*** want to do.
- The plan is achievable (something you can expect to be able to accomplish that week).
- The plan is action-specific.
- The plan answers the questions ***what, how much, when***, and ***how often?***
- You are certain that you will complete your entire plan at a level of 7 or higher on a scale from 0 = not at all sure to 10 = absolutely sure.

Once you have made a plan you are happy with, *write it down* and post it where you will see it every day. Thinking through a weekly action plan is one thing. Writing it down makes it more likely you will take action. Keep track of how you are doing and the problems you encounter. (There is a blank action planning form at the end of this chapter. You may wish to make photocopies of it to use weekly.)

Carrying Out Your Action Plan

If your weekly action plan is well written and realistically achievable, completing it is generally not too difficult. There are a couple of strategies you can use to make it easier:

- Ask family or friends to check with you on how you are doing. Having to report your progress is good motivation.
- Keep track of your daily activities while carrying out your plan. Many caregivers have lists of what they want to accomplish.
- Check things off as they are completed. This will guide you on how realistic your planning was and will be useful in making plans. Plus, it is satisfying to make those check marks!
- Make daily notes, even of the things you don't understand at the time. Later, these notes may be useful in establishing a pattern to use for problem-solving.

Checking the Results

At the end of each week, see if you completed your action plan and if you are any nearer to accomplishing your goal. Are you able to walk farther? Have you lost weight? Are you less anxious? Taking stock is key. You might not see progress day by day, but you should see a little progress each week. At the end of each week, check on how well you have fulfilled your action plan. If you are having problems, this is the time to use your problem-solving tool.

For example, the sleep-deprived person we mentioned was not able to get more sleep during the first week of her action plan. Each day a different problem popped up: One night her care partner got up at night and needed help; the next night she woke to use the bathroom at three in the morning and could not go back to sleep; the next the cats jumped on the bed; and so on. When looking back at the notes, the real problem became clear: She was afraid that she would not hear her care partner if anything happened. Putting a baby monitor in her care partners room solved the problem.

How People Change

Thousands of studies have been done to learn how people change—or why they don't change. Here's what we have learned:

- Most people change by themselves, when they are ready. While physicians, counselors, spouses, and self-help groups coax, persuade, nag, and otherwise try to assist people to change their lifestyle and habits, most people do so without much help from others.
- Change is not usually an all-or-nothing process. It happens in stages. Most of us change one small step at a time: Each step is an improvement over the one before it.
- In most cases, change resembles a spiral more than a straight line, with people going back to previous stages before advancing. ("two steps forward, one step back"). Relapses are not failures but setbacks, which are a key part of change. Relapses provide feedback and help us figure out what doesn't work.
- Confidence in your ability to change is the key ingredient for success. Your belief in your own ability to succeed predicts whether you will attempt change in the first place, whether you will persist if you relapse, and whether you will ultimately be successful in making the change.

Making Midcourse Corrections (Back to Problem-Solving)

When you are trying to overcome obstacles to make real changes, the first plan is not always the most workable plan. If something doesn't work, don't give up. Try something else: Modify your short-term plans so that your steps are easier; give yourself more time to accomplish difficult tasks; explore new options for reaching your goal; or check with your consultants for advice and assistance.

Please note: Not all goals are achievable. All caregivers know that caregiving means giving up some options. If this is true for you, don't dwell too much on what you can't do. Rather, start working on another goal you would like to accomplish. One caregiver we know talks about the 50% of things accomplished and the new skills learned.

Rewarding Yourself

The best part of managing caregiving well is the reward that comes from accomplishing your goals and living a fuller and more comfortable life. However, there are other special ways to reward yourself on your path to improvement. Don't wait until your goal is reached; rather, reward yourself frequently for your short-term successes. For example, decide that you won't read the paper until after you exercise. Thus, reading the paper becomes your reward. One caregiver put a dollar in a jar each time they got through a half day without an upset. When there was enough money, they went out for ice cream. To begin with, this was only once every ten days or so, but as time went on, they were having ice cream more and more often. In fact, the caregiver had to change the reward to a dollar a day. And the reward doesn't have to be ice cream. It can be a trip to the park or a cup of herbal tea in an outdoor café. There are many healthy pleasures that can add enjoyment to your life.

You can use the form on page 22 to start your own action plan.

My Action Plan

In writing your action plan, be sure it includes all of the following:

1. What you are going to do (a specific action).
2. How much you are going to do (time, distance, portions, repetitions, etc.).
3. When you are going to do it (time of the day, day of the week).
4. How often or how many days a week you are going to do it.

Example: This week, I will walk (what) around the block (how much) before lunch (when) three times (how many).

This week I will ________________________________ (what)

______________________________________ (how much)

______________________________________ (when)

______________________________________ (how often)

How sure are you? (0 = not at all sure; 10 = absolutely sure) ______

Comments

Monday ______________________________________

Tuesday ______________________________________

Wednesday ____________________________________

Thursday _____________________________________

Friday _______________________________________

Saturday _____________________________________

Sunday ______________________________________

Suggested Further Reading

Lake, Nell. *The Caregivers: A Support Group's Stories of Slow Loss, Courage, and Love*. New York: Scribner, 2014. Chronicles the experiences of a group of long-term caregivers and discusses critical issues of old age, end-of-life care, medical reform, and social policy. http://amzn.to/2EudQE4

Lauber, Rick. *The Successful Caregivers Guide*. Bellingham, WA: Self-Counsel Press, a subsidiary of International Self-Counsel Press Ltd., 2015. Provides practical tips, realistic guidance, encouragement, and insight into eldercare. http://amzn.to/2Clx0tS

Philo, Jolene. *The Caregiver's Notebook: An Organizational Tool and Support to Help You Care for Others*. Grand Rapids, MI: Discovery House Publishers, 2014. Offers caregivers a helpful and portable organization tool, as well as spiritual comfort. http://amzn.to/2HfNTK8

Porter, Robin. *The Complete Caregiver's Organizer: Your Guide to Caring for Yourself While Caring for Others*. Ann Arbor, MI: Spry Publishing LLC, 2015. Direct and attainable strategies for managing common issues that all caregivers face, from basic health and safety concerns to complex medical and legal questions, in addition to invaluable checklists, journaling components, and activities. http://amzn.to/2sx0PYI

Other Resources

AARP has a "Caregiving Question and Answer Tool" to easily search their site at https://www.aarp.org/caregiving/answers/

The **Aging Care** website's caregiving section includes information on individual health conditions, caregiver support, money and legal issues, recommended products, and a blog. https://www.agingcare.com/articles/make-caregiving-easier-141826.htm

Cancer.net features the American Society of Clinical Oncology's tips for being a successful caregiver. https://www.cancer.net/coping-with-cancer/caring-loved-one/tips-being-successful- caregiver

Caregiving 101: On Being a Caregiver is a printable guide for new caregivers. https://www.caregiver.org/caregiving-101-being-caregiver

This **Health.com Blog** outlines the 13 things you should know before becoming a caregiver. http://www.health.com/health/gallery/0,,20949560,00.html#caring-for-loved-ones-0

This post on **Mental Health America** lists what you can do to become an effective caregiver. http://www.mentalhealthamerica.net/conditions/being-effective-caregiver

Secure Aging is a financial and care management website for seniors. This blog entry offers tips to become a better caregiver. https://secureaging.com/tips-to-become-a-better-caregiver

The **U.S. Veterans Affairs (VA)** hospitals all provide caregiver support services for U.S. military veterans. https://www.caregiver.va.gov/

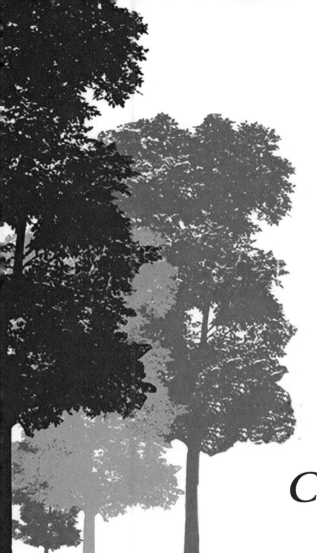

Chapter 3

Dealing with Stress and Difficult Care Partner Behavior

In Chapter 1, Introduction: A Blueprint for Better Caregiving, you learned that when you have a stressor, both your body and mind react. Stress can result in anger, frustration, slow thinking, tight muscles, and stomach upset—in fact, stress can affect almost any part of our minds or bodies.

Let's explore this idea a bit more. Imagine that you are on an elevator and feel someone or something poke you from behind—first reaction: You are startled; you may feel fear. What's going to happen. Am I going to be robbed? What is going on? You tense up; you may start to breathe faster. You are stressed. You turn around and see a woman who is blind with a cane who didn't judge distance well. You are relieved. You no longer feel threatened and breathe a sigh of relief. Your body relaxes. This example shows that stress comes from how you *interpret* the event, not the event itself.

Identifying Stress

When we ask caregivers what their biggest problem is, the reply is usually, "Stress." Then we ask what causes this stress and often hear things like:

- *"My care partner found the car key and went for a drive. He got lost."*
- *"My care partner refuses to take a shower."*
- *"My care partner wants to be with me all the time."*
- *"My care partner refuses to get in the car to go to medical appointments."*

All of these are annoying or difficult care partner behaviors. Take a moment and think of one or two of your care partner's annoying or difficult behaviors. Write them down here:

1. ______________________________________

2. ______________________________________

Check your body. Our guess is that just thinking about these has caused some stress.

First, let's look at your stress level. Circle the number in the diagram that describes your stress level right now. Then, you can do the same thing after you tried a stress breaker.

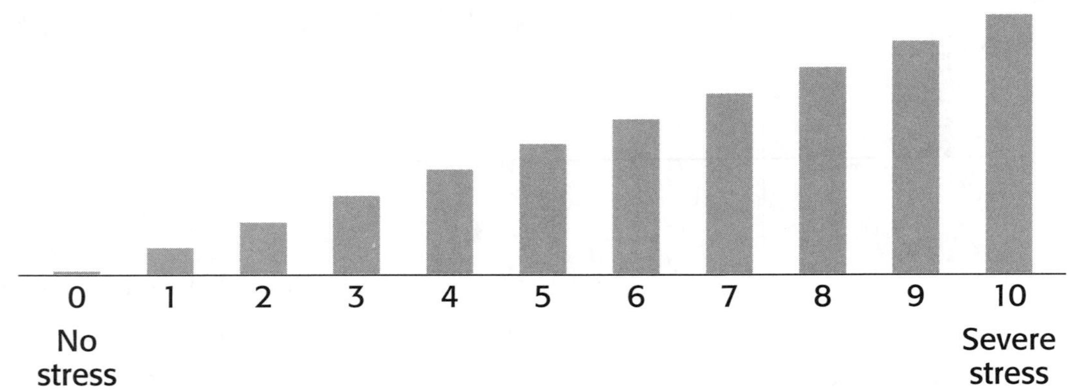

Before you can do anything about stress, you must notice stress building. Your body may get tense, your voice may get louder, and you may feel it in your gut. Each of us reacts to stress a little differently. You job is to know when this is happening. Pay attention to your body. You do not have to wait until you have a headache or a gut ache, or until you lose your temper or start crying. As soon as you notice stress starting to build, you can use thoughtful breathing as a quick stress breaker.

Breaking the Stress Cycle with Thoughtful Breathing

Thoughtful breathing is easy. We do not usually think about breathing but thoughtful breathing is something you do on purpose. You think about breathing to help you relax. It is like a time out. All you do is take three or four deep breaths down to your stomach. You will know they are deep breaths if your stomach moves more than your chest. Check this by putting one hand on your chest and one on your stomach. Take three or four deep breaths. If your lower hand is moving more than your upper hand, you are on target. If this does not happen right away, do not worry. It will with time. Right now, check with yourself. Are you feeling a little less stress?

Another time you can use thoughtful breathing is in the midst of a stressful situation. Maybe your care partner is refusing to get out of bed. Somehow, this has escalated into a struggle. You can use thoughtful breathing to break the cycle—literally to catch your breath. Sometimes all it takes is a small thing to de-escalate.

While thoughtful breathing is a stress breaker, it is even better if you can keep stress from escalating in the first place. One way of doing this is to identify and learn more about annoying or difficult care partner behaviors. Often, we do not want to discuss these behaviors. Just the same, we know that many (if not most) care partners do have behaviors that their caregivers finding annoying, difficult, or just plain maddening. These behaviors are a major cause of caregiver stress. We also know that these behaviors usually happen for a reason and, as a caregiver, you can change at least some of the. The starting point is to break this problem into smaller parts.

Addressing Difficult Care Partner Behaviors

There are eight steps in dealing with difficult care partner behaviors:

Step 1. Name the difficult behavior.

Step 2. If possible,determine the cause of the difficult behavior.

Step 3. Identify what happened before the behavior. This is the "trigger."

Step 4. Identify what you did during and after the behavior.

Step 5. Identify what your care partner did after the behavior.

Step 6. Determine how this made you feel.

Step 7. Evaluate your progress. Is the behavior changing? Are you feeling less stressed?

Step 8. Try something different.

Step 1: Name the Difficult Behavior

It is not always easy to define frustrating or difficult care partner behaviors, but most people tell us that they know it when it happens. It may be that you ask your care partner what she wants for dinner and she answers, "Ice cream." It may be that your care partner follows you around all the time. It may be that your care partner gets very angry any time you go out and leave him with someone else. It may be that your formerly clean and neat care partner now refuses to take a shower. If the behaviors cause either you or your care partner problems or stress, then they are probably difficult behaviors. You wrote down some difficult behaviors of your care partner on page 24. Look at these again. If you want to add or change something, do it now.

Step 2: Determine the Cause of the Difficult Behavior

Ask yourself, what are the reasons for difficult behaviors? There are several reasons for difficult care partner behaviors, and they may include the following:

1. Your care partner wants attention.
2. Your care partner needs stimulation or is bored.
3. Your care partner wants to escape or avoid something unpleasant.
4. Your care partner needs to go to the bathroom.
5. Your care partner is hungry, is in pain, or feels anxious or lonely.

This list can go on and on, and if your care partner cannot communicate well, then you may have to guess. After a while, the clues may become more obvious.

Notice that being angry or trying to "get you"/"get your goat" is not usually a reason for a difficult behavior. Trying to "get you" is something someone does on purpose. This is usually not possible for someone with dementia or other brain injuries. Typically, what care partners are trying to do when they engage in difficult behavior is to express themselves. They are hoping you understand their needs. Since people who need caregiving don't communicate well verbally, caregivers must observe their behavior and try to figure out what it *could* mean and then act accordingly. While it is very easy to take care partner behavior personally and then to feel guilty, in fact, most care partner behavior is not personally aimed at you or anyone else.

Consider this example. Myra does not communicate much and usually does not know where she is. Her husband, Richard, often sits her in front of the TV so he can get some work done. In just a few minutes, she is at his desk, calling out his name. This occurs many times a day. While we do not know the exact cause of this behavior, we can guess that Myra may be bored and she may want attention. Guessing this, Richard decides to spend short periods with Myra every hour and change her activities once or twice an hour. He discovers that the behavior disappears once he makes these changes. He also knows that he cannot spend every minute with Myra and decides that taking her to a senior day health program for a half day a few times a week may be a good solution.

Here is another example. See if you can spot the cause. Several times a day, Keenan follows Mitch around. He even wants to be there when he takes a shower. This drives Mitch up the wall and stresses him out. Mitch also notices that Keenan often soils himself during or after this behavior. What do you think might be the cause of Keenan's behavior?

Boredom may be causing Keenan's behavior. This is often a cause for difficult behaviors.

Acting out (soiling himself) provides some excitement. Alternatively, Keenan may be trying to avoid soiling himself. However, he does not know how to express this or what to do about it. He may be following Mitch around to get his attention and seek his help in using the bathroom. Mitch can try a few things. He can structure several activities for Keenan during the day. He might fold the clothing, work on a hooked rug, or watch a baseball game, and the two of them can go for a daily walk. Activity relieves boredom. He may also try leading Keenan to the bathroom every time the behavior occurs. With a little trial and error and some keen observation, Mitch may stop or lessen the behavior.

Once you think you know a little about what is causing difficult behaviors, it is much easier to find a solution.

Step 3: Identify What Happened Before the Behavior

What are the triggers for difficult behaviors? Often something happens before the difficult behavior that triggers the behavior. Here are some examples.

John asks Julianna what she wants for dinner. Julianna answers, "Ice cream." John does not think that ice cream is an appropriate dinner and sees this as a difficult behavior. The trigger was the open-ended question. What John really wanted to know was if Julianna wanted chicken or pasta. By using an open-ended question instead of giving a choice of two things, he inadvertently triggered the behavior. It is likely that Julianna thought of the food she liked best or the first thing that came into her mind.

In this example, it is clear that John does not like the idea of Julianna having ice cream for dinner. He might think that she is trying to annoy him. There are two things to consider with this example. First, why did John ask an open-ended question? The answer is often that John is trying to maintain Julianna's dignity by giving her choices. Unfortunately, sometimes the opposite occurs when she is frustrated at not being able to make a choice or her choice is unacceptable to John.

Another way of looking at this is that sometimes there is no good reason why Julianna should not have ice cream for dinner. John does not have to eat it. Perfect nutrition may not be important and maybe she will eat some pasta after the ice cream. Is this a behavior about which John should be concerned? There is no right or wrong answer, but it is good to remember that a behavior is difficult only if the caregiver sees it as difficult.

Here is another example. Rose is a full-time caregiver for her father Marcos. She has arranged to have someone from church come in and sit with Marcos for a couple of hours three times a week so she can shop and have lunch with a friend. However, when she comes home, Marcos shouts at her and says she does not care about him and that she is no good. Rose ends up in tears.

The trigger is easy to spot. It is Rose's leaving Marcos. However, taking a break is necessary and healthy. The difficult behavior needs to be addressed, but not by Rose never leaving the house.

Here are some ideas for dealing with triggers.

- **Eliminate the trigger.** If the dog jumping up on your care partner's lap makes him angry or agitated, then the dog's jumping will have to be stopped. The dog can be trained, you can get rid of the dog, or make sure that the dog and your care partner are never together. These are not easy decisions or choices, but the dog's behavior must be addressed in order to address your care partner's difficult behavior.
- **Arrange life so the trigger does not bother your care partner.** If a 3:00 a.m. train always wakes you or your care partner, you cannot get rid of the train. Earplugs, a sound track of white noise (recordings of the ocean or wind, for example), or double-paned windows may help.
- **Avoid the trigger.** If bright light is a trigger, offer your care partner dark glasses and help choose seats that face away from windows. If loud noises are a trigger, avoid places where these noises are likely to occur.
- **Distract your care partner.** Camille told Sally that it was time to take a shower. Sally hated showers and threw a fit. Camille realized that this was a familiar personality trait and an old trigger because Sally has never liked being told what to do. She suggested that they could go for a ride or work on a new puzzle after Sally's shower.
- **Tolerate the behavior or think about it in a different way.** Consider the example of Marcos shouting at Rose whenever she returned from a short time away from the house. It may not be possible or healthy to change the trigger, Rose's leaving, but it is possible for Rose to react differently or to think differently about the behavior. It is not her beloved father speaking but rather his illness.
- **Talk with your doctor or mental health professional about the trigger.** Professionals have techniques to help people become less sensitive to triggers. Sometimes consulting with a professional and learning new techniques is worth the effort, especially if the triggers cause very disruptive behavior.

Step 4: Identify What You Did during and after the Behavior

Often, we cannot prevent difficult behavior, but we can almost always change how we react. To do this, we have to decide if the behavior really makes any difference. If the behavior does make a difference, then changing your reaction may break a cycle. Let us return to Rose and Marcos. When Rose returns home, Marcos gets mad and says things that hurt Rose. What does this accomplish? Marcos gets Rose's attention and establishes an emotional connection even if it is a negative one. Rose feels hurt and guilty. She ends up crying.

In this situation, Rose can do several things. She can tell Marcos how much she loves him before leaving while also making sure that he knows she is leaving. When she returns she can immediately reassure him that she is now back and she still cares for him. She can point out to him that she did not leave permanently but was gone only for a short while. She can tell him how much she missed him and maybe bring him a small treat. Rose could set a timer for however long she will be gone. These will reassure Marcos that she is coming back.

If Marcos still responds angrily to her absence, Rose can sit quietly, not doing anything, until Marcos calms down or excuse herself and leave the situation for a few minutes. The important thing is that Marcos does not get attention by behaving negatively.

Step 5: Identify What Your Care Partner Did after the Behavior

Rose was always so upset with Marcos's reactions that she never really thought about what he did after the blow up. When she thought about it, she realized that he was always very quiet and almost reserved. It took them several hours or a day to get back to "normal."

Once she realized this, she thought that at some level he might be sorry or at least uncomfortable about his actions. She decided that if the behavior happened again, she would leave the room for a few minutes and when she returned she would say to him that she realized that this was hard for him. She would explain that it was also hard for her and tell him that they could work together to figure out how to get through the difficulty.

Step 6: Determine How This Made You Feel

For John, the consequence was that he was unhappy because Julianna wanted ice cream. After he stopped to think a moment he realized that there was no reason not to give her ice cream for dinner occasionally. He also knew her well enough to know that if she saw him eating pasta, she might want some as well. This is a win-win. Julianna gets what she wants and John gets his pasta.

By looking at the consequences for both parties, it is easier to determine what to do or sometimes not do. For Rose and Marcos, the consequence is lose-lose if Marcos gets angry and makes Rose cry. Both Rose and Marcos are unhappy. If Rose doesn't cry and instead leaves the room, it is a win for her even though it is a loss for Marcos. If she is able to reassure Marcos before and after she leaves that she is still going to be his caregiver and he does not lose his temper, it is a win-win. If Sally throws a fit about taking a shower and Camille decides it is not worth the effort to fight, the situation is a win for Sally (no shower) and a loss for her caregiver. If Camille convinces Sally to take a shower and they both enjoy a ride after the shower, it is a win-win.

Step 7. Evaluate Your Progress

There are many ways to deal with difficult care partner behaviors. To do so successfully means to step back a little and figure out how things are going and how you are feeling. Is the behavior getting better? How do you feel? Are you feeling less stressed? If so, you may be on the right path. If not, it may be time to move on to step 8 and try something different. One of the best ways to track your efforts is by starting a difficult behavior diary. A sample appears on the next page.

Behavior Diary

Remember, you have two places you can act to change a difficult behavior:

1. You can change or avoid the trigger.
2. You can change your reaction to the behavior.

Date:	
Behavior:	
Trigger:	
What, if anything, I did to change the trigger:	
What I did after the behavior:	
What my care partner did after the behavior:	
Results:	
Stress level: (circle number)	No stress 0 1 2 3 4 5 6 7 8 9 10 Extreme stress

Feel free to copy this and use it often. It is one of your most useful caregiver tools.

Step 8. Try Something Different

Don't be discouraged if bad behaviors don't go away immediately. Not all your attempts will work, and sometimes it will take more than one try. If something doesn't work, try something else, and always evaluate if the behavior reduced your stress. Things change and something that once worked may not work all of the time. It may take a few different approaches to change the triggers or change your reactions. Experimenting with new solutions is a worthwhile way to spend your time. As you experiment, you will become a better caregiver. Both you and your care partner will benefit.

Getting Help: Dangerous Care Partner Behaviors

So far, we have reviewed difficult, frustrating, or annoying care partner behaviors. Unfortunately, some care partner behaviors can be more than just annoyances, they can be dangerous for the care partner or for others. These behaviors include drug and/or alcohol abuse, hitting, biting, and kicking. You should know that you usually cannot change these behaviors. In fact, the harder you try to change a behavior, the worse it may get. What you can do is put safety first. Protect yourself and others who might be hurt. Get help.

Seek Safety

We will start with the most difficult advice. **If you feel that you or others in your household are in danger, get out.** You may need to have an escape plan ready. If it is warranted, have some clothing packed, money put away in a safe place, and gas in the car. You also need to think about where you would go. Maybe you can go to the home of a friend or relative. If you do not know where to go, call your local law enforcement or the Salvation Army. We know that this may sound drastic, but you cannot help your care partner if you or others in your family are in danger or are injured. If you do leave, and you fear for your care partner, call Adult Protective Services. You can also call 911 and ask them to call adult protective services or send an officer who has special mental health training.

Enlist the Help of Others

When you need to talk to a healthcare professional about dangerous behaviors, you can start by making an appointment with your care partner's healthcare provider. Do this without your care partner with you. This is also something you may be able to do with a telephone call or even a letter, email, or fax. When you talk with the provider, be as specific as possible. Focus on reporting the dangerous behavior with factual statements. For example, "My care partner drinks a six pack of beer every afternoon." Or "My care partner got so angry, he put a hole in the wall with his fist." Or "My care partner insists on keeping a loaded gun in the house."

You can also add your own concerns. For example, "After about three beers he becomes very angry, yells and shouts. I am afraid he will hit me or one of the children." Or "My care partner has never hit me but I am afraid that someday he will. I am also afraid that he will hurt himself." Or "Having a loaded gun around frightens me. I am afraid that my care partner will shoot me or shoot himself. He might even go off and use it in public."

Finally, ask the provider for advice. Listen carefully. What you hear may not be something you want to hear, such as the need for you to get out of the house or call law enforcement. Maybe the behavior can be stopped, but it might be that the behavior will continue. You should never put yourself or your family at risk. Your primary responsibility is to protect yourself and your family.

When talking to the provider there are a couple of things you need to know. The provider can listen to you and make suggestions to you about what you can do but may not be able to tell you anything about your care partner. The provider cannot tell you anything about your care partner unless your care partner has previously given permission to do so or you have conservatorship. (We explain more about conservatorship in Chapter 14, Planning for the Future: Fears and Reality.) U.S. law protects patient–provider relationships and discussions.

Sometimes your partner's provider may not know how to help or is not approachable. If this is the case, you need to find other support. You can start at the Alzheimer's Association or the social worker at the local senior center. You and your care partner do not need to be seniors and your care partner does not have to have Alzheimer's to use these services. Try the caregiver support person at the local Veterans Affairs (VA) Hospital or clinic. If your care partner ever served in the armed services (even 60 years ago and even if they never received services from the VA), you can still get great help from the VA caregiver support services. You can usually call these organizations and tell them your problem. They may not be able to help, but they often can refer you to some place that can. You will find helpful organizations, phone numbers, and websites at the end of most chapters in this book.

Finally, remember that if you feel like you or those around you are in danger, get out. Do not wait.

Suggested Further Reading

Boss, Pauline. *Loving Someone Who Has Dementia: How to Find Hope While Coping with Stress and Grief*. San Francisco: Wiley Books, 2011. Guidelines to stay resilient while caring for someone who has dementia. http://amzn.to/2ErTYkC

Jacobs, Barry J., and Julia L. Mayer. *AARP Meditations for Caregivers: Practical, Emotional, and Spiritual Support for You and Your Family*. Boston: Da Capo Life Long, 2016.

Emotional and spiritual motivation organized by theme, including topics such as accepting your feelings, knowing your limits, seeking support, and managing stress. http://amzn.to/2GgkJce

Manteau-Rao, Marguerite. *Caring for a Loved One with Dementia: A Mindfulness-Based Guide for Reducing Stress and Making the Best of Your Journey Together*. Oakland, CA: New Harbinger Publications, Inc., 2016.

Mindfulness-based dementia care (MBDC) guide to help reduce stress. http://amzn.to/2EJrYwi

Stafford, Rachel Macy. *Only Love Today: Reminders to Breathe More, Stress Less, and Choose Love*. Grand Rapids, MI: Zondervan, 2017.

Other Resources

Alzheimers.net is a blog on new approaches for dealing with difficult dementia behaviors. https://www.alzheimers.net/1-6-15-new-approaches-difficult-behaviors

American Academy of Cognitive Therapy. http://www.academyofct.org

This **Helpguide.org** article addresses caregiver stress and burnout. https://www.helpguide.org/articles/stress/caregiver-stress-and-burnout.htm

This **Mayo Clinic** blog on caregiver stress provides tips for taking care of yourself. https://www.mayoclinic.org/healthy-lifestyle/stress-management/in-depth/caregiver-stress/art-20044784

Womenshealth.gov describes caregiver stress, how it affects health, and how to prevent or relieve it. https://www.womenshealth.gov/a-z-topics/caregiver-stress

Chapter 4

Dealing with Difficult Emotions

DIFFICULT EMOTIONS AND CAREGIVING OFTEN GO TOGETHER. Having these emotions is perfectly normal. Many caregivers experience feelings of sadness, irritability, anxiety, grief, and/or guilt. Having such feelings is normal and understandable. Caregiving is often stressful and, for most of us, negative emotions are part of the stress response.

These feelings tend to ebb and flow over time. Often in the early stages, caregivers are angry about the changes that their loved one is experiencing and are not sure what to do to improve things. They often ask why did this happen? He did everything "right" and still he is very ill. Questions like this are common. Caregivers in the earlier stages also tend to be anxious about the future and wonder when will the next decline happen? How bad will it be? What can I do to cope?

As diseases progress, and our care partner is less able to function, anger and anxiety can change to sadness. Many caregivers become depressed. Some feel as if they have done all they can do and ask why doesn't my loved one improve? Is there nothing more that can be done? Others feel guilty and think they haven't done enough and think if only I had done X or Y, he would have improved, or at least not declined as rapidly. Growing awareness of the losses that have occurred (and the future losses ahead) can result in feelings of grief.

In the final stages of illness, some caregivers report feeling more "at peace"—they have reconciled themselves to what is next and have come to terms with what they did (and didn't) do for their loved one. But this is not always the case: Other caregivers become very depressed at the impending loss of their loved one and do all that they can to prolong life.

Depression

Of all these emotions, depression is the one that's probably most difficult for caregivers. Several studies found that up to 50% of caregivers (particularly those caring for a relative with Alzheimer's disease or other forms of dementia) report symptoms of depression some time during their caregiving career. Depression is not the same as stress: Stress is something one experiences in response to specific situations (like your loved one repeatedly asking you "What's for lunch?" (within an hour after having lunch). Stress is something that comes and goes over the course of a day, while depression often hangs over your head "like a black cloud" for days or weeks at a time. You know you have a problem when your usual ways of coping, of feeling better, don't work anymore. Or they work for just a short time and then you're downhearted and blue again.

Depression is problematic if it continues over time and is accompanied by other symptoms such as overeating or loss of appetite, sleeping too much or too little, having trouble concentrating, feeling hopeless about the future, and losing interest or pleasure in your usual activities. When this cluster of symptoms is present more or less every day for at least two consecutive weeks, it is helpful to make an appointment to discuss these feelings with your primary care provider and/or a trusted friend, clergyperson, or counselor. Most caregivers wait much longer than a few weeks to seek help for themselves. They are so used to putting their care partner first that they neglect their own well-being. But waiting is often unwise. Untreated depression reduces your quality of life, is associated with many physical health problems, and (over time) results in your being a less effective caregiver. If you think you are depressed (or others you trust have told you they are worried about this), please take time to get help for yourself.

Many different approaches to treating depression are effective. These include appropriate medications (which can only be prescribed by a physician) and various forms of psychotherapy. In particular, cognitive behavioral therapy (CBT), a short-term, problem-focused form of talking therapy, is as effective as medication for mild to moderate levels of depression. Persons specially trained and skilled in CBT can be found online through the Academy of Cognitive Therapy website. Just enter your zip code and you can receive information about practitioners in your region.

Embarrassment

Embarrassment is another feeling commonly reported by caregivers. Maybe your care partner eats with his hands. People often lose social skills when they lose some of their cognitive ability (their brains do not function as well as they did before). Most of us were taught that what other people think is important. But sometimes, as a caregiver, you have to put your old beliefs behind you and learn new techniques for interacting with the world.

You can also take active steps to deal with your own embarrassment. You can ask to sit in a corner with your partner facing the wall, thus, others will probably not notice. Or the Alzheimer's Association has business-type cards you can get or make yourself that say something like, "This person has Alzheimer's or dementia; his/her brain doesn't work like yours or mine. Thank you for understanding." The idea is that you slip this to a server in a restaurant, to someone next to you in church, or to a clerk/salesperson, etc. This can help lessen your embarrassment and helps the other person know what's going on. You will probably find that folks are kind. They have probably faced similar situations or know of someone who has.

Grief and Guilt

We often think of grief as something that happens when someone dies. When someone we care about, be it a family member or friend, changes or becomes ill, we also grieve. We grieve for the lives we used to have together, and we grieve for the future we could have had together. The reality of the present is not what we wanted or expected. Folks that are grieving sometimes deny what is happening. Instead of facing a loved one's decline or realizing their behavior is resulting from an illness, they may say things like, "Cherise is just having a bad day and will get better," or "She is acting that way because I am not a good enough caregiver and she is angry."

Sometimes grief is expressed as anger. A caregiver may say, "It's not fair that our lives were disrupted," or "It is all the hospital's fault for not catching this sooner." Bargaining is yet another way of expressing grief. "If you will just let us have a few good days, I will be happy."

Many caregivers feel guilty that they feel this sense of loss and grief! They think they are betraying their partners, or it's a sign they don't love them anymore. This is not the case. Experiencing a sense of loss and feelings of grief are perfectly normal. These feelings are common, particularly as dementia progresses and there is "less of a person" left in your loved one. After a time, most grief works itself out and we gain acceptance and peace. But this does not happen all at once, and the path can be difficult and painful.

Dealing with Difficult Emotions

It is often difficult to put a name on a difficult emotions. The names do not matter. What does matter is that you are feeling them and that there are things you can do about them. We will start with some things you can do for all difficult emotions, and then we will explain a few specific emotions.

Step 1: Acknowledge What You Are Feeling

We often go through life acting as though nothing is bothering us. At the same time, we have all kinds of feelings inside. Sometimes they bubble up and show themselves at inopportune times. For example, you may be angry with your care partner or worried about your own health. Instead of acknowledging these feelings, you yell at the dog or become angry with a salesclerk.

Step 2: Give the Feelings a Name, Such as Anger or Guilt

Do not worry about giving your feeling the "right" name. There is no right or wrong. Naming an emotion and acknowledging you feel it does not make you a bad person. It makes you a strong and thoughtful person. It is alright to say that you are angry about your condition, about having to be a caregiver, and having your life disrupted. Almost all caregivers tell us that they feel this way at one time or another.

Step 3: Try to Identify What Is Causing the Feeling

See if you can state how you feel in a sentence. For example, "I feel resentment that my sister does not help more," or "I worry that my care partner will get worse and I will not be able to cope."

Sometimes there is more than one cause for a feeling. When it comes to guilt, there may be many reasons. You might feel guilty for not being kinder to your care partner before you understood their problems. You might feel guilty that your care is not good enough. You may feel guilty because you feel trapped. It is also common for people to feel guilty because they want more time for themselves or because caregivers hope that the caregiving will soon end.

Step 4: Take Action

So far, we have been naming and explaining difficult emotions. Now it is time to do something about them. The following ideas are things you may want to try. You do not need to do all of them. Look over the list and decide where you want to start.

- **Talk with someone**. Talking to someone about what you are feeling often softens the feelings. You can talk to a professional, such as a social worker, psychologist, a health care provider, or the leader of your religious community. You can also talk with your family as well as with friends. You can talk to more than one person. Depending on whom you talk with, you can expect different outcomes. A professional may be very good at giving you suggestions, and friends and family may offer love and sympathy. By talking with people honestly, you may get some help you did not expect.

You might want to talk to a group of peers—other people who are caregivers. They will know exactly what you are talking about and understand your situation. You can find such groups online, through organizations such as the Alzheimer's Association, or groups at your local senior center. Many people shy away from such groups because they think that a group meeting is just a "pity party." This is not the case at all. At meetings like these, people share experiences as well as what has worked and what has not worked.

- **Write in a journal**. Thanks to good science, we now know that sometimes just writing down your feelings helps you to feel better. You do not need to show what you write to anyone—just write. You do not even have to think much about your writing. Sit down with paper and pen, or at a computer, and start a journal. Write down the date and then any feelings that come into your head and anything else you want to express. Five minutes is enough, but if you want to write longer, fine. Try to do this every day, even if you write only a line or two. You can find more details about this on pages 66–67 in Chapter 5.

Several things happen when people write like this. First, they feel better just getting their emotions expressed in writing. Second, over time they are surprised when they look back. Your journal acts like a road map to help you see where you have been. It may also offer insights into the future. For example, you might begin to see patterns. You might feel really down every time your care partner gets a little worse. You may also note that after a day or two, you adjust and life goes on. This may help the "downs" not to be so deep in the future. We cannot tell you what you will learn or how you will feel. We do know that keeping a journal has had many benefits for many people.

Writing is powerful so we want to offer word of caution. Journaling might stir up some thoughts and emotions that make you more feel depressed, stressed, or frightened. If this occurs, it can be a sign that you need help. Seek out an expert such as psychologist or social worker.

Adaptive Thinking

Another way of dealing with difficult emotions is adaptive thinking. This means changing the way you look at things to include thoughts that are more helpful to you. When you think adaptively, you still see the negatives but you don't dwell on them. These negative thoughts can get you down, but if you take a broader view that lets you look and think of things in different ways. Adaptive thoughts help to reduce your stress. You feel better and can go on more easily day to day. Sometimes we cannot change things, but we can change the way we think about things.

There are some special adaptive thinking hints that can be helpful for you as a caregiver. Focus on being the best caregiver you can be today. Do not reflect on what might have been or what the future might hold. Face the facts of the current situation and work within it.

Unfortunately, there might be very little that you can do as a caregiver to make your care partner better. But you can make each day the best it can be for both of you. To do this, you may need to rethink about what caregiving means to you. Take a minute and complete the following sentence. For me caregiving is ______________

____.

Now look at what you wrote. Is it largely negative? If so, you should change your statement to be a bit more positive. Can you think of any small joys you have gotten from caregiving? You do not want to be a Pollyanna or false in your definition. What you want to do is to think about caregiving in the most positive, neutral, or least negative way possible. For example, instead of "Caregiving is ruining my life; nothing will ever be the same," you might think, "Caregiving is really hard and I am doing the best I can." Here is another example: "For me caregiving is so frustrating. He can't do anything. All he does is shout and whine. He does not appreciate anything I do." You might change this to: "For me caregiving is a challenge. His condition is hard for both of us. I will do what I can to make him comfortable. I know he would thank me if he could."

Adaptive thinking takes practice. It does not come easily. However, it is worth the effort. The following four steps will help you adapt your thoughts:

1. Identify your frequent reoccurring negative thoughts.
2. Write these thoughts down.
3. Think how you might change each thought.
4. Every time you catch yourself having a negative thought, change it to your less negative or more positive choice.

With practice, your thinking will adapt, and, as this happens, you may well find yourself with fewer difficult emotions. Adaptive thinking is also called "positive thinking", and discussed in more detail on page 52 of Chapter 5.

You can start working on changing these unhelpful thoughts on page 56 of this book. Sometimes it takes more than just adapting our thinking. It takes action, especially setting priorities and not trying to do it all.

Establishing Priorities

We often hear from caregivers that they are overwhelmed. There is too much to do. What they do is never good enough. The work is never-ending. It is not surprising that you may be angry, depressed, and stressed. Caregiving is never-ending work, but so is life.

An important caregiver tool is establishing priorities. A good way to start is to write down all the things that *have to be done* and then add to this a list of all the things *you would like to do*.

Here is an example of a form:

Priorities Worksheet

Things That Have to Be Done	Things I Would Like to Do

Go through the list and mark everything that is important to your care partner's health and safety, and mark the three or four things that you would like to do most. Next, look at the list and see if there are items that are nice, but not necessary. Do not cross out the things you would like to do. Have you been able to find a few things that you do not need to do or that you can do less often?

Now, look at the list. Are there some things that could be done more easily? Can some of the things be done by someone else? If so, then come up with an action plan to make that happen.

Finally, look at the things you would like to do. Choose at least one and see if there is any way that this might happen. Sometimes this means changing your thinking. For example, a caregiver visits her husband in a nursing home for three hours every day. She would like to take a short trip to see her grandchildren but thinks she can't because she would miss her regular visits to her husband for a few days. The visits are her duty. Her visits do not add to the health or safety of her care partner. To try to figure out a way to make the trip to her grandchildren's, she might try some adaptive thinking. "If I visit my grandchildren, I will have more to talk about with my husband. He will enjoy hearing about them and looking at the photos I will take. Maybe, I can get someone at the nursing home to help him with Skype or FaceTime and we can all be together for a short time."

With so much to do, it is hard to establish priorities. However, you are doing this every day. This exercise makes you really think about your priorities. You might decide not to change a thing. That is OK, but until you look at what you are doing, it is hard to make this decision.

Facing the Facts

No matter how much we set priorities or adapt our thinking, life is not always as we would like it to be. This is especially true when you are a caregiver. Sometimes we put a rosy glow on reality (this is another way of saying we are in denial). "There is nothing much wrong. He cannot find the bathroom at night, has frequent falls, and eats with his hands, but these are little things. We do not need any extra help. He will get better and I can handle everything."

When you are denying the facts, you can pretend that nothing has changed and that life will return to the "way it used to be." You also can preserve your pride in being the perfect family member and caregiver. These "advantages," however, come at a high price. You are unhappy or depressed, and because you are so busy pretending everything is perfect, you can't talk to anyone about your problems. And on top of being isolated, you and your care partner might both be in physical or emotional danger. Your care partner's falls may result in injury. Your attempts to keep everything as it has been puts your care partner in more danger. It also puts you in danger. You may hurt yourself trying to help your partner.

Emotionally, your care partner might be very willing to admit that life has changed and find relief in giving up some of the pretenses of the "old normal." For the care partner, it can become more and more of a burden to pretend, until there comes a time when this is no longer possible.

Unfortunately, not facing the facts often leads to a crisis. You or your care partner breaks a hip. Your care partner leaves the house and the police find him the next day. You alienate family members and friends because they clearly see the facts and probably are willing to help but they become angry with your constant denials. Not knowing what to do or how to help, they stop coming around.

The big advantage to facing the facts is that it gives you control. No longer scrambling to hide from reality, you can have time to plan, time to get help, and have time to find small joys with your care partner. Facing the facts allows you to explore a new phase of life.

Sometimes it is difficult to know where to start in facing the facts. Friends, family members, and your health care providers can help. Ask them what they see when they look at your care partner. Ask how you can be a good caregiver. The hard part is that you must listen carefully, not interrupt or try to tell them they are wrong, and, most importantly, not get angry. You may not like what you hear. Denial is very powerful. You can overcome it. The good news is that facing the facts usually leads to a better quality of life for both the caregiver and care partner.

Dealing with Peer Pressure

Although your own feelings and thoughts can get in the way of facing the facts, peer pressure can be troubling and difficult to deal with, too. You might know people who fall into the following types:

- **The happy warriors.** Sometimes, well-meaning friends will tell you how they took care of their mothers for 15 years and that every day was a blessing and a joy. You may find caregiving difficult and not very joyful. Hearing this from a friend makes you feel guilty because you are not enjoying caregiving as she did. Worse, you might feel you are a bad person, because sometimes you do not much like being a caregiver.
- **The experts.** There are also "helpful friends." They have never been caregivers but they tell you exactly what you should and should not do. Sometimes these experts are family members. Experts can cause stress because they do not know what they are talking about or because you do not want to offend them. They can also make you feel guilty because their advice implies that you are not the best possible caregiver.
- **The doomsayers.** These people have been caregivers. It was a terrible experience. Doomsayers are more than happy to tell you all the gruesome details and to end every conversation by saying, "Just wait, it will get worse." Doomsayers give voice to your anxiety and uncertainty and cause stress, anger, and fear.

These are just a few of the "helpful" people you may meet. They usually mean well but, in fact, cause you extra problems.

One technique for dealing with not so helpful people is called the Broken Record Tool. You find a phrase such as "Thank you for your input," "Let me think about this," or "I would rather talk about something else." No matter what they say, you repeat your phrase. You just don't engage in a conversation or an argument about these topics with them. It is best to keep your phrase neutral. Just keep repeating your phrase. Usually, what happens is that, after hearing this phrase three or four times, the other person gives up.

You will find more ideas about how to communicate with not-so-helpful people as well as those from whom you need or want something in Chapter 6, Communicating Effectively.

Letting Go of What You Cannot Control

There are many things that you cannot control as a caregiver. This lack of control can make you feel guilty, sad, frightened, and angry. Recognizing and accepting what you cannot control is a great caregiver skill. Some caregivers find the serenity prayer used by Alcoholics Anonymous helpful:

God, grant me the serenity to accept the things I cannot change,
The courage to change the things I can,
And wisdom to know the difference.

So far, in this book, we have spent a lot of time encouraging you to recognize things you can change and offering various tools so that you can make changes. But we realize that not all things can be changed or improved. When you encounter things that you cannot change, you need to accept them and then let them go. Each of us only has so much energy and emotional capacity. You are certainly not alone in your feelings. If the tools in this book are not enough to help you with acceptance, we suggest that you talk with a counselor or spiritual leader. This is especially important if you are so frustrated that you feel you might lash out at your care partner.

Addressing Difficult Care Partner Emotions

Like you, your care partner also has difficult emotions. Unlike you, they might not be able to name them or have any idea how to manage them.

Many conditions impair cognition (memory) such as stroke, traumatic brain injury (TBI), Alzheimer's, post-traumatic stress disorder (PTSD), or Parkinson's. These same conditions can also change emotions.

People who have had strokes may cry or become very angry for what appears to you to be no reason or inappropriate reasons. They may lash out. They might experience rapid mood changes, and the person's mood may not correspond to what is happening around them. In addition, someone who has had a stroke may be frustrated or depressed. The American Stroke Association has the following tips for caregivers:

- Always treat your care partner with respect.
- Give praise when your care partner is acting appropriately.
- When giving choices, let the person choose between two safe and appropriate alternatives.
- When necessary, set limits.

Someone with Alzheimer's might become more confused and agitated as the day goes on. This "sundowning" effect often accompanies the disease. It is especially common during the middle stages of Alzheimer's as well as for people with some other types of dementia. Sundowning behavior tends to lessen as dementia increases. The Alzheimer's Association recommends the following suggestions for dealing with sundowning:

- As frustrating as this may be for you, always approach your care partner in a calm way and reassure them that they are in a safe place.
- Check triggers. Your care partner might need something or there may be a specific trigger.
- Sometimes it is helpful to remind your care partner of today's date and time.
- Don't argue or ask for an explanation.
- Do not take the actions personally.

People with Parkinson's-related dementia might have hallucinations or become paranoid or depressed. The recommendations just listed may be helpful in dealing with these situations. In addition, sometimes antidepressants or antipsychotic medications can be helpful. Check with your care partner's primary health care provider.

People with post-traumatic stress disorder (PTSD) commonly experience three primary difficult emotions:

1. **Hyperarousal, such as a very strong reaction to a common noise like the backfiring of a car.** Having trouble sleeping, being easily startled, anger, problems concentrating, panic, and always being alert to danger are signs of hyperarousal.
2. **Re-experiencing or going over an experience repeatedly, such as a battle or other traumatic experience.** Flashbacks are a more common name for re-experiencing. These can include bad memories, nightmares, or exaggerated reactions.
3. **Numbing, not having much emotion about anything.** Numbing is a bit like depression. The person does not feel much of anything and may not be interested in anything. Numbing usually is accompanied by withdrawal. At the same time, the person might focus on avoiding any trauma or feelings that might be a reminder of trauma.

PTSD is usually treated by psychotherapy. As a caregiver, you can urge your care partner to get mental health treatment and be supportive should they choose to do so. If possible, ask to be part of the treatment. If your care partner talks of suicide, take it seriously and seek immediate help. Remember, you are not the cause of the problem.

People with traumatic brain injury (TBI) may feel many of the same emotions discussed in this section. Just like people who have had a stroke, they may experience mood swings. For example, people who have TBI might break out laughing or become angry for no obvious reason. These usually last a very short period. Someone with TBI may also be anxious or depressed or have outbursts of anger.

Here is a list of things that you as a caregiver can do to help your care partner with TBI:

- Do not take the actions and words of your care partner personally. The TBI is the cause of the difficult emotions, not you.
- Remain calm. Work hard at not over reacting or becoming emotional.
- When possible, take your care partner to a quiet place to calm down.

- Tell your care partner that TBIs can cause difficult emotions and give your care partner a chance to talk about these.
- When appropriate, gently redirect the discussion or activity to another topic. For example, if talking about the news is a trigger for difficult emotions, change the conversation to talk about hobbies or the family.
- Let your care partner know that some behaviors such as yelling or threatening are not acceptable. If these occur, refuse to engage. You may even want to leave the room.
- Learn more about TBI at http://braininjury education.org.

You will note that depression is common for all of these conditions.

In this chapter, we have talked about some common caregiver stressors and given you some specific tools for dealing with these. We will continue with this same theme in the next chapter.

Suggested Further Reading

Ellison, Koshin Paley. *Awake at the Bedside: Contemplative Palliative and End-of-Life Care.* Somerville, MA: Wisdom Publications, 2016. Offers wisdom about death from pioneers of palliative and end-of-life care as well as doctors, chaplains, caregivers and poets. http://amzn.to/2Giechn

Jacobs, Barry J. *The Emotional Survival Guide for Caregivers Looking After Yourself and Your Family While Helping an Aging Parent*. New York: Guilford Press, 2006. Helps family members navigate tough decisions, avoid burnout, and preserve bonds. http://amzn.to/2o9cOBl

Karp, David Allen. *The Burden of Sympathy: How Families Cope with Mental Illness*. Oxford: Oxford University Press, 2004. Experiences of family members of the mentally ill and advice about how to draw boundaries of sympathy. http://amzn.to/2Ev3Cmw

Langshur, Sharon, Eric Langshur, and Mary Beth. Sammons. *We Carry Each Other: Getting through Life's Toughest Times*. San Francisco: Conari Press, 2007. A resource on what to say and do when you or a loved one suffer illness or loss. http://amzn.to/2Ggu4B0

Lebow, Grace, and Kane, Barbara. *Coping with Your Difficult Older Parent: A Guide for Stressed-Out Children*. New York: HarperCollins, 2011.

Lebowitz, Eli R., and Haim Omer. *Treating Childhood and Adolescent Anxiety: A Guide for Caregivers*. Hoboken, NJ: Wiley, 2013. Offers practical, evidence-based, and theory-driven strategies for helping children to overcome anxiety. http://amzn.to/2C69ZiW

Merkin, Daphne. *This Close to Happy: A Reckoning with Depression*. New York: Farrar, Straus and Giroux, 2017.

Scott, Paula Spencer. *Surviving Alzheimers: Practical Tips and Soul-Saving Wisdom for Caregivers*. San Francisco: Eva-Birch Media, 2014. How to defuse resentment, guilt, anger, and family friction and lifesaving insights from a team of top dementia-care experts from geriatrics, psychiatry, social work, law, dementia therapy, and caregiver advocacy. http://amzn.to/2BZsrcU

Yonover, Robert. *Caregivers Survival Guide*: *Step-by-Step Help from the Trenches*. New York: Skyhorse Publishing, 2018. Equips other caregivers who face similar physical, mental, social, and financial challenges with tips and guidelines from his own experiences and other experts. http://amzn.to/2BZVwoq

Other Resources

Caring.com lists the seven deadly emotions of caregiving and how to cope with them. https://www.caring.com/articles/7-deadly-emotions-of-caregiving

Family Caregiving Alliance provides a printable list of common emotions experienced by caregivers. https://www.caregiver.org/emotional-side-caregiving

See Chapter 11, Understanding Your Care Partner's Brain, for disease-specific references.

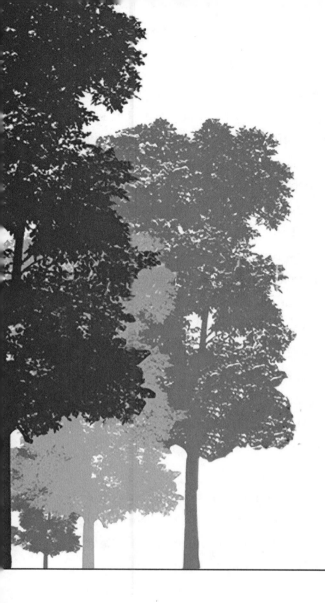

Chapter 5

Using Your Mind to Manage Stress

BEFORE WE SAY ANYTHING ELSE, we want to be clear—caregiving is stressful. Your caregiving stress is not all in your head, nor is the stress your fault. The goal of this chapter, like the last one, is to provide you with stress-managing tools. We know that no one can manage the stress of caregiving with just happy thinking. But we also know that there are many effective ways your mind can help you deal with stress. In this chapter, we introduce you to some of these mental tools.

Stress, the Mind, and the Body

There is a strong link between our thoughts, attitudes, and emotions and our mental and physical health. As one of our caregivers so truly said, "It's not always mind over matter, but mind matters." Although thoughts and emotions do not always cause stress, thoughts and emotions have a big influence on how we handle and respond to stressors. Research has shown that thoughts and emotions trigger certain hormones and other chemicals that send messages throughout the body. These messages affect how our body functions; for example, thoughts and emotions can affect our heart rate, blood pressure, breathing, blood sugar levels, muscle responses, concentration, ability to get pregnant, and our ability to fight off illness.

All of us, at one time or another, have experienced the power of the mind and its effects on the body. Both pleasant and unpleasant thoughts and emotions can cause the body to react in different ways. Our heart rate and breathing can increase or slow down; we may experience sensations such as sweating (warm or cold), blushing, tears, and so on. Sometimes just a memory or an image can trigger these responses.

For example, try this simple exercise: Imagine that you are holding a big, bright yellow lemon slice. You hold it close to your nose and smell its strong citrus aroma. Now you bite into the lemon. It's juicy! The juice fills your mouth and dribbles down your chin. Now you begin to suck on the lemon and its tart juice. What happens? Even though you are not actually biting into a lemon slice, the body responds. Your mouth puckers and starts to water. You might even smell the scent of the lemon. All of these reactions are triggered by the mind and its memory of your experience with a real lemon.

This example shows the power the mind has over the body. It also gives us a good reason to work to develop our mental abilities to help us manage our symptoms. With training and practice, we can learn to use the mind to relax the body, to reduce stress and anxiety, and to reduce the discomfort or unpleasantness caused by physical and emotional symptoms. In this chapter, we describe several ways in which you can begin to use your mind to manage stress and other symptoms. These are sometimes referred to as "thinking" or "cognitive" techniques because they involve the use of our thinking abilities to make changes in the body.

As you read, keep the following key principles in mind:

- Stress can have many causes. Because it can be caused by so many things, there are many ways to manage stress. If you understand the nature and causes of your stress or other symptoms, you will be able to manage them better.
- Not all management techniques work for everyone. It is up to you to experiment and find out what works best for you. Be flexible. This includes trying different techniques and checking your results to determine which management tool is most helpful under which circumstances.
- Learning new skills and gaining control of the situation take time. Give yourself several weeks to practice before you decide if a new tool is working for you.
- Don't give up too easily. As with exercise and other new skills, using your mind to manage stress requires both practice and time before you notice the benefits. So even if you feel you are not accomplishing anything, don't give up. Be patient and keep on trying.
- Stress reduction techniques should not have negative effects. If you become frightened, angry, or depressed when using one of these

tools, do not continue to use it. Try another tool instead.

- Stress is not all bad. In fact, we need stress to help us prepare for challenging situations. Stress can make us tougher and more resilient. Learning new things and overcoming challenges often involves some positive stress.

Relaxation Techniques

Many of us have heard and read about relaxation, yet some of us are still confused as to what relaxation is, its benefits, and how to do it. Simply stated, relaxation involves using thinking techniques to reduce or eliminate tension from both the body and the mind. Relaxation usually results in less stress, improved sleep, less frustration, and might also help with pain and shortness of breath. Relaxation is not a cure-all, but it can be a beneficial life skill.

The goal of relaxation is to turn off the outside world so that the mind and body are at rest. This allows you to reduce the tensions that can increase the intensity or severity of symptoms.

There are different types of relaxation techniques. Each has specific guidelines and uses. Some techniques are used mostly to achieve muscle relaxation. Others are aimed at reducing anxiety and emotional stress or diverting attention, all of which aid in stress management.

Quick and Easy Relaxation

Some types of relaxation are so easy, natural, and effective that people do not think of them as "relaxation techniques." They include the following:

- Take a nap or a warm, soothing bath.
- Curl up and read or listen to a good book.
- Watch a funny movie or a favorite TV show.
- Make a paper airplane and sail it across the room.
- Get a massage.
- Enjoy an occasional glass of wine or beer.
- Start a small garden or grow a beautiful plant indoors.
- Do crafts such as knitting, pottery, or woodworking.
- Read a poem or an inspirational saying.
- Go for a walk.
- Start a collection (for example, coins, folk art, shells, or something in miniature) and add to it.
- Listen to your favorite music.
- Sing around the house.
- Crumble paper into a ball and use a wastebasket as a basketball hoop.
- Look at water (for example, ocean waves, a lake, or a fountain).
- Watch the clouds in the sky.
- Put your head down on your table and close your eyes for five minutes.
- Rub your hands together until they're warm, and then cup them over your closed eyes.
- Vigorously shake your hands and arms for 10 seconds.

- Call a friend or family member to chat.
- Smile and introduce yourself to someone new.
- Do something nice and unexpected for someone else.
- Stroke or play with a pet.
- Go to a vacation spot in your mind.

Relaxation Tools That Take 5 to 20 Minutes

These techniques take a bit longer but are quite effective. The following are some guidelines to help you get the most out of these relaxation tools:

- Pick a quiet place and time when you will not be disturbed for at least 15 to 20 minutes. (If this seems too long, start with five minutes. By the way, in some homes the only quiet place is the bathroom. That is just fine.)
- Try to practice the technique once or twice daily and not less than four times a week.
- Don't expect instant success. Your mind way wander. This is normal. Most of these techniques take practice. Sometimes it takes three to four weeks of consistent practice before you start to notice benefits.
- Relaxation should be helpful. At worst, you may find it boring, but if it is an unpleasant experience or makes you more nervous or anxious, switch to a different stress management tool described in this chapter.

Body Scan

To relax your muscles, it is helpful to know how to scan your body and recognize where you are tense. Then you can release the tension. The first step is to become familiar with the difference between the feeling of tension and the feeling of relaxation. This exercise allows you to compare those feelings and, with practice, spot and release tension anywhere in your body. It is best done lying down on your back, but any comfortable position can work. A body scan script can be found on page 49.

Relaxation Response

In the early 1970s, physician Herbert Benson studied what he calls the "relaxation response." According to Benson, our bodies have several natural states. One example is the "fight or flight" response experienced by people when faced with a great danger. During the fight or flight response the body becomes quite tense as it prepares to "fight" or to "flee." This tension is eventually followed by the body's natural tendency to relax; this is the relaxation response. As our lives become more and more hectic, our bodies tend to stay tense for long periods. We lose our ability to relax. Practicing the relaxation response helps change this pattern.

Find a quiet place where there are few or no distractions. Get in a comfortable position. You should be comfortable enough to remain in the same position for 20 minutes.

Choose a word, object, or pleasant feeling. For example, repeat a word or sound (such as the word *one*), gaze at an object or symbol (perhaps a flower), or concentrate on a feeling (such as peace).

Adopt a passive attitude. A passive attitude is very important for this exercise. Empty all thoughts and distractions from your mind. You might become aware of thoughts, images, and

Body-Scan Script

As you get into a comfortable position, allowing yourself to begin to sink comfortably into the surface below you, you may perhaps begin to allow your eyes gradually to close. . . . From there, turn your attention to your breath. . . . Breathing in, allowing the breath gradually to go all the way down to your belly and then breathing out . . . and again, breathing in . . . and out . . . noticing the natural rhythm of your breathing. . . .

Now, allowing your attention to focus on your feet. Starting with your toes, notice whatever sensations are there—warmth, coolness, whatever's there . . . simply feel it. Using your mind's eye, imagine that as you breathe in, the breath goes all the way down into your toes, bringing with it new refreshing air. . . . And now noticing the sensations elsewhere in your feet, not judging or thinking about what you're feeling, but simply becoming aware of the experience of your feet as you allow yourself to be fully supported by the surface below you. . . .

Next focus on your lower legs and knees. These muscles and joints do a lot of work for us, but often we don't give them the attention they deserve. So now breathe down into the knees, calves, and ankles, noticing whatever sensations appear. . . . See if you can simply stay with the sensations . . . breathing in new, fresh air, and, as you exhale, releasing tension and stress and allowing the muscles to relax and soften. . . .

Now move your attention to the muscles, bones, and joints of the thighs, buttocks, and hips . . . breathing down into the upper legs, noticing whatever sensations you experience. It may be warmth, coolness, a heaviness or lightness. You may become aware of the contact with the surface beneath you, or perhaps the pulsing of your blood. Whatever's there . . . what matters is that you are taking time to learn to relax . . . deeper and deeper, as you breathe . . . in . . . and out.

Move your attention now to your back and chest. Feeling the breath fill the abdomen and chest. . . . Noticing whatever sensations are there . . . not judging or thinking, but simply observing what is right here right now, allowing the fresh air to nourish the muscles, bones, and joints as you breathe in, and then exhaling any tension and stress.

Now focus on the neck, shoulders, arms, and hands. Inhaling down through the neck and shoulders, all the way down to the fingertips. Not trying too hard to relax, but simply becoming aware of your experience of these parts of your body in the present moment. . . .

Turning now to your face and head, notice the sensations beginning at the back of your head, up along your scalp, and down into your forehead. . . . Then become aware of the sensations in and around your eyes and down into your cheeks and jaw. . . . Continue to allow your muscles to release and soften as you breathe in nourishing, fresh air, and allow tension and stress to leave as you breathe out. . . .

As you drink in fresh air, allow it to spread throughout your body, from the soles of your feet all the way up through the top of your head. . . . and then exhale any remaining stress and tension. . . . And now take a few moments to enjoy the stillness as you breathe in . . . and out . . . Awake, relaxed, and still . . .

Now as the body scan comes to a close, coming back into the room, bringing with you whatever sensations of relaxation . . . comfort . . . peace, whatever's there . . . knowing that you can repeat this exercise at any appropriate time and place of your choosing. . . . And when you're ready, open your eyes.

▸ To order the *Relaxation for Mind & Body* CD, go to www.bullpub.com/catalog/relaxation-for-mind-and-body

feelings, but don't concentrate on them. Just allow them to pass on.

To elicit the relaxation response, take the following steps:

- Sit or lie quietly in a comfortable position.
- Close your eyes.
- Relax all your muscles, beginning at your feet and progressing up to your face. Keep them relaxed.
- Breathe in through your nose. Become aware of your breathing. As you breathe out through your mouth, if you chose a word, say it silently to yourself. Try to empty all thoughts from your mind; concentrate on your word, sound, or symbol. When your mind wanders, as it certainly will, just gently guide your attention back to your chosen word, sound, or symbol.
- Continue this for 10 to 20 minutes. You can open your eyes to check the time, but do not use an alarm. When you finish, sit quietly for several minutes, at first with your eyes closed. Do not stand up for a few minutes.
- Maintain a passive attitude, and let relaxation occur at its own pace. When distracting thoughts occur, ignore them by not dwelling on them, and return to repeating the word you chose. Do not worry about whether you are successful in achieving a deep level of relaxation.
- Practice this once or twice daily.

Distraction

Our minds have trouble focusing on more than one thing at a time; therefore, we can lessen the intensity of stress symptoms by training our minds to focus attention on something other than our bodies and their sensations. This technique, called distraction or attention refocusing, is particularly helpful for those people who feel that their stress symptoms are painful or overwhelming. (It is important to mention that with distraction you are not ignoring the stress but choosing not to dwell on it.)

Sometimes it is difficult to put anxious thoughts out of your mind. When you try to suppress any thought, you may end up thinking more about it. For example, try not thinking about a tiger charging at you. Whatever you do, don't let the thought of a tiger enter your mind! You'll probably find it nearly impossible not to think about the tiger.

Although you can't easily stop thinking about something, you can distract yourself and redirect your attention elsewhere. Think about the charging tiger again. Now stand up suddenly, slam your hand on the table, and shout *"Stop!"* What happened to the tiger? Gone—at least for the moment.

Distraction works best for short activities or times in which stress is anticipated. For example, if you know a certain caregiving job will cause discomfort or that falling asleep at night is difficult, you might try one of the following distraction techniques:

- Make plans for exactly what you will do after the unpleasant activity passes. For example, if getting your care partner to take a shower is a challenge, think about what you can do after the shower is over. If you have trouble falling asleep, try making plans for some future event, being as detailed as possible.
- Think of a person's name, a bird, a flower, or whatever, for every letter of the alphabet. If you get stuck on one letter, go on to the next. (These are good distractions for pain and for sleep problems.)
- Challenge yourself to count backward from 100 by threes (100, 97, 94, . . .).
- To get through unpleasant daily chores (such as sweeping, mopping, or vacuuming), imagine your floor as a map of a country or continent. Try naming all the states, provinces, or countries, moving east to west or north to south. If geography does not appeal to you, imagine your favorite store and where each department is located.
- Try to remember words to favorite songs or the events in an old story.
- Try the "*Stop!*" technique. If you find yourself worrying or entrapped in endlessly repeating negative thoughts, stand up suddenly, slap your hand on the table or your thigh, and shout "*Stop!*" You can practice this technique whenever your mind endlessly repeats negative thoughts. With practice, you won't have to shout out loud. Just whispering "*Stop!*" or tightening your vocal cords and moving your tongue as if saying "*Stop!*" will often work. Some people imagine a large stop sign. Others put a rubber band on their wrist and snap it hard to break the chain of negative thought. Do anything that redirects your attention.
- Redirect your attention to a pleasurable experience:
  - Picture something outside, such as your garden or the seashore.
  - Remember Thanksgiving at Grandma's house.
  - Think about how you felt when your team won the Super Bowl.
  - Picture your children or grandchildren when they were babies.
  - Remember a time when your pet did something funny.

There are, of course, many variations to these examples, all of which help you refocus attention away from your problem.

So far, we have discussed short-term refocusing strategies that involve using only the mind for distraction. Distraction also works well for long-term projects or stress symptoms that tend to last longer, such as depression.

In these cases, the mind is focused not internally but externally on some type of activity. If you are somewhat depressed or have continuous unpleasant feelings, find an activity that interests you, and distract yourself from the problem. The activity can be almost anything, from gardening to cooking to reading or going to a movie. One of the marks of successful caregivers is that they have a variety of interests and take time to restore themselves.

Positive Thinking and Self-Talk

We all talk to ourselves all the time. For example, when waking up in the morning, we may think, "I really don't want to get out of bed. I'm tired and I don't think I can be a caregiver one more day." Or at the end of an enjoyable evening, we think, "Gee, that was fun. I had forgotten that my care partner and I could still have fun." What we think or say to ourselves is called our self-talk. The way we talk to ourselves tends to come from how and what we think about ourselves. Our thoughts can be positive or negative, and so is our self-talk. Therefore, self-talk can be an effective self-management tool (if it's positive thinking) or a weapon that hurts or defeats us (if it's habitually negative thinking).

Our self-talk is usually learned from others and becomes a part of us as we grow up. It comes in many forms; unfortunately, these forms are often negative. Negative self-statements usually take the form of phrases that begin with something like, "I just can't do . . . ," "If only I could . . . ," "If only I didn't . . . ," "I just don't have the energy . . . ," or "How could I be so stupid?" This type of negative thinking represents the doubts and fears we have about ourselves in general and about our abilities to deal with our role as a caregiver and our care partner's condition and its symptoms. Negative thinking damages our self-esteem, attitude, and mood. Negative self-talk makes us feel bad and undermines our ability to deal with stressful challenges.

What we say to ourselves plays a major role in determining our success or failure in becoming effective caregivers. Negative thinking tends to limit our abilities and actions. If we tell ourselves "I'm not very smart" or "I can't" all the time, we probably won't try to learn new skills because this just doesn't fit with what we think about ourselves. Soon we become prisoners of our own negative beliefs. Fortunately, self-talk is not something fixed in our biological makeup, and therefore it is not completely out of our control. We can learn new, healthier ways to think about ourselves so that our self-talk can work for us instead of against us. By changing the negative, self-defeating statements to positive ones, we can manage stress and other symptoms more effectively. This change, like any habit, requires practice and includes the following steps:

1. **Listen carefully to what you say to or about yourself, both out loud and silently.** If you find yourself feeling anxious, depressed, or angry, try to identify some of the thoughts you were having just before these feelings started. Then write down all the negative self-talk statements. Pay special attention to the things you say during times that are particularly difficult for you. For example, what do you say to yourself when you start to get annoyed with your care partner or when you do not think you are doing enough? Challenge these negative thoughts by asking yourself questions to identify what about the statement is really true or not true. Are you exaggerating the situation, generalizing, worrying too much, or assuming the worst? Are you thinking in terms of black and white? Could there be gray? Maybe you are making an unrealistic or unfair comparison, assuming too much

responsibility, taking something too personally, or expecting perfection. Are you making assumptions about what other people think about you? What do you know for a fact? Look at the evidence so that you are better able to change these negative thoughts and statements.

2. **Work on changing each negative statement to a more positive one, or think up a positive statement to replace the negative one.** Write the positive statements down so you can get in the habit of repeating them instead of the negative statements. For example, negative statements such as "I don't want to get up," "I'm too tired and it will just be another awful day," "I can't do anything that pleases my care partner, so why bother?" or "I'm good for nothing" become positive messages such as "I'm feeling pretty good today and I'm going to do something I enjoy," "I might not be able to do everything but I know that my care partner appreciates the effort even if she cannot express appreciation," or "My care partner needs and depends on me; what I do is worthwhile and important."
3. **Read and rehearse these positive statements, silently to yourself or with another person.** This conscious repetition or memorization of the positive self-talk will help you replace those old, habitual negative statements.
4. **Practice these new statements in real situations.** This practice, along with time and patience, will help the new patterns of thinking become automatic.
5. **Rehearse success.** When you aren't happy with the way you handled a particular situation, try this exercise:
   - Write down three ways that it could have gone better.
   - Write down three ways it could have gone worse.
   - If you can't think of alternatives to the way you handled it, imagine what someone whom you greatly respect would have done.
   - Think what advice you would give to someone else facing a similar situation.

Remember that mistakes aren't failures. They're opportunities to learn. Mistakes give you the chance to rehearse other ways of handling things. This is great practice for future crises.

As you first do this, you may find it hard to change negative statements into more positive ones. A shortcut is to use either a thought stopper or a positive affirmation. A thought stopper can be anything that is meaningful to you (for example, a puppy, a polar bear, a rose or an oak tree). When you have a negative thought, replace it with your thought stopper. It might sound silly, but try it. It works for some people and you may be one of them.

A positive affirmation is a positive phrase that you can use over and over. It's ready to use when you need it. For example, "I am getting better every day," "I can do this," or "God loves me." Like the positive statements, use this to replace negative thoughts.

Imagery

You may think that "imagination" is all in your mind. But the thoughts, words, and images that flow from your imagination can have very real effects on your body. Your brain often cannot distinguish whether you are imagining something or if it is really happening. Perhaps you've had a racing heartbeat, rapid breathing, or tension in your neck muscles while watching a movie thriller. These sensations were all produced by images and sounds on a film. During a dream, maybe your body responded with fear, joy, anger, or sadness—all triggered by your imagination. If you close your eyes and vividly imagine yourself by a still, quiet pool or relaxing on a warm beach, your body responds to some degree as though you were actually there.

Guided imagery and visualization allow you to use your imagination to relieve stress symptoms. These techniques will help you focus your thoughts on healing images and suggestions.

Guided Imagery

This tool is like a guided daydream. It allows you to divert your attention, refocusing your mind away from your symptoms and transporting you to another time and place. It has the added benefit of helping you achieve deep relaxation by picturing yourself in a peaceful environment.

With guided imagery, you focus your mind on a particular image. Imagery usually involves your sense of sight, focusing on visual images. Adding other senses—smells, tastes, and sounds—makes the guided imagery especially vivid and powerful.

Some people are highly visual and easily see images with their "mind's eye." But if your images aren't as vivid as scenes from a great movie, don't worry; it's normal for the intensity of imagery to vary. The important thing is to focus on as much detail as possible and to strengthen the images by using all your senses. Adding real background music can also increase the impact of guided imagery.

With guided imagery, you are always completely in control. You're the movie director. You can project whatever thought or feeling you want onto your mental screen. If you don't like a particular image, thought, or feeling, you can redirect your mind to something more comfortable, or you can open your eyes and stop the exercise and use a different script next time.

The guided imagery scripts presented on pages 59 and 62 can help take you on this mental stroll. Here are some ways to use imagery:

- Read the script over several times until it is familiar. Then sit or lie down in a quiet place and try to reconstruct the scene in your mind. The script should take 15 to 20 minutes to complete.
- Have a family member or friend read you the script slowly, pausing for about 10 seconds wherever there is a series of periods (. . .).
- Make a recording of the script, and play it to yourself whenever convenient.
- Use a prerecorded tape, CD, or digital audio file that has a similar guided imagery script (see examples in the Other Resources section at end of this chapter).

Guided-Imagery Script: A Walk in the Country

Begin by getting into a comfortable position, whether you are seated or lying down. Loosen any tight clothing to allow yourself to be as comfortable as possible. Uncross your legs and allow your hands to fall by your sides or rest in your lap, and, if you are at all uncomfortable, shift to a more comfortable position.

You're giving yourself some time to quiet your mind and body. Allow yourself to settle comfortably, wherever you are right now. If you wish, you can close your eyes. Breathe in deeply, through your nose, expanding your abdomen and filling your lungs and, pursing your lips, exhale through your mouth slowly and completely, allowing your body to sink heavily into the surface beneath you. . . .

And once again breathe in through your nose and all the way down to your abdomen, and then breathe out slowly through pursed lips, letting go of tension, letting go of anything that's on your mind right now and just allowing yourself to be present in this moment. . . .

Imagine yourself walking along a peaceful old country road. The sun is gently warming your back . . the birds are singing . . . the air is calm and fragrant. . . .

With no need to hurry, you notice your walking is relaxed and easy. As you walk along in this way, taking in your surroundings, you come across an old gate. It looks inviting and you decide to take the path through the gate. The gate creaks as you open it and go through.

You find yourself in an old, overgrown garden, flowers growing where they've seeded themselves, vines climbing over a fallen tree, soft green wild grasses, shade trees.

You notice yourself breathing deeply . . . smelling the flowers . . . listening to the birds and insects . . . feeling a gentle breeze cool against your skin. All of your senses are alive and responding with pleasure to this peaceful time and place. . . .

When you're ready to move on, you leisurely follow the path out behind the garden, eventually coming to a more wooded area. As you enter this area, your eyes find the trees and plant life restful. The sunlight is filtered through the leaves. The air feels mild and a little cooler. . . . You savor the fragrance of trees and earth . . . and gradually become aware of the sound of a nearby stream. Pausing, you allow yourself to take in the sights and sounds, breathing in the cool and fragrant air several times. . . . And with each breath, you notice how refreshed you are feeling. . . .

Continuing along the path for a while, you come to the stream. It's clear and clean as it flows and tumbles over the rocks and some fallen logs. You follow the path easily along the creek for a way, and after a while, you come out into a sunlit clearing, where you discover a small waterfall emptying into a quiet pool of water.

You find a comfortable place to sit for a while, a perfect niche where you can feel completely relaxed.

You feel good as you allow yourself to just enjoy the warmth and solitude of this peaceful place. . . .

After a while, you become aware that it is time to return. You arise and walk back down the path in a relaxed and comfortable way, through the cool and fragrant trees, out into the sun-drenched, overgrown garden. . . . One last smell of the flowers, and out the creaky gate.

You leave this country retreat for now and return down the road. You notice you feel calm and rested. You feel grateful and remind yourself that you can visit this special place whenever you wish to take some time to refresh yourself and renew your energy.

And now, preparing to bring this period of relaxation to a close, you may want to take a moment to picture yourself carrying this experience of calm and refreshment with you into the ordinary activities of your life. . . . And when you're ready, take a nice deep breath and open your eyes.

▸ To order the *Relaxation for Mind & Body CD*, go to www.bullpub.com/catalog/relaxation-for-mind-and-body

Visualization

This technique is similar to guided imagery. Visualization allows you to create your own images. However, in guided imagery, the images are suggested to you. Visualization is another way of using your imagination to create a picture of yourself in any way you want, doing the things you want to do. All of us use a form of visualization every day—when we daydream, worry, read a book, or listen to a story. In all these activities the mind creates images for us to see. We also use visualization intentionally when making plans for the day, considering the possible outcomes of a decision we have to make, or rehearsing for an event or activity. Visualization can be done in different ways and can be used for longer periods or while you are engaged in other activities.

One way to use visualization to manage stress is to remember pleasant scenes from your past or create new scenes. To practice visualization, try to remember every detail of a special holiday or party that made you happy. Who was there? What happened? What did you do or talk about? You can also try this by remembering a vacation or some other memorable and pleasant event.

During visualization you can plan the details of some future event or fill in the details of a fantasy. For example, how would you spend a million dollars? What would your ideal home or garden look like? Where would you go and what would you do on your dream vacation?

Another form of visualization involves using your mind to think of symbols that represent stress-related discomfort or pain felt in different parts of your body. For example, a stiff neck might be red, or a tight chest might have a constricting band around it. After forming these images, you then try to change them. The red color might fade until there is no more color, or the constricting band will stretch and stretch until it falls off. These new images then cause the way you think of the pain or discomfort to change.

Visualization helps build confidence and skill and therefore is a useful technique to help you set and accomplish your personal goals (see Chapter 2, Becoming a Better Caregiver: The Basics). After you write your weekly action plan, take a few minutes to imagine yourself taking a walk, doing your exercises, or using a relaxation technique from this chapter. You are mentally rehearsing the steps you need to take in order to achieve your goal successfully.

Imagery for Different Conditions

You have the ability to create special imagery to help (though not cure) specific stress-related symptoms or feelings. Use any image that is strong and vivid for you—this often involves using all your senses to create the image—and one that is meaningful to you. The image does not have to be accurate for it to work. Just use your imagination and trust yourself. Here are examples of images that some people have found useful:

For Tension and Stress

A tight, twisted rope slowly untwists.

Wax softens and melts.

Tension swirls out of your body and down the drain.

For Fatigue

A light bulb is turned on and you feel a sudden burst of energy.

A puppy races around you with boundless energy and enthusiasm.

You slowly take off a heavy winter coat allowing you to feel lighter and more energetic.

For Pain

All of the pain is placed in a large, strong metal box that is closed, sealed tightly, and locked with a huge, strong padlock.

You grasp the TV remote control and slowly turn down the pain volume until you can barely hear it; then it disappears entirely.

The pain is washed away by a cool, calm river flowing through your entire body.

For Depression

Your troubles and feelings of sadness are attached to big colorful helium balloons and are floating off into a clear blue sky.

A strong, warm sun breaks through dark clouds.

You feel a sense of detachment and lightness, enabling you to float easily through your day.

Use any of these images, or make up your own. Remember, the most effective images are vivid and have meaning to you. Use your imagination for health and healing.

Prayer and Spirituality

There is strong evidence of the relationship between spirituality and health. Spirituality is one way we find meaning, hope, comfort, and inner peace in our lives. Many people find spirituality through religion. Some find it through music, art, or a connection with nature. Others find it in their values and principles.

Many people are religious and share their religion with others. Others do not have a specific religion but do have spiritual beliefs. Our religion and beliefs can bring a sense of meaning and purpose to our lives, help us put things into perspective, and set priorities. Our beliefs may help us find comfort during difficult times. They can help us with acceptance and motivate us to make difficult changes. A spiritual or religious community can serve as a source of support when needed and give us the opportunity to help others.

Recent studies find that people who belong to a religious or spiritual community, or who regularly engage in religious activities, such as prayer or study, have improved health. There are many types of prayer—any of which may contribute to improved health including asking for help, direction, and forgiveness and offering words of gratitude, praise, and blessing, among others. In addition, many religions have a tradition of contemplation or meditation. Prayer does not need a scientific explanation. It is probably the oldest of all self-management tools.

Although religion cannot be "prescribed," we encourage you to explore your own beliefs. If you are religious, try practicing prayer more consistently. If you are not religious, consider adopting some form of reflection or meditative practice. If you and your care partner have a prayer tradition, continue it. Say prayers out loud. You might not think your care partner is listening or understanding. Hospital chaplains will tell you that when they pray with unconscious patients, the patterns on heart monitors tend to slow and become more regular.

Guided-Imagery Script: A Walk on the Beach

Begin by getting into a comfortable position, whether you are seated or lying down. Loosen any tight clothing to allow yourself to be as comfortable as possible. Uncross your legs and allow your hands to fall by your sides or rest in your lap, and if you are at all uncomfortable, shift to a more comfortable position.

When you are ready, you allow your eyes gradually to close and turn your attention to your breathing. Allow your belly to expand as you breathe in, bringing in fresh new air to nourish your body. And then breathing out. Notice the rhythm of your breathing . . . in . . . and out . . . without trying to control it in any way at all. Simply attend to the natural rhythm of your breath. . . .

And now, in your mind's eye, imagine yourself standing on a beautiful beach. The sky is a brilliant blue, and as some fluffy white clouds float slowly by, you drink in the beautiful colors. . . . The temperature is not too hot and not too cold. The sun is shining, and you close your eyes, allowing the warmth of the sun to wash over you. . . . You notice a gentle breeze caressing your face, the perfect complement to the sunshine.

Then you find yourself turning and looking out over the vastness of the ocean . . . you become aware of the sound of the waves gently washing up on shore . . . You notice the firmness of the wet sand beneath your feet, or if you decide to take off your shoes, you may enjoy the feeling of standing, in the cool, wet sand. . . . Perhaps you allow the surf roll up and gently wash across your feet, or perhaps you stay just out of its reach. . . .

In the distance, you hear some seagulls calling to one another and look out to see the birds gracefully gliding through the air. And as you stand there, notice how easy it is to be here, perhaps noticing some sensations of relaxation, comfort, or peace . . . whatever's there. . . .

Now take a walk along the shore. Turn and begin to stroll casually along the beach, enjoying the sounds of the surf, the warmth of the sun, and the gentle massage of the breeze. As you move along, taking your time, your stride becomes lighter, easier. . . . You notice the scent of the ocean. . . . You pause to take in the freshness of the air. . . . And then you continue on your way, enjoying the peacefulness of this place.

After a time, you decide to rest a while and find a comfortable place to sit or lie down . . . and simply allow yourself to take some time to enjoy this, your special place. . . .

And now, when you feel ready to return, you stand and begin walking back down the beach in a comfortable, leisurely way, taking with you any sensations of relaxation, comfort, peace, joy . . . whatever's there . . . noticing how easy it is to be here. Continue back until you reach the place where you began your walk. . . .

And now pausing to take one last long look around. Enjoying the vibrant colors of the sky and the sea . . . the gentle sound of the waves washing up on the shore, the warmth of the sun, the cool of the breeze. . . .

And as you prepare to leave this special place, taking with you any sensations of joy, relaxation, comfort, peace . . . whatever's there . . .knowing that you may return at any time appropriate time and place of your choosing.

And now bringing your awareness back into the room, focusing on your breathing . . . in and out . . . taking a few more breaths . . . and when you're ready, opening your eyes.

▸ To order the *Relaxation for Mind & Body* CD, go to www.bullpub.com/catalog/relaxation-for-mind-and-body

Also, if you or your care partner is religious, consider telling the caregivers who are part of the care team. Most won't ask. Help them understand the importance of religious beliefs in managing your and your care partner's health and life. Most hospitals have chaplains or pastoral counselors. Even if you are not in the hospital, these spiritual advisers will probably be willing to talk with you. Most respite and hospice services have chaplains. Ask for that person to visit at least once. You might find new support and, if not, they do not have to come again. Their advice and counsel can supplement your medical and psychological care.

Other Techniques for Managing Stress

There are additional valuable techniques you can consider which can clear your mind, positively shift your emotional state, as well as reduce tension and stress.

Mindfulness

Mindfulness involves simply keeping your attention in the present moment, without judging what is happening as happy or sad, good or bad. It encourages living each moment—even painful ones—as fully and as mindfully as possible. Mindfulness is more than a relaxation technique; it is an attitude toward living. It is a way of calmly and consciously observing and accepting whatever is happening, moment to moment.

This sounds simple enough, but our restless, judging minds make it surprisingly difficult. Just like a restless monkey jumps from branch to branch, our mind jumps from thought to thought.

Mindfulness practice is one form of meditation. In mindfulness, you focus the mind on the present moment. The "goal" of mindfulness is simply to observe—with no intention of changing or improving anything. But people are positively changed by the practice. Observing and accepting life just as it is, with all its pleasures, pains, frustrations, disappointments, and insecurities, often enables people to become calmer, more confident, and better able to cope with whatever comes along.

To develop your capacity for mindfulness, sit comfortably on the floor or on a chair with your back, neck, and head straight, but not stiff. When you are comfortable, begin the following practice:

- Concentrate on a single object, such as your breathing. Focus your attention on the feeling of the air as it passes in and out of your nostrils with each breath. Don't try to control your breathing by speeding it up or slowing it down. Just observe it as it is.
- Even when you resolve to keep your attention on your breathing, your mind will quickly wander off. When this occurs, observe where your mind went: perhaps to a memory, a worry about the future, a bodily ache, or a feeling of impatience. Then gently return your attention to your breathing.
- Use your breath as an anchor. Each time a thought or feeling arises, momentarily acknowledge it. Don't analyze it or judge it. Just observe it, and return to your breathing.

- Let go of all thoughts of getting somewhere, or having anything special happen. Just keep stringing moments of mindfulness together, breath-by-breath.
- At first, practice this for just five minutes, or even one minute at a time. You may wish to gradually extend the time to 10, 20 or 30 minutes.

Because the practice of mindfulness is simply the practice of moment-to-moment awareness, you can apply it to anything: eating, showering, working, talking, running errands, or playing with your children. Mindfulness takes no extra time. Considerable research has demonstrated the benefits of mindfulness practice in relieving stress, easing pain, improving concentration, and relieving a variety of other symptoms.

Quieting Reflex

The "quieting reflex" technique was developed by physician Charles Stroebel. It can help you deal with short-term stress, such as the urge to eat, yell at your care partner, road rage, or other annoyances. It relieves muscle tightening, jaw clenching, and holding your breath by activating the sympathetic nervous system.

The quieting reflex technique should be practiced frequently throughout the day, whenever you start to feel stressed. It can be done with your eyes opened or closed.

1. Become aware of what is annoying you: a ringing phone, an angry comment, the urge to smoke, a worrisome thought—whatever.
2. Repeat the phrase "Alert mind, calm body" to yourself.
3. Smile inwardly with your eyes and your mouth. This stops facial muscles from making a fearful or angry expression. The inward smile is a feeling. It cannot be seen by others.
4. Inhale slowly to the count of three, imagining that the breath comes in through the bottom of your feet. Then exhale slowly. Feel your breath move back down your legs and out through your feet. Let your jaw, tongue, and shoulder muscles go limp.

With several months' practice the quieting reflex becomes an automatic skill.

Nature Therapy

Many of us suffer from what has been called "nature deficit disorder," but it can be readily cured with regular doses of the outdoors. For thousands of years, exposure to natural environments has been recommended for healing. Taking a break from artificial lighting, excessive computer and TV screen time, and indoor environments can be restorative. A brief walk, if only to the corner newspaper box or a visit to a nearby park, can restore the mind and body. Or bring nature indoors with plants, pets, and nature photography. Even a few minutes of playing with or stroking a pet can lower blood pressure and calm a restless mind. An added benefit of these examples is that even though you might be doing them for yourself, they can work for your care partner at the same time!

Worry Time

Worrisome negative thoughts feed anxiety. Ignored problems have a way of thrusting themselves back into our consciousness. You'll find it easier to set aside worries if you make time to deal with them.

Set aside 20 to 30 minutes a day as your "worry time." Whenever a worry pops into your mind, write it down and tell yourself that you'll deal with it during worry time. Jot down the little things ("Will my care partner eat dinner?") along with the big ones ("What will I do if my care partner gets worse?"). During your scheduled worry time, don't do anything except worry, brainstorm, and write down possible solutions. For each of your worries, ask yourself the following questions:

- What is the problem?
- How likely is it that the problem will occur?
- What's the worst that could happen?
- What's the best that could happen?
- How would I cope with the problem?
- What are possible solutions?
- What is my plan of action?

Be specific. Instead of worrying about what might happen if you cannot keep your job, ask yourself how likely it is that you will lose your job. And if you do, what will you do, with whom, and by when? Write a plan on how you might balance your job and caregiving or how you might take a leave of absence.

If you're anxious about possibly having to clean a care partner who cannot make it to the bathroom in time, imagine how you would manage the situation. Ask yourself if any of this is really unbearable. Tell yourself you might feel uncomfortable or embarrassed, but you'll survive.

Remember, if a new worry pops up during the rest of the day, jot it down and save it to address during worry time. After you jot it down, distract yourself by refocusing intently on whatever you were doing before the worry interrupted you.

Scheduling a definite worry time cuts the amount of time you spend worrying by at least a third. If you look at your list of worries later, you'll find that the vast majority of them never became realities. Or if they did really happen, they were not nearly as bad as you had anticipated.

Change Your Perspective

Sometimes you can relieve stress and break the cycle of negative thoughts by shifting your perspective. If you find yourself upset, ask, "How important will this be in an hour, a day, a month, or a year?" Or you might consider how important this stress is compared to natural disasters or other calamities. This reframing often helps us sort out the things that are really important and need action versus the more minor annoyances that capture our attention.

Practice Gratitude

One of the most effective ways to improve your mood and overall happiness is by focusing your attention on what's going well in your life. What makes you feel grateful? Psychologists have done research to demonstrate that people can increase their happiness by gratitude exercises. We encourage you to try these three:

- **Write a letter of thanks.** Write and then deliver a letter of gratitude to someone who was especially kind to you but has never been properly thanked. Perhaps it's a teacher, a mentor, a friend, or a family member. Express your appreciation for the person's help and kindness. The letter will have more impact if you include some specific examples of what the recipient has done for you. Describe how the actions made you feel.

Ideally, read your letter out loud to the person and, if possible, face-to-face. Be aware of how you feel, and watch the other person's reaction.

- **Acknowledge at least three good things every day.** Each night before bed, write down at least three things that went well on that day. No event or feeling is too small to note. By putting your gratitude into words, you increase appreciation and memory of your blessings. Knowing that you will need to write each night changes your mental filters during the whole day. You will seek out, be more aware of, and specially note the good things that happen. If doing this daily is too much or begins to seem like a routine chore, do it once a week.
- **Make a list of the things you take for granted.** Perhaps you can celebrate a day in which your care partner smiles or remembers your name. Counting your blessings can add up to a better mood and more happiness.

Compile a List of Strengths

Make a personal inventory of your talents, skills, achievements, and qualities, big and small. Celebrate your accomplishments. When something goes wrong, consult your list of positives, and put the problem in perspective. It then becomes just one specific experience, not something that defines your whole life.

Practice Kindness

This world is plagued by acts of violence. When something bad happens, it's front-page news. As an antidote to this misery, despair, and cynicism, practice acts of kindness. Look for opportunities to give without expecting anything in return. Here are some examples of small acts that can make you and others feel better in a very real way:

- Hold the door open for the person behind you.
- Give an unexpected gift of movie or concert tickets.
- Send an anonymous gift to a friend who needs cheering up.
- Lend a hand to someone who is carrying a load.
- Tell positive stories you know of helping and kindness.
- Cultivate an attitude of gratefulness for the kindness you have received.
- Plant a tree.
- Smile and let people cut ahead of you in line or on the freeway.
- Pick up litter.
- Give another driver your parking space.

Be creative. Kindness is contagious and has a ripple effect. In one study, the people who were given an unexpected treat (cookies) were later more likely to help others.

Write Away Stress

It's hard work to keep our deep negative feelings hidden. Over time, the cumulative stress of hiding our emotions undermines our body's defenses and can weaken our immunity. Confiding our feelings to others or writing them down puts them into words and helps us sort them out. Words help us understand and absorb a traumatic event and eventually put it behind us. Putting something in writing can give us a sense of release and control.

The psychologist Jamie Pennebaker in his books *Opening Up* and *Expressive Writing: Words That Heal* describes a series of studies looked at the healing effects of confiding or writing. One group was asked to express their deepest thoughts and feelings about something bad that had happened to them. Another group wrote about ordinary matters such as their plans for the day. Both groups wrote for 15 to 20 minutes a day for three to five consecutive days. No one read what either group had written.

The results were striking. The writing "therapy" was surprisingly powerful. When compared with the people who wrote about ordinary events, the ones who wrote about their bad experiences reported fewer symptoms, fewer visits to the doctor, fewer days off from work, improved mood, and a more positive outlook. Their immune function was enhanced for at least six weeks after writing. This was especially true for those who expressed previously undisclosed painful feelings in their writing.

Try the "write thing" when something is bothering you: when you find yourself thinking (or dreaming) too much about an experience; when you avoid thinking about something because it is too upsetting; or when there's something you would like to tell others but don't for fear of embarrassment or punishment.

Here are some guidelines for writing as a way to help you deal with any unpleasant or traumatic experience:

- Set a specific time aside for writing. For example, you might write 15 minutes a day for four consecutive days, or one day a week for four weeks.
- Write in a place where you won't be interrupted or distracted. This might have to be at night or early in the morning.
- Don't plan to share your writing—that could stop your honest expression. Save what you write or destroy it, as you wish.
- Explore your very deepest thoughts and feelings and analyze why you feel the way you do. Write about your negative feelings such as sadness, hurt, hate, anger, fear, guilt, or resentment.
- Write continuously. Don't worry about grammar, spelling, or making sense. If clarity and coherence come as you continue to write, so much the better. If you run out of things to say, just repeat what you have already written.
- Even if you find the writing awkward at first, keep going. It gets easier. If you cannot write, try talking into a tape recorder for 15 minutes about your deepest thoughts and feelings.
- Don't expect to feel better immediately. You may feel sad or depressed when your deepest feelings begin to surface. This usually fades within an hour or two or a day or two. The overwhelming majority of people report feelings of relief, happiness, and contentment after writing for a few consecutive days.
- Writing might help you clarify what actions you need to take, but don't use writing as a substitute for taking action or as a way of avoiding things.

Once established, relaxation, imagery, and positive thinking can be some of the most powerful tools you can add to your caregiver tool box. They will help you manage symptoms as well as master the other skills discussed in this book.

As with exercise and other acquired skills, using your mind to manage your stress and other symptoms requires both practice and time before you begin to notice the benefits. So, if you feel you are not accomplishing anything, don't give up. Be patient and keep on trying.

Suggested Further Reading

Abbit, Linda. *Conscious Caregiver: How to Take Care of Mom and Dad without Losing Yourself.* New York: Adams Media Corporation, 2017. How to talk to your loved ones about their situation, handle the emotional stress, stay financially secure, and take the time to care for yourself. http://amzn.to/2o63eE4

Ben-Shahar, Tal. *Happier: Learn the Secrets to Daily Joy and Lasting Fulfillment.* New York: McGraw-Hill, 2007.

Benson, Herbert, and Miriam Z. Klipper. *The Relaxation Response.* San Francisco: Quill, 2000.

Boroson, Martin. *One Moment Meditation.* New York: Winter Road Publishing, 2009.

Craze, Richard. *Teach Yourself Relaxation.* 3rd ed. New York: McGraw-Hill, 2009.

Davis, Martha, Elizabeth Eshelman, and Matthew McKay. *The Relaxation and Stress Reduction Workbook.* Oakland, CA: New Harbinger, 2008.

Diener, Ed, and Robert Biswas-Diener. *Happiness: Unlocking the Mysteries of Psychological Wealth.* Malden, MA: Blackwell, 2008.

Emmons, Robert A. *Gratitude Works! A 21-Day Program for Creating Emotional Prosperity.* San Francisco: Jossey-Bass, 2013.

Kabat-Zinn, Jon. *Wherever You Go, There You Are: Mindfulness Meditation in Everyday Life.* New York: Hyperion, 2005.

Lyubomirsky, Sonia. *The How of Happiness: A New Approach to Getting the Life You Want.* New York: Penguin, 2008.

McGonigal, K. *The Upside of Stress: Why Stress Is Good for You, and How to Get Good at It.*

New York: Avery, 2015.

Neff, Kritin. *Self-Compassion: The Proven Power of Being Kind to Yourself.* New York: HarperCollins, 2011.

Ornstein, Robert, and David Sobel. *Healthy Pleasures.* Cambridge, MA: Perseus, 1990.

Pennebaker, James, and John Evans. *Expressive Writing: Words That Heal.* Enumclaw, WA: Idyll Arbor, 2014.

Rezek, Cheryl A. *Mindfulness for Carers: How to Manage the Demands of Caregiving While Finding a Place for Yourself*. London: Jessica Kingsley Publishers, 2015. Includes easy-to-use and enjoyable mindfulness exercises for all those involved in caring for people with acute or long-term health and mental health conditions, disabilities, and other support needs, including relatives and other informal carers, adoptive parents and foster carers, as well as professional medical, health, and social care staff. http://amzn.to/2Es85ux

Selhub, Eva M., and Alan C. Logan. *Your Brain on Nature*. Ontario: John Wiley & Sons Canada, Ltd., 2014.

Sobel, David, and Robert Ornstein. *The Healthy Mind, Healthy Body Handbook* (also published under the title *The Mind and Body Health Handbook*). Los Altos, CA: DRX, 1996.

Stahl, Bob, and Elisha Goldstein. *A Mindfulness-Based Stress Reduction Workbook*. Oakland, CA: New Harbinger, 2010.

Strecher, Victor. *Life on Purpose: How Living for What Matters Most Changes Everything*. San Francisco: HarperOne, 2016.

Wiseman, Richard. *59 Seconds: Think a Little, Change a Lot*. New York: Borzoi Books, 2009.

Other Resources

Association of Cancer Online Resources (ACOR). http://www.acor.org

Greater Good Magazine. http://greatergood.berkeley.edu

Mental Health America, Live Your Life Well. http://www.mentalhealthamerica.net/live-your-life-well

Naparstek, Belleruth. *Health Journeys Guided Imagery* [audio CDs]. https://www.healthjourneys.com (See "A Guided Meditation to Help with Caregiver Stress.")

National Institute of Mental Health. http://www.nimh.nih.gov

Regan, Catherine, and Rick Seidel. *Relaxation for Mind and Body: Pathways to Healing*. Boulder, CO: Bull Publishing Company, 2012. Audio CD.

Rubin, Gretchen, **The Happiness Project.** http://www.happiness-project.com

StressStop.com. http://www.stressstop.com

Weil, Andrew, and Martin L. Rossman. *Self-Healing with Guided Imagery: How to Use the Power of Your Mind to Heal Your Body*. Louisville, CO: Sounds True, 2006. Audio CD.

Online support groups

Family Caregiver Alliance Support Groups. https://www.caregiver.org/support-groups

National Alliance on Mental Illness (NAMI) Family-to-Family. https://www.nami.org/FindSupport/NAMI-Programs/NAMI-Family-to-Family. (For those whose care partner has a mental health condition.)

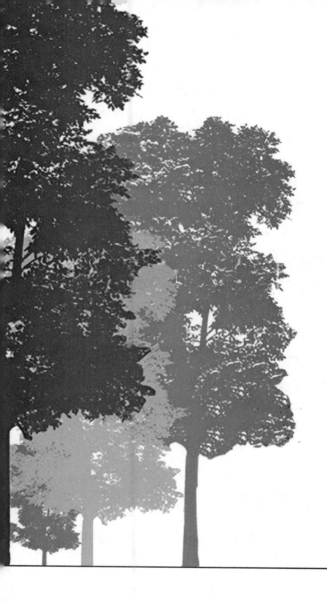

Chapter 6

Communicating Effectively

"I FEEL SO ALONE." "No one understands what it is like to be a caregiver." "My family and friends are no help." Being a caregiver is stressful and frustrating, but good communications can help with this frustration. Whenever we talk with someone, we want them to understand, and we are frustrated when we feel we have not been understood. Failure to communicate effectively can lead to anger, helplessness, isolation, and depression. For caregivers, these feelings can be even worse.

Healthy communication is the lifeblood of relationships, and relationships are a lifeline to healthy coping. Poor communication is the biggest reason for poor relationships between spouses or partners, or relationships with family members, friends, coworkers, or members of our health care team. We have already touched on communicating with your care partner when we explained about emotions and stress in Chapter 4, Dealing with Difficult Emotions. In this chapter, we share some ideas for communicating with family, friends, and members of the health care team.

Your community of support (family, friends, and your own health care providers) and the health care team of your care partner must "understand" you. And when you don't understand advice or recommendations from your doctor or your care partner's doctor, the results can be life threatening. As a caregiver, effective communication skills are essential. In this chapter, we discuss tools to improve communication. Specifically, these are tools to express your feelings in a positive way, to minimize conflict, to ask for help, and to say no. We will also discuss how to listen, how to recognize body language and different styles of communication, and how to get more information.

Keep in mind that communication is a two-way street. As uncomfortable as you may feel about expressing your feelings or asking for help, chances are that others are also feeling this way. It might be up to you to make sure the lines of communication are open. Here are two fundamental keys to better communication:

1. Do not feel uncomfortable or avoid communicating with others because "they should know . . ." People are not mind readers.
2. Remember that you cannot change the communication of others. What you can do is change your communication to be sure you are understood.

Communicating Thoughtfully

When communication is difficult, take the following steps. First, review the situation. Exactly what is bothering you? What are you feeling? Here is an example. Neema is a caregiver and needed someone to cut the lawn. She called her brother-in-law, Malcolm, for help. The following conversation took place:

Neema: Malcolm, our yard is really a mess. Could you help?

Malcolm: Uh, maybe. When would be a good time?

Neema: Terrific. How about Sunday morning?

Malcolm: You know we go to church on Sundays.

Neema: Oh, never mind. Everything else is always more important.

Malcolm: Well, if you cannot be reasonable, I cannot help.

In this conversation, neither Neema nor Malcolm stopped to think about what was really happening. The conversation ended with both feeling out of place and the yard work did not get done.

The following is the same conversation but with both people using more thoughtful communications:

Neema: Malcolm, our yard is really a mess. It would help a lot if you could come over and cut the grass.

Malcolm: I can probably do that. When would be a good time?

Neema: Terrific! How about Sunday morning?

Communicating with Care Partners

Before starting with this topic, we have another special note for caregivers. These suggestions are for communicating with family, friends, and health care professionals. They may or may not work with your care partner. This is especially true if your care partner has cognitive problems (problems thinking clearly). In this case, your care partner might not be able to respond like a person without these problems can respond. This behavior is not being mean or manipulative, and the person does not have bad intentions. It is just that the disease or condition does not allow your partner to communicate in the same way as before. It may be unfair to care partners to expect them to communicate as they would have before needing care. You can certainly try these techniques with your care partner, but do not be disappointed if they are not successful.

Malcolm: Gosh, I'm sorry, but we go to church on Sunday mornings. Would Sunday afternoon be OK, or maybe I could come over some evening after work?

Neema: I'm sorry, I totally forgot about church. Anytime in the afternoon would be fine. Thanks!

Malcolm: See you at about two. Maybe I will bring Paul to help. He would love to see his aunt.

In this dialog, Neema was more specific about what she wanted done. This made it clear to Malcolm that she wanted an hour or so of grass cutting, not a whole day of weeding. Notice that after Neema mentioned coming on Sunday, Malcolm did not say "you know"; he said, "we go." Malcolm did not consider this a thoughtless request and he made some alternative suggestions.

Neema admitted she was not thinking when she asked about Sunday morning and they reached a happy conclusion. Neither blamed the other or took offense. This is thoughtful communication.

Unfortunately, we are often in situations where the other person uses blaming communication. Maybe we are not listening, get caught, and then we also use blaming communication. This is what happened to Malcolm and Neema in the first scenario. In the second scenario, neither blamed the other. You should know that even if the other person uses blaming communication, you can use thoughtful communication and save the day. Look at the following example:

Jan: Why do you always spoil my plans? At least you could have called. I am really tired of trying to do anything with you.

Neema (the caregiver): I understand. When Raj [her care partner] gets into one of his moods, I just can't leave him. When my anxiety acts up at the last minute, I am confused. I keep hoping I can go and so I don't call you because I don't want to disappoint you. I really want to go. I keep hoping things will get better.

Jan: Well, I hope that in the future you will call. I don't like being caught by surprise.

Neema: I understand. If it is OK with you, let's go shopping now. I think I can leave Raj for a couple of hours today. I will call him while we are out. I do want us to keep making plans. In the future, if things do not go the way I planned, I will let you know sooner.

In this example, only Neema is using thoughtful communication. Jan continues to blame. The outcome, however, is still positive. Both people got what they wanted.

The following are some suggestions for using good communication and creating supportive relationships:

Show respect. Always show respect and regard for the other person. Try not to preach or be excessively demanding. Avoid demeaning or blaming comments, such as "Why do you always spoil my plans?" The use of the word *you* is a clue that your communication might be blaming. A bit of tact and courtesy can go a long way in defusing sensitive situations.

Be clear. Describe a specific situation or your observations using the facts. Avoid words like "always" or "never." For example, Neema said, "When my anxiety acts up at the last minute, I am confused. I keep hoping things will get better, so I don't call." This is specific and clear communication about her feelings and the reason behind her actions.

Check assumptions. Ask for more detail. Jan did not do this. She assumed that Neema was rude because she did not call. It would have been better if she asked Neema why she hadn't called earlier. Assumptions are the enemy of good communication. Many arguments arise from people expecting the other people to read their minds. One sign that you are making assumptions is when you are thinking, "They should know what I need . . ." Direct, specific expression of needs and feelings is key. It is also important that you ask questions if you don't understand. Gathering more information is more effective than mindreading.

Open up. Try to openly and honestly express your feelings. Don't make the other person guess what you are feeling—chances are they are off-base. Neema did this. She talked about wanting to go, not wanting to disappoint Jan, and hoping that Raj's mood would get better.

Accept and recognize others' feelings. Try to understand what other people are feeling. This is not always easy. Sometimes you need to think about what was said instead of answering right away. You can always stall a bit by saying, "I understand," or "I don't fully understand; could you explain some more?"

Use humor. Sometimes gently introducing a bit of humor works wonders. But don't use sarcasm or demeaning humor and know when to be serious.

Don't be a victim. You deserve respect, and you have a right to express your wants and needs. You become a victim when you expect that someone else "should" act in a certain way. Unless you have done something to hurt another, you should not apologize. Apologizing all the time is a sign you might be feeling and acting like a victim.

Listen. Good listeners seldom interrupt. Wait a few seconds until someone is finished talking. They may have more to say.

Using "I" Messages

Many of us are uncomfortable expressing our feelings, especially when it seems we are being critical of someone else. When emotions are high, attempts to express frustration can be full of "you" messages. "You don't understand," "you make me so frustrated," "you never listen," and "you never call" are some examples of "you" messages. Using the word "you" can suggest blame, causing the other person to feel under attack. Suddenly, the other person is on the defensive and barriers go up. Situations can just escalate from there, leading to anger, frustration, and bad feeling.

"I" statements are direct, assertive (but not aggressive) expressions of your views and feelings, whereas "you" sentences are accusative and confrontational. For example: "I try very hard to do the best work I can," not, "You always criticize me." Or "I appreciate it when you turn down the television while I talk," not, "You never pay attention."

Here are some more examples:

"You" message: Why are you always late? We never get anywhere on time.

"I" message: I get upset when I'm late. It's important to me to be on time.

"You" message: There's no way you can understand how hard it is to be alone with Raj all day.

"I" message: Being alone with Raj all day is hard. I could use a little help. Watch out for hidden "you" messages. These are "you" messages with "I feel . . ." stuck in front of them. Here's an example:

"You" message: You always walk too fast.

Hidden *"You"* message: I feel angry when you walk so fast.

"I" message: I have a hard time walking fast.

"I feel that you are not treating me fairly" is a "you" statement disguised as an "I" statement. A true "I" statement is, "I feel angry and hurt."

The trick to "I" messages is to avoid the use of the word "you" and, instead, report your personal feelings using the word "I." Of course, like any new skill, using "I" messages take practice. Start by really listening, to yourself and to others. (Grocery stores are a good place to hear lots of "you" messages as parents talk to their children.) In your head take some of the "you" messages and turn them into "I" messages (see box "Exercise—'I' Messages" on the next page). You'll be surprised at how fast "I" messages become a habit. If using "I" statements seems difficult, try this format:

- I observe (state just the facts).
- I think (state your opinions).
- I feel (say what your feelings are).
- I want (state exactly what you'd like the other person to do).

Imagine that because you cannot go to a birthday party, you made a cake for a friend to take along. One of your kids comes along in the kitchen, sees it on the counter, and cuts out a large slice. You're upset because, with a piece missing, the gift is ruined. You might say, "You ate the cake. You should have asked me about it first (opinion). I'm really upset and disappointed

Exercise—"I" Messages

Change the following statements into "I" messages. (Watch out for hidden "you" messages!)

You expect me to wait on you hand and foot!

You never have enough time for me and my care partner. You're always in a hurry.

You hardly ever touch me anymore. You don't pay any attention to me anymore.

Doctor, you didn't tell me the side effects of all these drugs or why my care partner must take them.

because I can't give it as a gift now (feeling). I'd like an apology and for you to ask me first next time (want)."

By the way, there is one more thing to learn from this example. The cake-maker made an assumption that a cake with one missing piece would not be appreciated. Telling the story about what happened to that slice could be fun to hear.

Here are some "I" message cautions. First, "I" messages are not a cure-all. Sometimes, the listener needs time to really "hear" them. This is especially true if listeners are used to hearing blaming "you" messages from you. If "I" messages do not work at first, continue to use them. Things will change as you gain skill and old patterns of communication are broken.

Second, some people use "I" messages as a means of manipulation. They may often express that they are sad, angry, or frustrated to gain sympathy from others. If used in this way, problems can escalate. Effective "I" messages must report honest feelings.

One last note: "I" messages are an excellent way to express positive feelings and compliments! "I really appreciate that you sent the cake. Everyone loved it and the story about the missing piece made everyone laugh."

Minimizing Conflict

In addition to using "I" messages, there are other ways to reduce conflict.

Shift the focus. If a discussion gets off topic and emotions are running high, shift the focus of the conversation. That is, bring the discussion back to the topic you agreed to talk about. For example, you might say something like, "We're both getting upset now and drifting away from the topic we agreed to discuss." Or, "I feel like we are bringing up other things than what we agreed to talk about, and I'm getting upset. Can we discuss these other things later and just talk about what we originally agreed to discuss?"

Buy time. For example, you might say, "I think I understand your concerns, but I need more time to think about it before I can respond." Or, "I hear what you are saying, but I am too frustrated to respond now. I need to find out more about this before I can respond."

Make sure you understand each other's viewpoints. You can do this by summarizing what you heard and asking for clarification. You can also switch roles. Try arguing the other person's position as thoroughly and thoughtfully as possible. This will help you to understand all the sides of an issue, as well as to respect and value the other's point of view. It will also help you to develop tolerance and empathy for others.

Look for compromise. You might not always find the perfect solution to a problem or reach complete agreement. When this happens, it may be possible to compromise. Find something on which you can both agree. For example, you can do it your way this time and the other person's way the next time. Agree to part of what you want and part of what the other person wants. Or decide what you'll do and what the other person will do in return. These are all forms of compromise that can help you through some difficult times.

Say you're sorry. We have all said or done things that have, intentionally or unintentionally, hurt others. Many relationships are hurt—sometimes for years—because people have not learned the powerful social skill of apologizing. Often, all it takes is a simple, sincere apology to restore a relationship.

Rather than a sign of weak character, an apology shows great strength. To be effective, an apology must:

- Admit the specific mistake, and accept responsibility for it. You must name the offense; no glossing over with just, "I'm sorry for what I did." Be specific. You might say, for example, "I'm very sorry that I was angry and hung up on you. I was at my wits' end." Explain the particular circumstances that led you to do what you did. Don't offer excuses or sidestep responsibility.
- Express your feelings. A genuine, heart-felt apology involves some suffering. Sadness shows that the relationship matters to you.
- Acknowledge the impact of wrong-doing. You might say, "I know that I hurt you and that my behavior cost you a lot. For that, I am very sorry."
- Offer to make amends. Ask what you can do to make the situation better, or volunteer specific suggestions.

Making an apology is not fun, but it is an act of courage, generosity, and healing. It brings the possibility of a renewed and stronger relationship, and it can also bring peace within yourself.

Do not assume the worst about people. Many caregivers discover that people in their lives whom they expected to be helpful are not. These people do not call or offer help. A common caregiver response is to be angry and to write these people off as not caring. In fact, a person might not call because they don't know what to do or say. They are afraid to approach you because they know that the relationship has changed or that you might ask them to do something they cannot do or are not willing to do. As hard as it might be, if the relationship is important to you, reach out. Call the person, suggest you get together for coffee or the person come over for coffee while your care partner is sleeping. People do not "just know" what to do. Sometimes, they need to be guided. Give them the benefit of the doubt and make sure you treat them as "innocent unless proven guilty."

Receiving and Giving Help

Receiving and giving help are a part of being human and especially critical for caregivers. Learning how to effectively ask for and accept help and learning how to request help are worthwhile goals for caregivers.

Asking for and Accepting Help: Be Specific

Even though most of us sometimes need help, few of us like to ask for it. We might not want to admit that we are unable to do things for ourselves. We might not want to be a burden on others.

When we finally do ask for help, we may hedge or make a very vague request: "I'm sorry to have to ask this . . .," "I know this is asking a lot . . .," or "I hate to ask this, but . . ." Hedging tends to put the other person on the defensive: "Gosh, what's he going to ask that's such a big deal, anyway?" To avoid this response, be specific. A general request can lead to misunderstanding. The person being asked to help may react negatively because not enough information was given. This leads to a further breakdown in communication and no help. A specific request is more likely to have a positive result. Consider the following examples:

General request: I know this is the last thing you want to do, but I need help shopping. Will you help me?

Reaction: Uh . . . well . . . I don't know. Um . . . can I get back to you after I check my schedule? (probably next year!)

Specific request: I need help shopping. Would you call me when you are going to the grocery and I can give you a short list? Then either I or Elena will pick them up at your house. Of course, I will pay you.

Reaction: Of course, I am happy to do this, and I can just drop your things off as you are right on my way home. Would once a week be often enough?

We often hear "How can I help?" Our answer is often "I don't know" or "Thank you but I do not need any help." All the time, we are thinking "They should know . . ." or "If they cared, they would know . . ." Be prepared to respond to offers of help by expressing a specific request. For example, "It would be great if we could go for a walk together once a week" or "Could you please take the garbage can to the curb tonight? I can't lift it."

Just remember that most people cannot read your mind, so you'll need to tell them what help you want and thank them for it. Think about how each person can help. If possible, give them a task that they can easily accomplish. You are giving them a gift when you accept their help. People like being helpful and feel rejected when they cannot assist. It is also beneficial to be grateful for the help you receive (see "Practice Gratitude" in Chapter 5, Using Your Mind to Manage Stress, pages 61 and 62).

But there will be times when you do not want or need help. Caregivers sometimes deal with offers of help that are not needed or desired. In most cases, these offers come from important people in your life. These people care for you and genuinely want to help. A well-worded "I" message allows you to decline the help without embarrassing the other person. "Thank you for being so thoughtful, but today I think I can handle it myself. I hope I can take you up on your offer another time."

Let's look at the other side of requests for assistance. How should you respond when you are the one being asked for help? It is probably best not to answer right away. You might need more information. If a request leaves you feeling negative, trust your feelings.

The example we just discussed about helping a person shop is a good one. "Help me shop" can mean anything from picking up a few groceries to being responsible for all their clothing, pharmacy, and grocery shopping all the time. Using skills that get at the specifics will avoid problems. It is important to understand fully any request before responding. Asking for more information or restating the request in your own words will often bring more clarity: "Before I answer . . ." (this will hopefully prevent the person whose request you are paraphrasing from thinking that you are immediately going to say yes).

Saying No: Ask for Information

If you decide to say no, you should acknowledge the importance of the request. In this way, the person will see that you are rejecting the request rather than the person. Your turn-down should not be a put-down. "I would like to help you with your shopping, but I will be away this week." Again, specifics are the key. Try to be clear about the conditions of your turn-down: Will you always turn down this request, or is it just that today, this week, or right now is not convenient? If you are feeling overwhelmed and put upon, saying no can be a useful tool. You could make a counteroffer like, "I won't be able to drive today, but I will next week." But remember, you have a legitimate right to decline a request, even if it is a reasonable one.

Listening

Good listening is probably the most critical communication skill. Most of us are much better at talking than we are at listening. When others talk to us, we are often preparing a response, instead of just listening. There are several steps to being a good listener.

1. **Listen to the words and tone of voice, and observe body language** (see the next section). There might be times when the words don't tell the whole story. Is the voice wavering? Is the speaker struggling to find "the right words"? Do you notice body tension? Does the person seem distracted? Is the tone sarcastic? What is the facial expression? If you pick up on some of these signs, speakers may have more on their minds than the words alone express.
2. **Let people know you heard them.** This might be a simple "uh huh." Many times, the only thing the other person wants is

acknowledgment, or just someone to listen, Sometimes, it is helpful just to talk to a sympathetic listener,

3. **Let people know you understand both the content and emotional impact of what they are saying.** You can do this by restating the content. For example, "You are planning a trip." Or you can respond by acknowledging the emotions: "That must be difficult" or "How sad you must feel." When you respond on an emotional level, the results are often startling. These responses tend to open the gates for more expression of feelings and thoughts. Responding to either the content or emotion can help communication. They discourage the other person from simply repeating what has been said. But don't try to talk people out of their feelings or tell them that they "shouldn't feel that way." They are real to them. Just listen and reflect.
4. **Get more information.** This is especially important if you are not completely clear about what was said or what is wanted.

Getting More Information: Asking Questions

Getting more information is a bit of an art. It can involve both simple and more complicated techniques.

The simplest way to get more information is to ask. "Tell me more" will probably get you more, as will "I don't understand . . . please explain," "I would like to know more about . . .", "Would you say that another way?", "How do you mean?", "I'm not sure I got that," or "Could you expand on that?"

Be specific when you are asking for more information. If you want specific information, you must ask specific questions. We often speak in generalities. For example:

Doctor: "How has you care partner been feeling?"

Caregiver: "Not so good."

The doctor has not gotten much information. "Not so good" isn't very useful. Here's how the doctor gets more information:

Doctor: Has your care partner been sleeping any better?

Caregiver: Not really.

Doctor: Could you tell me more?

Caregiver: Well, he goes to sleep but gets up four or five times a night and never goes back to sleep after 5:00 a.m.

Doctor: What time does he go to sleep then?

Caregiver: About 7:30. Then I have three or four hours to get things done.

Doctor: Does he also take a nap?

. . . and so on.

Health care providers are trained to get specific information from caregivers and patients, although they sometimes ask general questions. Most of us are not trained, but we can learn to ask specific questions. Simply asking for specifics often works: "Can you be more specific about . . .?","Are you thinking of something special?"

A word of caution: avoid asking "Why?" This is a general, not a specific, question. "Why" makes a person think in terms of cause and effect and can make people feel responsible and defensive. A person might respond at an entirely different level than you had in mind.

Most of us have had the experience where a three-year-old just keeps asking "Why?" over and over and over again. This goes on until the child gets the wanted information (or the parent runs from the room, screaming). The poor parent doesn't have the faintest idea what the child has in mind and answers, "Because . . ." in an increasingly specific order until the child's question is answered. Sometimes, however, a parent's answers are very different from what the child really wants to know and children never get the information they wanted. Rather than "why," begin your queries with "who," "which," "when," or "where." These words promote a specific response.

One last note about getting information: Sometimes we do not get the correct information because we do not know what question to ask. For example, you may be seeking legal services from a senior center. You call and ask if they have a lawyer and you hang up when the answer is no. If, instead, you had asked, "I need to ask a lawyer about getting power of attorney for my mother, so can you give me some suggestions on where I can find a low-cost one?" you might have gotten two or three referrals for low-cost legal advice. Maybe you don't need a lawyer to get the document done after all.

Getting More Information: Paraphrasing

Another way to get more information is to paraphrase, or to repeat back what you heard in your own words. This is a good tool if you want to make sure you understand what other people meant—not just what they said, but what they intended and meant. Paraphrasing can either help or hinder effective communication. It depends on the way the paraphrase is worded. Remember to paraphrase in the form of a question, not a statement. Consider the following example:

Caregiver: I don't know. Josephine [care partner] is so messy when she eats and she sometimes eats with her hands. I want to go to dinner, but I think everyone in the restaurant will be looking at us.

Paraphrasing as a statement: Obviously, you're telling me you don't want to go to dinner.

This response might provoke an angry response such as, "No, I didn't say that! If you're going to be that way, we'll stay home for sure." Or the response might be no response—a total shutdown because of either anger or despair ("he just doesn't understand"). People don't like to be told what they meant.

Paraphrasing as a question: Are you saying that you'd rather stay home than go to dinner?

Response to the second paraphrase (the question): That's not what I meant. I just think that we might do better at a restaurant where we would be less noticeable. How about that new Italian place?

As you can see, the second paraphrase helps communication. The questioner has discovered the real reason for expressing doubt about going to dinner. In short, you get more information when you paraphrase with questions.

Paying Attention to Body Language and Conversational Styles

Part of listening to what others are saying includes observing how they say it. Even when we say nothing, our bodies are talking; sometimes they are even shouting. Research shows that our body language is responsible for more than half of what we communicate.

If we want to communicate really well, we must be aware of body language, facial expressions, and tone of voice. These should match what we say in words. If we do not do this, we are sending mixed messages and creating misunderstandings. For example, if you want to make a firm statement, look at the other person and keep your expression friendly. Stand tall and confident; relax your legs and arms and breathe. You might lean forward to show your interest. Try not to sneer or bite your lips; this might indicate discomfort or doubt. Don't move away or slouch, as these communicate disinterest and uncertainty.

When you notice that the body language and words of others are sending message you do not think are positive do not match, gently point this out. Ask for clarification. For example, you might say, "I hear you saying that you would like to go with me to the family picnic, but you look tired and you're yawning as you speak. Would you rather stay home and rest, while I go alone?"

In addition to reading people's body language, it is helpful to recognize and appreciate that we all express ourselves differently. Our conversational style varies according to where we were born, how we were raised, our occupation, our cultural background, and especially our gender. For example, some people tend to ask questions that are more personal than the questions others ask. These show interest and help to form relationships. Others are more likely to offer opinions or suggestions and state facts. They tend to discuss problems just to find solutions not to share their feelings and experiences. No one style is better or worse, just different. By acknowledging and accepting these differences, we can reduce some of the misunderstanding, frustration, and resentment we feel in our communications with others. Recognizing these differences is especially important when we are communicating with people from different cultures. Hand gestures, eye contact, and posture, for example, might have very different meanings in one culture than another. If you are confused, just ask.

Communicating with Members of Your Health Care Team

One of the keys to getting good health care for yourself and your care partner is to communicate well with health care providers. This can be a challenge. We may be afraid to talk freely, or we think there is not enough time. Health professionals might use words we do not understand; we may not want to share personal and possibly embarrassing information. These fears and feelings can block communications with providers and jeopardize your care partner's health and your own health.

Providers share the responsibility for poor communication. They sometimes feel too busy to take the time to talk with and know their patients and their caregivers. They may ignore or not "hear" our questions. Their actions or inaction might offend us.

While we do not have to become best friends with our providers, we should expect that they are attentive, caring, and able to explain things clearly. This is especially important if we are caregivers and we or our care partners have an ongoing health condition. We might think that we can only get the "best" care by going to specialists. While this can sometime be true, it can also greatly complicate care. You may be seeing several specialists. They may not know you and might not be aware of what the other care providers are doing, thinking, or prescribing. These are good reasons to have a primary provider or a medical "home." A relationship with a provider is much like a business partnership or even a marriage. This long-term relationship will probably take some effort, but it can make a large difference to your health and that of your care partner.

Your provider probably knows more intimate details about you and your care partner than you do. In turn, should feel comfortable expressing your fears, asking questions that you think are "stupid," as well as negotiating a satisfactory treatment plan.

Two things will help keep the lines of communication open. First, we must be clear about what we want from our providers. Many of us would like warmhearted computers—gigantic brains, stuffed with knowledge about the human body and mind. We want our providers to analyze the situation, read minds, make a perfect diagnosis, create a treatment plan, solve all problems, and tell us what to expect. At the same time, we want them to be warm and caring and make us feel as though we are special patients.

Most providers wish they were just that sort of person. Unfortunately, no one provider can be all things to all patients. Providers are human. They have bad days, they get headaches, they get tired, and they get sore feet. They have families who demand their time and attention, they might be caregivers themselves, and they may get frustrated by paperwork, electronic record keeping, and large bureaucracies.

Most doctors and other health care professionals received grueling training. They entered the health care system because they wanted to help sick people. They are frustrated when they cannot cure someone with a chronic condition. Many times, they must take their satisfaction from improvements rather than cures, or from slowing the decline of some conditions. Undoubtedly, you have been frustrated, angry, or depressed from time to time about your care partner, but bear in mind that your doctors have probably felt similar emotions about their inability to make your care partner well. In this, you are truly partners.

Time is the second threat to a good relationship with health care professionals. If you or your provider had a fantasy about the best thing that could happen in your relationship, it would probably involve more face-to-face time. When time is short, the resulting anxiety can bring about rushed communication. "You" messages and misunderstood messages are common.

Most physicians and other providers are on very tight schedules. This becomes painfully clear when you have had to wait in the doctor's office because an emergency or late patient has delayed your appointment. Doctors try to stay on schedule. This sometimes causes both patients and doctors to feel rushed. One way to help you to get the most from your visit is to take P.A.R.T.

Take P.A.R.T.

P = Prepare
A = Ask
R = Repeat
T = Take action

Prepare

Before visiting or calling your health care provider or that of your care partner, prepare your agenda. What are the reasons for your visit? What do you expect from your doctor?

Take some time to make a written list of your concerns or questions. Have you ever thought to yourself, after you walked out of the doctor's office, "Why didn't I ask about . . . ?" or "I forgot to mention . . . ."? Making a list beforehand helps you ensure that your main concerns get addressed. Be realistic. If you have 13 different concerns, your provider probably cannot deal with all of them in one visit. Star or highlight your two or three most important items.

Give the list to your doctor at the beginning of the visit, pointing out that you have starred your biggest concerns. By giving your doctor the whole list, you highlight which items are your priorities and also let the doctor see everything in case there is something medically significant that is not starred. If you wait until the end of your appointment to bring up concerns, there will not be time to discuss them. Here is an example:

The provider asks, "What brings you in today?" and you might say something like, "I have a lot of things I want to discuss this visit (looking the clock and appointment schedule, the doctor immediately begins to feel anxious), but I know that we have a limited amount of time. The things that most concern me is that Emiko (your care partner) is not sleeping and can no longer find the toilet." The doctor feels relieved because the concerns are focused and potentially manageable within the appointment time available.

There are two other things to prepare before your visit. Bring a list of all your (or your care partner's) medications and the dosage. If you have a patient portal, such as MyHealth, you might find the information there. If this is difficult, then put all the meds in a bag and take them to the appointment. Do not forget vitamins and over-the-counter (OTC) medications.

The final thing to prepare is your story. Visit time is short. When the provider asks how you are doing, some people will go on for several minutes about this and that concern. It is better to say, "I think that overall my anxiety is less, but now I have more trouble sleeping." You should be prepared to describe your (or your care partner's) symptoms:

- When they started
- How long they last
- If they are always there or come and go
- Where they are located
- What makes them better or worse
- Whether you have had similar problems before
- Whether there have been any changes in diet, exercise, or medications that might contribute to the symptoms

- What worries you most about the symptoms
- What you think might be causing the symptoms

If you (or your care partner) are on a new medication or treatment, be ready to report how it went. If you are going to several providers and they are not all using the same electronic medical record take with you any tests results from the past six months.

In telling your story, talk about trends (are things getting better or worse, or are they the same?). Also talk about tempo (are symptoms more or less frequent or intense; for example, "In general, Emiko is slowly getting better; although today she does not seem well").

Be as open as you can in sharing your thoughts, feelings, and fears. Remember, your provider is not a mind reader. If you are worried, explain why: "I am worried that my care partner will get worse and I may not be able to work," or "My father had similar symptoms before he died." The more open you are, the more likely it is that your provider can help. If you have a problem, don't wait for the provider to "discover" it. State your concern immediately (for example, "I am worried about this mole on Emiko's back").

The more specific you can be (without overdoing it with irrelevant details), the clearer a picture the doctor will have of your problem, and the less time will be wasted for both of you.

Share your hunches or guesses about what might be causing the symptoms, as they often provide vital clues to an accurate diagnosis. Even if it turns out your guesses are not correct, it gives your doctor the opportunity to reassure you or address your hidden concerns.

Ask

Your most powerful tool in the doctor–patient partnership is the question. You can fill in vital missing pieces of information and close critical gaps in communication with your questions. And asking all your questions reflects your active participation in the process of care. Getting answers and information is a cornerstone of self-management and good caregiving. Be prepared to ask questions about diagnosis, tests, treatments, and follow-up:

1. **Diagnosis**. Ask what's wrong, what caused it, if it is contagious, what's the outlook (or prognosis), and what can be done to prevent or manage it.
2. **Tests.** If the doctor wants to do tests, ask how the results are likely to affect treatment and what will happen if the test is not done. If you decide to go forward with a test, find out how to prepare for the test and what it will be like. Also ask how and when you will get the results.
3. **Treatments.** Ask if there are any choices in treatments and the advantages and disadvantages of each. Ask what will happen if no treatment is chosen instead. (See Chapter 12, Managing Medications.)
4. **Follow-up.** Find out if and when you should call or return for a follow-up visit. What symptoms should you watch for, and what should you do if they occur?

Repeat

One way to check that you have really heard and understood everything is to briefly report back key points (for example, "You want my care partner to take this three times a day with meals"). Repeating back also gives the provider a chance to quickly correct any misunderstandings and miscommunications.

If you don't understand or remember something the provider said, admit that you need to go over it again (for example, "I'm pretty sure you told me some of this before, but I'm still confused about it"). Don't be afraid to ask what you might consider a "stupid" question. These questions should be asked and may prevent a misunderstanding.

Sometimes it is hard to remember everything. You can take notes or bring another person to important visits, and you can record the visit with your smartphone. If your provider uses an electronic medical record, you can also ask to have a copy printed of the doctor's notes to take with you.

Take Action

At the end of a visit, you need to clearly understand what to do next. This includes which treatments and tests should be performed and when to return. You should also know any danger signs you should look out for and what you should do if they occur. If necessary, ask your provider to write down instructions, recommend reading material, or other places you can get help.

If, for some reason, you can't or won't follow providers' advice, let them know (for example, "I didn't take the aspirin because it gives me stomach problems," "My care partner's insurance doesn't cover that much therapy, so I can't afford it," or "I've tried to exercise, but I can't seem to keep it up"). If providers know why you can't or won't follow advice, they may be able to make other suggestions. If you don't share the barriers to taking actions, it's difficult for your providers to help. If you or your care partner don't take your medication or follow providers' recommendations, it is also difficult for them to know which treatments work or don't work and what to recommend in the future.

Asking for a Second Opinion

Sometimes, you might want to see another provider or have a second opinion. Asking for this can be hard. This is especially true if you or your care partner have had a long relationship with your provider. You could worry that asking for another opinion will anger your provider or that the provider will take your request in the wrong way. Providers are seldom hurt by requests for a second opinion. If a condition is complicated or difficult, the doctor may have already consulted with another doctor (or more than one). This is often done informally. However, if you find yourself asking for third, fourth, and fifth opinions, this may be unproductive.

Asking for a second opinion is perfectly acceptable. This is an expected part of a provider's work life. Ask for a second opinion by using a nonthreatening "I" message: "I'm still feeling confused and uncomfortable about this treatment. I feel another opinion might reassure me. Can you suggest someone I could consult?"

In this way, you have expressed your own feelings without suggesting that the provider is at fault. You have also confirmed your confidence by asking that this health care professional suggest another provider. (However, you are not bound by the suggestion; you can choose anyone you wish.)

Give Positive Feedback to Providers

Let your providers know about how satisfied you are with the care they are providing. If you do not like the way you or your care partner have been treated by any of the members of your health care team, let this person know. In the same way, if you are pleased with the care, also let your providers know. Everyone appreciates compliments and positive feedback, especially members of a health care team. They are human, and your praise can help nourish and console these busy, hardworking professionals. Letting them know that you appreciate their efforts is one of the best ways to improve your relationship with them. Plus, it makes them feel good!

Share in Medical Decisions

Many decisions in medical care are not clear-cut, and often there is more than one option. The best decisions, except in life-threatening emergencies, depend on your values and preferences and should not be left solely to a doctor. For example, if you have high blood pressure, you might say, “I’m very conservative about taking medications. What’s a reasonable period of time for me to try exercise, diet, and relaxation first, before I start taking the medication?” You might also say, “I know that my care partner is not going to get better. Will this medication really help his quality of life? If not, will *not* taking it harm his quality of life?”

To make an informed choice about any treatment, you need to know the cost and risks of the proposed treatment. This includes the likelihood of possible complications, such as drug reactions, bleeding, infection, injury, or death. It also includes the personal costs, such as lost time from work, and financial considerations such as how much of the proposed treatments your insurance will cover.

You also need to understand how likely it is that the proposed treatments will offer benefits. Sometimes, the best choice may be not to treat or to delay a decision about treatment in favor of “watchful waiting.”

No one can tell you which choice is right for you and your care partner. But to make an informed choice, you need information about the treatment options. Informed choice, not merely informed consent, is essential to quality medical care. The best medical care for you and your care partner combines a doctor’s medical expertise with your own knowledge, skills, and values.

Making decisions about treatments can be difficult. For some suggestions on how make decisions see “Making Decisions: Weighing the Pros and Cons” on page 12 in Chapter 2, Becoming a Better Caregiver: The Basics, and see “Asking Questions about New Treatments” on page 232 in Chapter 13, Making Treatment Decisions, for help on how to evaluate new treatments.

Working with the Health Care System

So far, we have discussed communication with providers. Today, most providers work in a larger system, such as clinics. Policies relating to appointments, billing, telephone, and electronic messaging use are usually decided by someone other than your provider.

If you are unhappy with your health care system, don't just steam and get angry. Do something about it. Find out who is running the organization and who makes decisions. Then share your feelings in a constructive way by letter, phone, or email. Most health care systems want to keep you as a client, and, therefore, usually respond. The problem is that the people who make the decisions tend to isolate themselves. It is easier to express our feelings to the receptionist, nurse, or doctor. Unfortunately, these people have little or no power in the system. However, they can tell you whom to write. The more closely you can form a partnership with your providers, the more responsive all of you will be to each other.

If you do decide to write or send a message through your health care organization's electronic portal (email is not secure and providers generally are forbidden using it), keep your letter short and factual, and tell what actions you would find helpful. Here is an example:

> Dear Ms. Brown:
>
> Yesterday, my mother and I had a 10 a.m. appointment with Dr. Zim. She did not see us until 12:15, and our total time with the doctor was eight minutes. I was told to make another appointment so we could get our questions answered.
>
> I know that sometimes there are emergencies. I would appreciate being called if my doctor is running late or told when to return. We would also like 15 or more minutes with my mother's doctor.
>
> Please reply within two weeks.
>
> Thank you.

The following are a few common complaints and some hints for working with the health care system to address these issues. Not all of these problems and suggestions will apply to all systems, but most do.

- "I hate the phone system." Often, when we call for an appointment or information, we reach an automated system. This is frustrating. Unfortunately, we cannot change this. However, phone systems do not change often. If you can memorize the numbers or keys to press, you can move more quickly from one part of the system to another. Sometimes, pressing the pound key, #, or 0 will get you to a real person. Once you do get through, ask if there is a way to navigate the automated system faster next time.

- "It takes too long to get an appointment." Ask for the first available appointment. Take it. Then ask how you can learn about cancellations and getting on a "wait list" for appointments. Some organizations are happy to call you when they have an empty spot, but you might have to call others once or twice a week to check on cancellations. Ask the person making the schedule what you can do to get an earlier appointment. Ask for a telephone number so you can reach the person making appointments directly. Some systems are now setting time aside each day for "same day" appointments. If this is an option with your health care system, ask when is the best time to call to get one of those appointments. It is usually early in the morning of that day. If you are in distress or believe that you must see a doctor soon, tell the scheduler. If nothing is available, ask what you can do to see someone soon. No matter how frustrated you are, be nice. The scheduler has the power to either give you an appointment or not.

- "Between myself and my care partner we have so many providers; I do not know who to ask for what." One of those providers must be in charge. Your job is to find out which one. Ask each provider who is in charge of coordinating your care or that of your care partner. When you get a name, it is most likely your primary care doctor or general practitioner (GP). Call or email doctors to confirm that they are coordinating your care. Ask how you can help make communication and care smoother between providers. One way might be to let the lead doctor know when someone else orders a test or new medication. Keeping the doctor informed is especially important when providers are not in the same system and are not sharing electronic medical records.

- "So, what is an electronic medical record (EMR) and what does it have to do with me?" Most of your medical information is on a secure computer. Your information can be seen by any provider in the same system. You should know what information is on the system. Sometimes the EMR has just test results, other times it has test results and medication information, and sometimes it has everything that is known about you. An electronic medical record is just like a paper record: It does no good if your providers don't read it. For example, when you have a test, the doctor ordering the test will know when the test results are ready. However, your other doctors will not know anything about the test unless you tell them to read the results. Learn about the medical records system so you can help all your providers use it more effectively.

  In the United States and many other countries, you have the right to a copy of almost everything in your record. Ask for copies of all your test results so that you can carry them with you from one provider to the next. In this way, you know that they will not get lost. This information can often be found in patient portals such as MyHealth or MyChart.

- "I can never reach the doctor to talk." It is hard to get a provider on the phone but you might be able to email. Many systems now have ways that doctors and patients can communicate by electronic messaging. The next time you see your provider, ask about this. One good thing about electronic communication systems is there is usually a way to get routine things, such as prescription refills, done quickly. It could mean calling a special number or talking to the nurse. Learn how to do this.

In a medical emergency, do not waste time trying to contact your doctor; rather, call 911 (in the United States), go to a hospital emergency department, or call the rescue squad.

- "I have to wait too long in the waiting room or the examination room." Emergencies happen sometimes, and this can cause a wait. More often, the system is not efficient. If your schedule is tight and it causes a problem if you are delayed at your appointment, you might try calling your doctor's office before you head to the appointment, and asking how long you will have to wait. If they report that the doctor running late, you can decide whether to make sure to bring a book or ask to reschedule. You can also show up with your book and ask about the wait. Rather than getting upset, let the receptionist know that you are going to step out for a little while to run a quick errand nearby, go for a cup of coffee, or do some shopping and that you will return within a specified amount of time.

- "My care partner and I don't have enough time with the provider." This is a system problem. The system decided how much time each patient should have. The decision is sometimes based on what you tell the scheduler. If you say your partner needs a blood pressure check, you will be given a short visit. If you say you are very depressed and cannot function, you might be given a longer appointment. When making the appointment, ask for time you want, especially if this is more than 10 or 15 minutes. Be prepared to state your reasons and make a case for more time. You can also ask for the last appointment in the day. You may have to wait a while, but at least the provider will not be pressured because there are more patients to see after you.

Once you are with a provider, and you request more time than is allotted, you make other people wait. An extra five minutes might not seem like much. However, a doctor often sees 30 patients a day. If each one takes five extra minutes, this means that the doctor has to work an extra two and a half hours that day. That little bit of extra time adds up.

If something in the health care system is not working for you, ask how you can help to make it work better. Very often, if you learn how to navigate the system, you can solve or at least partially solve your problems. Be nice—or at least as nice as possible. If the system or your provider sees you as a difficult patient, life will become more difficult. If you think that things should not be this way and that it is not fair to place this burden on the patient, we wholeheartedly agree. Health systems should change to be more responsive and patient-friendly. A few health care systems are already doing this. In the meantime, you can use the suggestions

Making Sure Your Communication Is Clear

Words That Help

Right now, at this time, at this point ("At this point, I do not need any help, but I might next week. Can I call you?")

Who, which, where, when ("What do you mean, please explain, tell me more, I don't understand).

Words That Hinder

Never, always, every time, constantly ("Every time I try to get out, it fails.")

You obviously ("You obviously have never been a caregiver.")

Why

in this chapter to communicate better and deal more effectively with difficult situations.

Good communication skills help make life easier for everyone, especially caregivers. The box "Making Sure Your Communication Is Clear" lists some words that can help or hinder communication.

Communicating with Young Children

Having a friend or relative with dementia is especially confusing to young children. Here are some tips that might help:

- Share the information clearly and in simple terms. Be truthful. Do not reassure that that everything will be OK.
- Remind the child that the person is still the same person but they have a disease.
- Prepare the child for the unexpected. Remind them that these behaviors are due to the condition.
- Make it clear that dementia is not contagious.
- The child is not to blame.
- Help them plan activities they can do with your care partner such as singing old songs, looking at old photos, doing a simple craft. Reading them a story.
- Most important, listen, reassure and answer questions.

The following is an excellent site for finding more resources in how to deal with children and teens. https://www.nia.nih.gov/health/resources-children-and-teens-about-alzheimers-disease.

Suggested Further Reading

Beck, Aaron T. *Love Is Never Enough: How Couples Can Overcome Misunderstandings, Resolve Conflicts, and Solve Relationship Problems through Cognitive Therapy*. New York: HarperCollins, 2010.

Chou, Calvin L., and Laura Cooley. *Communication Rx: Transforming Healthcare through Relationship-Centered Communication*. New York: McGraw-Hill Education, 2018. A practical guide by the Academy of Communication in Healthcare on teamwork, coaching, shared decision-making, feedback, conflict engagement, diversity, and more. http://amzn.to/2o312OL

Coste, Joanne Koenig. *Learning to Speak Alzheimers: A Groundbreaking Approach for Everyone Dealing with the Disease*. Milsons Point, N.S.W.: Transworld Publishing, 2004. An accessible and comprehensive method to enhance communication between care partners and patients. http://amzn.to/2Cmlqia

Davis, Martha, Patrick Fanning, and Kim Paleg. *The Messages Workbook: Powerful Strategies for Effective Communication at Work and Home*. Oakland, CA: New Harbinger Publications, 2004.

Feil, Naomi, and Vicki De. Klerk-Rubin. *The Validation Breakthrough: Simple Techniques for Communicating with People with Alzheimer's and Other Dementias*. Baltimore: Health Professions Press, 2012. An effective method of communication that alleviates distressing behaviors caused by Alzheimer's-type dementia. http://amzn.to/2EKxOxE

Gottman, John, M., and Joan DeClaire. *The Relationship Cure: A Five Step Guide to Strengthening Your Marriage, Family, and Friendships*. New York: Three Rivers Press, 2001.

Gottman, John M., and Nan Silver. *The Seven Principles for Making Marriage Work: A Practical Guide from the Country's Foremost Relationship Expert*. Amazon Digital Services, 2018.

McCarthy, Bernie. *Hearing the Person with Dementia: Person-Centered Approaches to Communication for Families and Caregivers*. London: Jessica Kingsley Publishers, 2011. A clear explanation of what happens to communication as dementia progresses, how this may affect an individual's memory, language and senses, and how care partners might need to adapt their approach as a result. http://amzn.to/2Cm4Wqc

McKay, Matthew, Martha Davis, and Patrick Fanning. *Messages: The Communication Skills Book*. Oakland, CA: New Harbinger, 2009.

National Institute on Aging. National Institutes of Health. "Talking with Your Doctor: A Guide for Older People." U.S. Department of Health and Human Services. NIH Publication No. 05-3452. August 2005; repr. April 2010. You can download or order a copy from this website: https://www.nia.nih.gov/health/doctor-patient-communication/talking-with-your-doctor

Tannen, Deborah. *You Just Don't Understand: Women and Men in Conversation*. New York: HarperCollins, 1991.

Other Resources

This **AboveMS** blog is from a care partner's perspective. https://www.abovems.com/en_us/home/team/team-members/care-partners-perspective.html

This **American Association of Retired Persons (AARP)** post teaches you how to become an effective advocate and communicate with your loved one's medical team. https://www.aarp.org/caregiving/health/info-2017/dealing-with-doctors.html

The **American Heart Association** gives communication tips for caregivers. http://www.heart.org/HEARTORG/Support/Communication-Tips-For-Caregivers_UCM_301841_Article.jsp#.WoZKEDPMw9c

The **American Heart Association** provides a printable fact sheet about how you should communicate as a caregiver. http://www.heart.org/idc/groups/heart-public/@wcm/@hcm/documents/downloadable/ucm_300661.pdf

This resource from **Medicare.com** outlines effective communication for health care providers and caregivers. https://medicare.com/caregiver-resources/pathways-to-effective-communication-for-health-care-providers-and-caregivers

Chapter 7

Getting Help

A major part of caregiving is knowing when you need help, what help you need, and how to find help. Seeking help is a sign of strength and one of the best things you can do to lower stress. Unfortunately, here is what too often happens to many caregivers. Minh is overwhelmed. She hasn't been sleeping much because her Tran has been getting out of bed in the middle of the night. She hasn't had time to do anything except to watch her care partner. She is stressed, angry, and may even have cross words with her care partner. Minh knows that she needs help. She then decides that no one can do a better job at caregiving, and besides, she knows that no help is available. At this point, she just continues doing what she is doing and becomes more and more overwhelmed until some crisis occurs.

This story could have a happier ending, and in this chapter, we will give you some of the tools to make a happier ending possible.

The first step is to figure out with what you need help. As we mentioned in Chapter 6, Communicating Effectively, being as specific as possible is important. Start by writing of a list of what help you would like. Do not worry if it is available or possible, just write the list.

Thinking about resources for getting that help is the second step. Who can help? As we begin to look for help, most of us start by asking family or friends. Sometimes this can be difficult. We are afraid that others will see us as weak. Sometimes our pride gets in the way. The truth is that most people want to be helpful but do not know how. Your job is to tell them what you need. Finding the right words to ask for help is discussed in Chapter 6, Communicating Effectively. You might protest that no one has offered help and assume that this means that no one wants to help. Sometimes this is because you have not asked or you have not asked for specific help. A good way to start is with a family meeting.

Holding a Family Meeting

Sometimes the best way to get help is to hold a family meeting. This could seem like a big step or like something that shows weakness on your part. While it might be a big step, it is not a sign of weakness. Calling a family meeting shows strength. The objective is care for your care partner while maintaining the mental and physical health of the caregiver(s). Remember that everyone does not have to be in the same place at the same time. You can hold the meeting by conference call or via a video calling program like Skype, FaceTime, or Google Hangouts. You will find tools for setting up family meetings on pages 96 and 97. The following are some additional tips:

- **Invite everyone who might be interested or helpful.** This may include extended family, such as in-laws and close friends. As you make the list of the people you want to invite, don't forget those who are far away. They might not be able to come to your house to help but they could have good ideas or be able pitch in to pay for help. Even if that is not possible, they are interested and part of the family. Do not exclude them. Invite them to sit in on the phone or computer video conferencing if they cannot attend the meeting in person. Most family meetings do not include the care partner. If that is the case, find a friend, volunteer or care companion (see page 102) to take your care partner out while you attend the meeting.
- **Find a professional to run the meeting.** This professional may be a social worker, a religious leader, or even a friend who has experience in running complex meetings. The person does not need to know much about you, your care partner, your family, or the situation. Their job is to facilitate. By having an uninvolved party run the meeting, there is more chance that everyone will

participate and be heard. It will also be easier to limit the input of any not-so-helpful family members. This might seem like a bother or unnecessary expense, but it is a good idea.

- **Avoid having alcohol available during the meeting.** Alcohol tends to change the thinking and emotions of even "social" drinkers and there always seems to be someone who has a little too much. Stick with nonalcoholic drinks. One way to make this easier is to hold the meeting in the morning or early afternoon.
- **Write an agenda and share it with everyone before the meeting.** Everyone then has a chance to prepare and avoid surprises. It can also help focus the discussion and keep the meeting from going off-topic.
- **Set ground rules.** Listening is hard and even harder when the topic is emotionally charged. Listening to everyone else may be the hardest part of the meeting for attendees. One way you can make this easier is with ground rules such as the following:
  1. Begin the meeting by allowing each person to talk in turn for as long as they want without interruption. At the end of this time, the person speaking says "I have spoken" and the others say "I have heard" (or some other pre-arranged phrases).
  2. There is no discussion until everyone has spoken. After everyone has said how they feel, then you can have a discussion but never an interruption.
  3. Use the words "our" and "we," not "me" and "I."
- **Start the meeting with a status report.** Tell the group about your care partner's present condition. Be specific and clear and factual. Unless the group sees your care partner every day, they may not know what is really going on. Short visits, as you know, can be deceiving.
- **Let all members of the group express how they feel about the situation.** Remember the ground rules. No interrupting.
- **Avoid expressing anger and pushing emotional buttons.** All families have emotional issues, and many family members are experts on how to "get to" another family member. Other family members may be likely to overreact because of the stress they are experiencing.
- **Clearly express the problem and the specific help that you want.** If there are distractions or excuses, use your Broken Record Tool (see page 43 in Chapter 4, Dealing with Difficult Emotions). You might have to do this several times. Remember, no anger.
- **Ask what each person can contribute.** Do not tell people what they should do.
- **As help is offered, write this down and repeat back to the group.** Be flexible. Say, for example, "Mary, I understand that you cannot come here to help, but your offer of paying for a housekeeper one day a week would be a great help."
- **After the meeting, send everyone a copy of the written plans agreed to in the meeting.**
- **At their best, family meetings are regularly scheduled.**

Family Meeting Checklist

- ☐ Invite everyone who might be interested or helpful. This may include in-laws and close friends.
- ☐ Find a professional to run the meeting.
- ☐ Don't serve alcohol.
- ☐ Write and share an agenda before the meeting.
- ☐ Establish ground rules and make sure everyone agrees to them.
- ☐ Start the meeting with a current report on your care partner's status.
- ☐ Let everyone express how they feel about the situation.
- ☐ Use the words "our" and "we," not "me" and "I."
- ☐ Avoid anger.
- ☐ Express the problem and the help that you want.
- ☐ Do not tell people what they should do.
- ☐ Ask for solutions.
- ☐ Record offers of help.
- ☐ Follow up by sending everyone a copy of the agreements.
- ☐ Regularly schedule your family meetings if possible.

Finding Resources in the Community

Unfortunately, some caregivers either do not have family or close friends or cannot bring themselves to ask family for help. More often, family or friends cannot provide all the help that is needed. Thankfully, we have another wonderful resource: our community.

Finding community resources can be a little like a treasure hunt. As in a treasure hunt, creative thinking wins the game. Finding what you need may be as simple as looking in the local newspaper or on the internet and sending a couple of emails or making phone calls. Other times it might require some sleuthing. The community resource detective must find clues and follow them. Sometimes this means starting over when a clue leads to a dead end.

The first step is defining the problem and then deciding what you want. For example, suppose you would really like to have an evening meal prepared three times a week. You might start by asking friends and neighbors. You could also call your local Area Agency on Aging (these are located in most communities across the United States). After a few days, you have a whole list. You learn that the Care and Share group at a local church has a program that supplies one meal a

Family Meeting Planning Tool

The following tool will help you plan a family meeting. On the form, give a name to each category, and under each category write what you need. Do not leave the meeting until the righthand column is filled out!

The following are sample categories of the help you may need:

- Household chores, such as repairs, grocery shopping, gardening, pet care, housekeeping
- Finances, such as paying the mortgage or rent, keeping track of financial records, paying bills, buying or renting equipment such as wheelchair
- Health, such as making medical appointments, submitting insurance forms and other forms related to medical care, drafting and executing durable power of attorney for health care, etc.
- Family communications, such as keeping family members informed, arranging family meetings

Family Meeting Planning Tool		
Category:		
Name of task	Who will do it	When they will do it
Category:		
Name of task	Who will do it	When they will do it
Category:		
Name of task	Who will do it	When they will do it
Category		
Name of task	Who will do it	When they will do it

week to local community members. You also learn that you can order delivery services from many local restaurants and grocery stores on the internet. The Area Agency on Aging shared information about Meal on Wheels, and also a program that serves lunch at your local community center every Monday, Wednesday, and Friday. Another friend told you about a business that allows you to order pre-prepared meal kits that you can cook at home. Finally, one of your neighbors talked about your need with a friend who is a teacher and said that providing some meals for you might be a good project for her middle school cooking class. You decide to go with Care and Share and one meal a week from Meals on Wheels. The last night you will order from some of your favorite restaurants.

There are people in every community who are natural resources. These "naturals" or "connectors" seem to know everyone and everything about their community. They tend to be folks who have lived a long time in the community and have been closely involved in it. They are also natural problem-solvers. These people are the ones that other people turn to for advice. They always seem to be helpful. Your connector might be a friend, a business associate, the mail carrier, your physician, your pet's veterinarian, the checker at the corner grocery, the pharmacist, a bus or taxi driver, a real estate agent, the Chamber of Commerce receptionist, or your librarian. Think of this person as an information resource and don't be shy about asking them about your particular need. Sometimes they will take on the thrill of the hunt and, like a modern-day Sherlock Holmes, announce that "the game is afoot!" and promptly join you in your search.

Many of us are members of neighborhood, school, or church groups on the Internet. These groups are terrific for finding resources.

As this example illustrates, the most important steps in finding community resources are:

1. Identifying the problem.
2. Identifying what you want or need.
3. Searching for resources.
4. Asking friends, family, and neighbors for ideas.
5. Contacting organizations that might deal with similar issues.
6. Identifying and asking "natural connectors."

One last note: The best sleuth follows several clues at the same time. This will save you time and shorten the hunt. Watch out, though—once you get good at thinking about community resources creatively, you will become a natural connector in your own right!

When we need to find goods or services, there are certain resources we can call on. One resource often leads to another. The natural connector is one of those resources, but our community resource "detective's kit" needs a variety of other useful tools. The local newspaper and internet search engines (such as Google or Bing) are the most frequently used tools. These are particularly helpful if you are looking for someone to hire. For most searches, this is where to start.

Organizations and Referral Services

Almost all communities have one or more information and referral services. Sometimes these are related to a geographic area such as a city or county. Other times they are specific to an age group, such as the Area Agency on Aging.

Sometimes they are specific to a condition such as Alzheimer's or Parkinson's disease.

There are several types of agencies offering these services. To find them in the United States, search "United Way Information and Referral," "Senior Information and Referral" (or "Area Agency on Aging" or "Council on Aging"), and "information and referral." Once you have an information and referral telephone number or email, your searches will become much easier. These services maintain huge files of referral addresses and telephone numbers for just about any help you might need. Even if they don't have the answer you seek, they are usually able to refer you to another agency.

Voluntary agencies such as the American Heart Association or Alzheimer's Association are great resources. There are similar organizations in most other countries as well as the U.S. These agencies, funded by contributions from individuals and from corporate sponsors, provide up-to-date information, as well as support and direct services to caregivers. They also fund research intended to help people live better with their illness and to research care and cure options. For a small fee, you can become a member of one of these organizations, entitling you to receive regular bulletins by mail or email. You do not, however, have to be a member to qualify for their services; they are there to serve you. Many of these organizations have wonderful websites. In our modern, globally connected world, you can live in rural North Dakota and access help on the internet from the Parkinson's Foundation in Victoria, Australia.

There are other organizations in your community offering information and referral services along with direct services. These include the local chapter of AARP (formerly known as the American Association of Retired Persons), senior centers, community centers, and religious and social service agencies. These organizations offer information, classes, recreational opportunities, nutrition programs, legal and tax help, and social programs. There is probably a senior center or community center close to you. Your city government office or local librarian knows where these resources are and how you can contact them.

Most religious groups offer information and social services to persons who need it, either directly through the place of worship or through organizations such as the Council of Churches, Catholic Diocese, or Jewish Family Services. To get help from religious organizations, start with a local place of worship. People there will either help you or refer you to someone who can help you. You usually need not be a member of the congregation or even of the religion to receive help.

Call your local hospital, clinic, or health insurance plan and ask to be connected to the social service department. The Veteran Administration offers services to those who are a U.S. military veteran or whose care partner is a veteran. Every Veterans Administration Hospital has a caregiving coordinator.

Libraries

Your public library is a particularly good resource if you are looking for information. Libraries are no longer just collections of books. Even if you think you are an excellent library detective, it's a good idea to ask the reference librarian to make sure you haven't overlooked something. These people see volumes of material cross their desks constantly and are knowledgeable about the community (they're probably among the ranks of the local natural connectors). And if you cannot get to the library, you can call or go online.

In addition to city or county libraries, there are other, more specialized health libraries. Ask your information and referral service if there is a health library in your community. Such libraries specialize in health-related resources and they typically have a computerized database search service available along with the usual print, audiotape, and videotape materials. These libraries are usually maintained by nonprofit organizations and hospitals and will sometimes charge a small fee for use. Again, thanks to the internet, you may be able to connect with a health library that is far away.

Universities and colleges also have libraries open to the public. By U.S. law, the regional "government documents" sections of these libraries must be open to the public at no charge. Government publications exist for just about any subject, and the health-related publications are particularly extensive. You can find everything from information on organic gardening to detailed nutritional recipes. The librarians are usually very helpful, and these publications represent "your tax dollars at work."

If you are fortunate enough to have a medical school in your community, you might be able to use its medical library. This, however, is a place to go to for information rather than to look for help with tasks. Naturally, you can expect to find a great deal of information about disease and treatment at a medical library. Unless you have special knowledge about medicine, however, the detailed information you find in a medical library can be confusing and even frightening. Use medical libraries with care.

Books

Books can be useful (indeed, you are reading a book now!). Many caregiving-related books contain reading and resource lists, either at the ends of chapters or at the backs of books. These lists can be very helpful. We list Suggested Further Reading and Other Resources at the end of each chapter of this book.

Newspapers

Your local newspaper, especially if you live in a smaller community, can be an excellent resource. Be sure to look in the calendar of events. Even if you are not interested in a particular featured event, calling the contact telephone number may help you find what you are looking for. Look in other logical places for news stories that might also be of interest. For example, if you are looking for an exercise program, check out the sports and fitness section.

Sometimes you can find clues in the classified section. Look under "announcements," "health," or any other heading that seems promising. Review the index of classified headings, which is usually printed at the front of the section near the rate information, to see which headings your newspaper uses. Most newspapers now also have websites as well. Often the website who are a veteran or can have more information than is in print.

The Internet

Today most people have access to the internet. Even if you are not an internet user, you know an internet user. If you do not have a computer, you can use one in your local library or ask a friend for help. The internet is the fastest-growing source of information currently available. More information is being added every second of every day. The internet offers information about caregiving and anything else you can imagine. It also provides several ways in which you can interact with people all over the world. For example, someone who has Gaucher disease, a rare health condition, might find it difficult to locate others with the same disease where they live. The internet can put a person in touch with a whole group of such people; it doesn't matter whether they are across the street or on the other side of the world.

The good thing about the internet is that anyone can maintain a website, a Facebook page, a Twitter account or other social network page, a blog, or a group. That is also the bad thing about the internet. There are virtually no controls over who is posting information or whether the information is accurate or safe. This can mean that although there is a lot of information out there that might be very useful, it also means that you might encounter incorrect or possibly dangerous information.

You should never assume that information found on the internet is entirely trustworthy. Approach information obtained online with skepticism and caution. Ask yourself, is the author or sponsor of the website clearly identified? Is the author or source reputable? Is the information contrary to what everyone else seems to be saying about the subject? Does common sense support the information? What is the purpose of the website? Is someone trying to sell you something or win you over to a particular point of view?

One way to start analyzing the purpose of the website is to look at the URL (the address, starting with http:// or https://). The URL will usually look something like this:

https://www.stanford.edu

At the end of the main part of a U.S.–based website's URL, you will most commonly see .edu, .org, .gov, or .com (or .info, .biz, and .co). This will give you a clue about the nature of the organization that owns the website. A college or university URL will end in .edu, a nonprofit organization will end in .org, a governmental agency will end in .gov, and a commercial organization will end in .com. As a general rule of thumb, .edu, .org, and .gov are trustworthy sites, although a nonprofit organization can be formed to promote just about anything. A website with .com is trying to sell a product or service or is selling advertising space on its site to others trying to sell you something. This doesn't mean that a commercial website can't be a good one. On the contrary, there are many outstanding commercial sites dedicated to providing high-quality, trustworthy information. They are often able to cover the costs of providing this service only by selling advertising or by accepting grants from commercial firms. The URLs for some of our favorite reliable websites are listed at the end of this chapter.

The Internet and Social Networking Sites

Social networking sites and blogs are exploding on the internet. Sites such as Facebook, Twitter, Instagram, Reddit, Tumblr, Google+, Snapchat, and Pinterest are currently very popular, but everything may change by the time this book is published. These sites enable the average person to communicate easily with others who want to listen (or read). Some sites, such as Facebook, require that users determine who will be allowed to read the thoughts they post on their page.

Many such sites have been started by caregivers or people living with particular health conditions, and the authors are eager to share their experiences. Some have discussion forums associated with them. The information and support offered can be valuable, but be cautious: Some sites can be proposing unproven and dangerous ideas.

Discussion Groups on the Internet

Yahoo, Google, and other websites host discussion groups for just about anything you can imagine. Anyone can start a discussion group about any subject. Groups are run by the people who start them. For any one health problem, you will probably find dozens of discussion groups. You can join them and the discussions if you wish, or just "lurk" (read without interacting). For caregivers, this may allow you to connect to people who share your experiences. This could be the only opportunity to talk with someone else. Smart Patients, for example, has an excellent online group at:

https://www.smartpatients.com

To find discussion groups, go to the Google or Yahoo (or other) home page and search for a link to "groups."

Keep in mind that the internet changes by the second. Our guidelines reflect conditions at the time this book was written. Things may have changed by the time you read this.

Getting Caregiving Help

One of the things that caregivers tell us they need the most help with is figuring how to actually get the help they need or want. Earlier in this chapter, we outlined how to ask for help from family and friends. Sometimes, however, more help is needed. The following section will help you decide what help you need and how to find it.

In-Home Care*

Many different types of people and organizations offer in-home help. The following list can help you think about what you and your care partner want and need.

- **Housekeeper/yard worker**: This is someone who can will help with the household and/or outdoors chores. These chores might include ironing, cleaning, cutting the grass, or shoveling the snow. These workers do not usually interact much with a care partner. They help to free up caregiver time and make your life less complicated.

- **Care companion:** A care companion provides an extra pair of eyes, ears, and hands. They can help your care partner do as much as possible for themselves and help out with the following tasks:
    - Drive your care partner on errands or to social outings
    - Grocery shop

*The material in this section was adapted from Caring.com's website.

- Take your care partner to the doctor
- Cook and/or fill the freezer with healthful, prepared meals
- Light housekeeping such as vacuuming, bathroom and kitchen cleaning
- Organizational projects such as cleaning your garage, closets, or junk drawer
- Keep your loved one company—playing cards, looking at photo albums, or even just sitting and chatting

- **Personal care assistant**: Personal care assistants give care that involves physical assistance. They usually have some training and can help your care partner with everyday tasks such as:
  - Bathing
  - Toileting
  - Getting dressed
  - Shaving
  - Dental hygiene
  - Nail care
  - Walking
  - Incontinence

If needed, most personal care assistants will also help with driving, shopping, cooking, light housekeeping, and keeping your care partner company.

- **Respite care in your home:** Sometimes you just need a break and a little time for yourself. Having someone come in just once or twice or on a regular basis can provide this help. This can be a friend or relative. You can check with your place of worship, senior center, or Area Agency on Aging to see if they have suggestions for people who can fill this role for you. If your care partner is a veteran, even if he or she does not use veteran's services, you can call the caregiver support person at your local Veterans Administration health care facility. In-home care agencies can also help. Call them to arrange care for a one-time event or to schedule someone to come on a weekly or monthly basis.
- **Live-in care**: Many in-home care agencies can help you arrange round-the-clock care. This protects your care partner and lets you get some sleep. This might be a single caregiver who lives in or a set of caregivers who work in shifts. You can find live-in care in the same ways we suggested for respite care.

Two types of organizations offer in-home services, **in-home care agencies** and **in-home care registries**.

- If you use an **agency**, then the agency carries all the employer responsibilities. It hires the caregiver, pays the payroll taxes, etc. It also provides some training and supervision. Be sure to get all the details about each agency's policies as these can differ from agency to agency.
- **Registries** are a referral service that helps you find a caregiver. People who are referred will usually have experience and may have required training. You will pay a fee to the registry for this service, but, unlike an agency, they do not employ care providers. If you hire someone from a registry, that person is your employee or independent contractor. This means that you might be responsible for paying taxes and social security and you must buy your own liability insurance. When you contact a

registry, ask about the training and experience of the people they refer and what you will be expected to do as the employer of an independent contractor.

- You can also hire someone **recommended by a friend** or found through a help wanted ad or posting on a website. If you go this route, you are responsible for checking all references and doing all the screening. The person can work for you as either an employee or an independent contractor. You will need to talk to your lawyer about the implications of both of these when you consider such things as taxes and insurance.

If you want to explore hiring in-home help, the Caring.com website can provide you with the information you need. They have advice on how to proceed, lists of agencies, reviews from families, and checklists to help you through the process (http://www.caring.com).

Adult Daycare

Not all help needs to be provided in your home. There are many adult day care centers throughout the country. These often provide transportation and are sometimes partially financed by various government programs. For example, your care partner attends an adult day care center for a half or full day one or more days a week. These centers are set up to have activities, including exercise and socialization. They can typically address the needs of adults that need continuing supervision, such as those with dementia. In addition to giving you some much needed private time, these centers provide your care partner with an opportunity to socialize and learn new skills.

One word of warning: Your care partner may not want to go to such a center. It is new, unknown, and does not include you. Before bringing this up with your care partner, talk with the center director or social worker about how to handle this. One thing to remember is that your care partner's mental functioning has probably changed. They might not be able to be an equal partner in decision-making, they might not be able to make rational decisions. For you, this could be very difficult. It is just another way in which you are reminded that things are not as they use to be. You may feel grief and loss. This is normal but can be difficult all the same.

Caring.com has information about this option as well.

Moving to a New Residence

The time may come when your care partner needs to move to a new residence. This might be due to your care partner's declining health or because of your own health needs. It may be because you find it too difficult to care for your care partner as you think you should. Perhaps you've reached the end of your physical or emotional energy. Whatever the reason, caregivers often feel guilty about this. Sometimes your care partner is upset about leaving familiar surroundings and will let you know, potentially adding to the guilt. In spite of this, you should recognize that your care partner will receive better care and that you will be able to take better care of yourself as well.

It's a difficult decision to make, but once you make it, there are care communities that offer several types of care. Chapter 2, Becoming a Better Caregiver: The Basics, has a tool that can help you with this decision-making process, as well as any other type of decision.

- **Independent living senior communities:** If either you or your care partner is a senior, this option is open to you. These communities usually offer meals in a dining room, weekly housekeeping, and sometimes laundry service and transportation. They often offer a wide selection of activities and field trips as well. This can be an option if you want to be free of cooking and cleaning and to be around others on a daily basis. These communities do not offer personal assistance to your care partner.
- **Assisted living:** An assisted living residence can offer all of the services that independent living residences do, plus some personal care assistance and/or medication dispensing assistance. Personal care assistance typically includes help with tasks such as showering and dressing. However, your care partner must be able to get to the bathroom, get in and out of bed, and get to the common dining room on their own. You can choose to live with your care partner in assisted living, but you may have to eventually move out if you care partner has to move to a skilled nursing facility or dies.
- **Skilled nursing:** For many, there are a lot of negative feelings around skilled nursing facilities. You might have seen negative stories in the press about bad "nursing homes." There is no doubt that some nursing homes have been caught giving poor-quality care, but these are outnumbered by the facilities that provide excellent care to their residents. Skilled nursing facilities have doctors, nurses, physical therapists, social workers, psychologists, occupational therapists, and nutritionists available on site. If your care partner must have 24-hour care from a professional staff, skilled nursing is usually the best option.

  Do your homework if you are considering skilled nursing. Tour the facility, ask questions, visit again, and look around more closely. Visit during a busy time like mealtime or a shift change. Is everything clean? How does it smell? How many beds are in each room? Is there space to do more than just sleep in the bedrooms? Is everyone in bed, or do you see many of the residents in common areas or outside on the patio? Does the staff seem happy? What is the facility's rating on the Five-Star Medicare Quality Rating system? To figure out your options, try contacting a local nursing-home ombudsman. Every state has ombudsmen to investigate residents' concerns and some help families evaluate facilities. Websites that offer directories and ratings of nursing homes can be found in the Other Resources section at the end of this chapter.

  Skilled nursing care can be expensive. Explore options for financial assistance and find out the facility's policy on taking Medicaid if your care partner's money runs out. If you or your care partner is a veteran, you may qualify for care and assistance funds from the VA.
- **Continuing care communities (CCRC):** There are facilities that offer all three of the above services (independent living, assisted

living, and skilled nursing) at one site. The advantage to these communities is that if you and your care partner need different levels of care, the facility can accommodate both of you. A second advantage is that should the care needs of you or your care partner change, you can remain in the same facility.

- **Board and care homes:** Board and care homes are usually small homes in residential areas that offer personal care, meals, housekeeping and sometimes transportation. They differ from assistant living in that they do not offer the wide range of activities found in assisted living. Most board and care homes have around six or so residents, who have their own rooms but eat together. It isn't likely that you would be able to live with your care partner in board and care. Board and care homes tend to be less costly than assisted living.

Whatever options you consider for your care partner, it requires a lot of thought and research. It's a big decision. You might want to use the decision-making tools on pages 12–14 and/or call a family meeting.

Suggested Further Reading

August, Yosaif. *Coaching for Caregivers: How to Reach Out before You Burn Out*. S.l.: Yes to Life Publishing, 2013. A how-to manual that coaches caregivers on how to reach out for help. http://amzn.to/2EHKKnQ

Emlet, Michael R. *Help for the Caregiver: Facing the Challenges with Understanding and Strength*. Greensboro, NC: New Growth Press, 2008. Practical ways to manage your caregiving role. http://amzn.to/2BuL5bE

Other Resources

Agingpro online directory offers access to professionals in aging, resources, educational articles, virtual classroom, ask the expert, and support groups. http://www.agingpro.com

Alzheimer's Association. http://www.alz.org/care

Association of Cancer Online Resources (ACOR). http://www.acor.org

Caregiver.com can help you to find a trusted in-home care provider. https://www.caregivers.com

CaringBridge. http://www.caringbridge.org. This site lets you post about your care partner and then your posts can be seen by those you designate. This way you do not have to keep up correspondence with so many friends and family members.

Center for Advancing Health. http://www.cfah.org

Centers for Disease Control and Prevention (CDC). http://www.cdc.gov

Daily Strength offers over 500 online support communities and information exchange on a variety of health and wellness issues, including caregiving. http://www.dailystrength.org

Eldercare Locator by the U.S. Administration on Aging connects you to services for older adults. https://eldercare.acl.gov/Public/Index.aspx

Family Caregiver Alliance's (FCA) Connections e-newsletter focuses on issues and information important to family caregivers. https://www.caregiver.org/connections-newsletter

FCA online caregiver support group: http://lists.caregiver.org/mailman/listinfo/caregiver-online_lists.caregiver.org

FCA online LGBTQ caregiver support group: http://lists.caregiver.org/mailman/listinfo/lgbt-caregiver_lists.caregiver.org

Family Caregiver Alliance's Family Care Navigator lists government health and disability programs, legal help, and advocacy, as well as resources on living arrangements for care recipients and more. https://www.caregiver.org/state-list-views?field_state_tid=152

HealthCentral. http://www.healthcentral.com

National Cancer Institute. http://www.cancer.gov

National Institutes of Health (NIH). http://www.nih.gov

MedlinePlus. http://www.nlm.nih.gov/medlineplus

National Library of Medicine (tutorial for evaluating internet health information). http://www.nlm.nih.gov/medlineplus/evaluatinghealthinformation.html

Parkinson's Foundation. http://www.pdf.org

Psych Central. http://www.psychcentral.com

Traumatic Brain Injury. http://traumaticbraininjury.com

Healthfinder. http://www.healthfinder.gov

Chapter 8

Preventing Injuries

As a caregiver, one of your primary goals is to prevent care partner injury. But injury isn't a problem just for care partners—injury is a concern for everyone. Statistics show that caregivers are at high risk of injuries too. Caregiver fatigue is very common and a major cause of injuries because mental and physical fatigue can result in inattention, distraction, and delayed physical reaction times. Your risk of injury increases if you are caregiving 20 or more hours per week. Helping your partner with activities of daily living (ADLs), such as getting out of bed, bathing, toileting, dressing, and taking care of your other responsibilities, such as preparing and eating meals, cleaning house, and shopping, can be a lot of work and can put you at risk for injury. When your care partner needs a lot of assistance, both during the day and overnight, the risk is even greater.

Poor posture, age-related physical changes, inactivity, and an unsafe environment are among factors that combine with fatigue and contribute to caregiver injury risk. It is typical for caregivers to experience back pain, muscular pain, joint pain, and injuries from falls. These injuries can affect your ability to provide care to your care partner as well as your mental health and well-being. Injury risk is something people would often like to ignore. However, by learning about your risks, you can make yourself and your care partner safer. Often, just by paying more attention to risks and making small changes, you can prevent injuries.

In this chapter, we outline ways to reduce injury risk and prevent injuries. The focus is on you, the caregiver, but we do not ignore potential care partner injuries. We also address ways to reduce care partner injury from combative behavior, choking, and poison exposure. If you have previously experienced injury as a caregiver, this chapter is designed to reduce additional future risk.

Understanding the Unintentional Injury Cycle

Many factors increase the risk of injury. The injury cycle (see Figure 8.1) illustrates various factors that can cause unintentional injuries for caregivers. As you can see in the illustration, physical and emotional caregiver burden/fatigue can cause poor body mechanics and deconditioning and physical changes that result in injury. For example, a caregiving task such as transferring can result in injury. You may be unaware of your awkward unbalanced body position until one day you experience back pain as you help your care partner dress. Similarly, you could reach out to catch your care partner, but due to slowed reaction time, both of you end up injured. Deconditioning and physical changes in both you and your care partner can result in decreased strength in legs and arms, decreased balance and endurance, dizziness, pain, and decreased vision, hearing, and sensory processing, which can increase the risk of a fall. For example, a caregiving task such as transferring, moving from one position to another, could have been easy yesterday but has become difficult today because you feel dizzy. An unsafe environment with hazards, like clutter

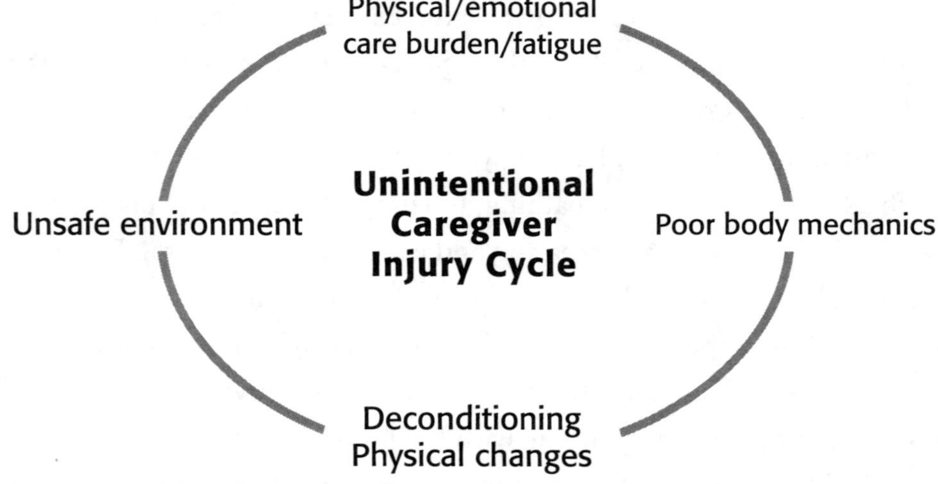

Figure 8.1 **Caregiver Injury Cycle**

and cords stretched across the floor, make it easy to trip, also contributing to the injury cycle risks.

Aspects of the injury cycle can increase risk of injuries by themselves or be related and influence each other. If your body is deconditioned and weaker, your posture will be worse and it will take more effort to perform caregiver activities. This increases the likelihood of poor posture and body mechanics, which in turn increases the risk of back and limbs strain. A weaker, tired caregiver is much more likely to sustain injury due to hazards in the environment. Factors in the cycle interact to increase risk of injuries.

While not all injuries can be prevented, the rate and severity of injury can be dramatically reduced. There are many tools you can use to break the unintentional injury cycle. The Injury Risk Assessment Exercise on page 112 is a list of questions you can ask yourself to determine your risks of injury. You will notice that the prevention tools listed in the last column overlap and often address more than one type of injury risk. In the next section, we will discuss these injury prevention tools in detail so you can use them as a daily part of your caregiving activities.

Reducing Injury Risk

Most caregivers are not trained to prevent injuries. The Toolkit for Reducing Injury Risk provides specific ways to interrupt the cycle of unintentional injury and make your caregiving less painful and dangerous. Furthermore, the toolkit strategies can reduce your care partner's injury risk by helping you both prevent injuries so you remain safer when working together. In the following sections, we describe each tool and how to use it to reduce your injury risk.

Toolkit for Reducing Injury Risk

- Exercise.
- Use proper body mechanics during caregiving activities.
- Emphasize your own self care needs.
- Build calm and positive connection with care partner.
- Use mindful movement approaches.
- Modify home and surroundings.
- Use special equipment.
- Seek health professional guidance.

Exercising and Being Physically Active to Address Physical Changes

You might have experienced physical limitations due to illness, chronic health conditions, and/or aging that affect your safety and increase your injury risks. Researchers have found that exercise can positively impact your physical abilities. However, finding the time and energy to exercise while caregiving is difficult. Given the pressures and responsibilities of caregiving, even regular exercisers may consider reducing or stopping their program. Non-exercisers might not ever start. Yet, even 30 minutes of exercise two or three times a week can make a difference in your physical abilities and health as a caregiver. In Chapter 9, Exercising for Health and Wellness, we explain the importance

Injury Risk Assessment Exercise

If you answered yes to the questions here . . .	Your injury risk is . . .	And here are prevention tools to reduce your injury risk:
◆ Are you edgy and short-tempered with your care partner due to fatigue and exhaustion? ◆ Do you have difficulty making enough time to care for yourself? ◆ Are you preoccupied and inattentive when assisting your care partner?	Physical and emotional care burden and fatigue	◆ Meet own needs. ◆ Promote calm and positive connections. ◆ Practice mindful movement. ◆ Use proper body mechanics. ◆ Modify your home and surroundings. ◆ Use special equipment. ◆ Seek health professional guidance. ◆ Exercise.
◆ Do you frequently get into awkward positions and experience body pain during caregiving activities? ◆ Do you do over 50% of the lifting during transfers with your care partner?	Poor body mechanics	◆ Exercise. ◆ Use proper body mechanics. ◆ Use special equipment. ◆ Modify home and surroundings. ◆ Seek health professional guidance. ◆ Promote calm and positive connections. ◆ Practice mindful movement.
◆ Are you afraid of falling? ◆ Have you noticed changes in your vision or hearing? ◆ Do you use your hands to push up from a chair? ◆ Do you take medications that increase your risk of a fall?	Deconditioning and body changes	◆ Exercise. ◆ Modify your home and surroundings. ◆ Seek health professional guidance. ◆ Use proper body mechanics.
◆ Are there hazards and clutter in your home that increase risk of fall or injury? ◆ Do you have furniture that is too low, too soft, or without arms? ◆ Do you frequently wear slippers and shoes with no backs? ◆ Do you think your care partner uses a cane or walker improperly?	Unsafe environment	◆ Use special equipment. ◆ Modify your home and surroundings. ◆ Seek health professional guidance. ◆ Promote calm and positive connections.

of physical activity in increasing energy level, managing stress, improving fitness, and controlling chronic health conditions. The health risks associated with inactivity are greater than the risks of injury during exercise.

Exercising to Decrease the Risk of Low Back Pain and Body Pain

Exercise can decrease your risk of low back and body pain. Back pain is more common among people who are not physically fit. When you bend and reach without noticing your body position, it puts you at further risk for increased back pain. For example, if your care partner is overweight, there is increased risk for pain and musculoskeletal discomfort for both the care partner and their caregiver. If your care partner "gets stuck" coming to stand, you might be required to grip hard with both hands and hold on tight, keeping your forearm muscles contracted, to keep your care partner from falling. Over time, gripping tight and holding muscles in a contraction can result in shortening of the muscles of your wrist at your forearm (near your elbow). This or similar situations might happen repeatedly over time. Short muscles put tension on ligaments and tendons and result in immediate or eventual pain. The pain can end up feeling like a severe muscle cramp.

Building flexibility, strength, and endurance reduces back injury and body pain. Flexibility or stretching exercises lengthen muscles and can reduce pain and tension. Generally, stretches need to be done gently and held for a few seconds so as not to force the muscle to lengthen. Find exercises to improve flexibility in Table 8.1 on page 114.

Strengthening the back and core muscles offers many benefits. Chest and back strengthening improve posture and alignment. If you have weak back and abdominal muscles, your spine is not properly supported during movement activities. Strong core muscles support the spine, absorb shock from movement, and protect other joints such as the knees and shoulders. Often muscles get sore or painful when the workload is heavier than your muscles can handle. With stronger muscles, you strain less easily. Table 8.1 lists several postural and core muscle strengthening exercises that are explained in detail in Chapter 9, Exercising for Health and Wellness.

Endurance activities, such as walking, bicycling, swimming and low impact aerobics, are good choices and described in more detail in Chapter 9. These exercises repetitively use large muscles to increase your heart rate. Studies show that low-impact aerobic exercise is beneficial for the maintaining the integrity of the discs between the bones of your spine.

Exercising to Reduce the Risk of Falls

Researchers have found that exercise to improve strength and balance is the most effective strategy to reduce risk of falls for you and your care partner. As we age, we have less coordination, flexibility, strength, and balance, and our reaction time diminishes. This is often due to inactivity. At any age, exercise can improve all of these.

One of the biggest risks for falls is muscle weakness. Stiff, weak muscles limit motion and increase risk of strain or pain. You can increase your stability by building strength in your leg muscles around the hips, knees, and ankles. (See Table 8.1, Exercises to Reduce Injury Risk. for specific exercises to build strength.) If you have poor balance, you can easily fall while exercising since you have difficulty changing positions. As you practice these exercises, be sure you have support, such as a chair, kitchen counter, or table.

Walking is often included as part of a fall risk reduction program to improve endurance, but walking alone won't reduce fall risk. See Table 8.1 for balance exercises to add to your plan such as heel and toe walking. Hold onto a counter or supportive surface or use a walking aid if you have difficulty with balance. If you have not been told to use a walking aid but feel you need one, review Table 8.2, Mobility Aids and Injury Prevention Tips, and talk to your health care practitioner. You can judge your improvement in balance by noticing your ability to hold a position longer or hold a position while using less support.

As you can see in Table 8.1, many exercises are recommended to improve flexibility, strength, and balance in order to reduce injury risk. If you are looking for general injury prevention, select exercises from all three areas. Tailor your program to meet your own needs. You can try a few and assess how you feel or use this list to determine if group exercise programs you participate in include exercises that have the potential to reduce your injury risk. You will know the exercises or physical activities made a difference if you can do more repetitions, use less support, and continue for longer with fewer rest breaks.

To work on your strength and balance, another option is to repeat a difficult daily task, such as getting up from a chair or climbing stairs. Repeatedly doing "chair squats" or "chair rises" by coming from sitting to standing without using your arms can improve your fitness. Walking and stair climbing can also improve with practice. Leisure activities such as tai chi, yoga, dancing, and gardening can improve your physical fitness too. Make sure to tune in to your posture, balance, and how you feel during daily tasks for safety and success.

If you have a history of body pain or falls, it is best to speak with your health practitioner and consider a consult with a physical therapist. Physical therapists can create and supervise an

Table 8.1 **Exercises to Reduce Injury Risk**
(The page numbers in this table refer to detailed descriptions of these exercises that you can find in Chapter 9, Exercising for Health and Wellness.)

Flexibility	
Back and Neck	
Heads up	p. 143
Neck stretch	p. 144
Cat and cow pose in seated position	p. 144–145
Knee-to-chest stretch	p. 145
Pelvic tilt	p. 145
Back lift	p. 145
Low-back rock and roll	p. 146
Arms and Legs	
Pat and reach	p. 146
Shoulder shape-up	p. 146
Good morning (with wrist stretch down and wrist stretch up)	p. 147
Hamstring stretch	p. 147–149
Achilles stretch	p. 148
Better posture	
Shoulder-blade pinch	p. 148–149
Curl-up	p. 149
Roll-out	p. 149
Leg strength	
Straight-leg raises	p. 150
Back kick	p. 150
Hip hooray	p. 150
Knee strengthener	p. 151
Power knees	p. 151
Ready-go	p. 151
Tiptoes	p. 151–152
Sit-to-stand	p. 152
Balance	
Beginning balance	p. 153
Swing and sway	p. 153
Toe walk	p. 154
Heel walk	p. 154
One-legged stand	p. 154
Walk-the-line	p. 154–155

exercise program and help you carry it out correctly. If you have injuries related to smaller muscles, such as arm and hand, occupational therapists are often more experienced and similarly can create and supervise your exercise program.

Finding Fall Prevention Programs

We know it may be hard to get out of the house, but you might prefer a group exercise program to exercising on your own. A Matter of Balance, Stepping On, Stay Active and Independent for Life (SAIL), Tai Chi for Arthritis, and Tai Ji Quan: Moving for Better Balance are group programs that have been studied and found effective in reducing risk of falls. They are offered in many U.S. locations but not in all states. If you are 60 or older and your concern is fall prevention, links to these programs are listed as resources at the end of this chapter. You can also find a locator map for programs near you at the Evidence-Based Leadership Council website:

http://www.eblcprograms.org/evidence-based/map-of-programs.

There are national senior exercise programs listed as references at the end of the Chapter 9, Exercising for Health and Wellness, and many include exercises to improve balance. The Otago Exercise Program offers individually tailored exercises taught by a physical therapist. If you are referred to a physical therapist for balance training, ask if this program would be beneficial for you.

Using Proper Body Mechanics during Caregiving Activities

Your care partner may have difficulty moving. This can come on slowly. For example, it could begin with your care partner just needing more help getting dressed. Or it can come on suddenly. All at once your care partner needs help with almost everything. The amount of help your care partner needs might be the same every day or it might vary day-to-day. One of the most common challenges for care partners is changing positions, such as getting on and off the toilet or getting in and out of bed. These position changes are referred to as transfers.

If you help your care partner transfer out of bed, your back is likely to twist in an unnatural direction. You might not be in this twisted position for a long period, but you might be doing it multiple times a day or week. Often caregivers sacrifice their own bodies to keep their care partners safe. The way you move while you are helping your care partner transfer or get up can not only hurt you (resulting in back pain, falls, or muscle pain), but it can also hurt your care partners. If you are not stable, your care partner might fall. Helping your care partner manage daily activities requires teamwork just like dancing does. To prevent injury to both you and your care partner, you need to establish ways to help your care partner that are consistent, safe, and efficient. The following sections on posture and body mechanics and care partner transfers can lead you in the right direction.

Practicing Good Posture and Body Mechanics

Good posture and body mechanics for you and your care partner will reduce risk of pain and injury. A good posture habit strengthens your body. Attention to posture and body mechanics (how you use your body) are especially important during transfers because this is when you or your care partner are likely to twist, get into awkward positions, and lose your balance.

Proper posture involves maintaining the three natural curves in the spine at the neck, upper back, and lower back. When these curves are maintained, the spine is the strongest. The natural curves help the body absorb the "shock of movement" and the strain of holding positions with the least strain. Proper posture also requires that all body parts are in alignment. This prevents strain on muscles, ligaments, tendons, and joints. Figures 8.2–8.4 illustrate good sitting and standing posture.

Good standing posture is characterized by the following:

- Ears over shoulders
- Shoulders over hips (shoulders even and relaxed)
- Hips over knees
- Knees over feet (knees straight but not locked)
- Feet shoulder width apart (even weight on both feet)

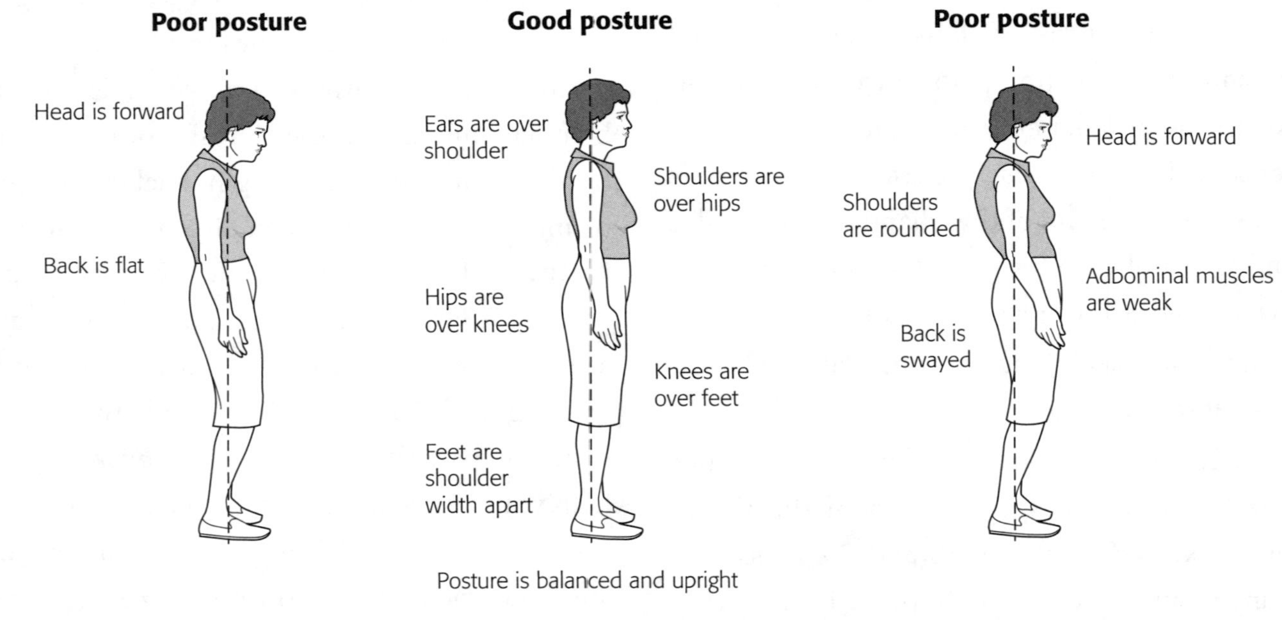

Figure 8.2 **Standing Posture**

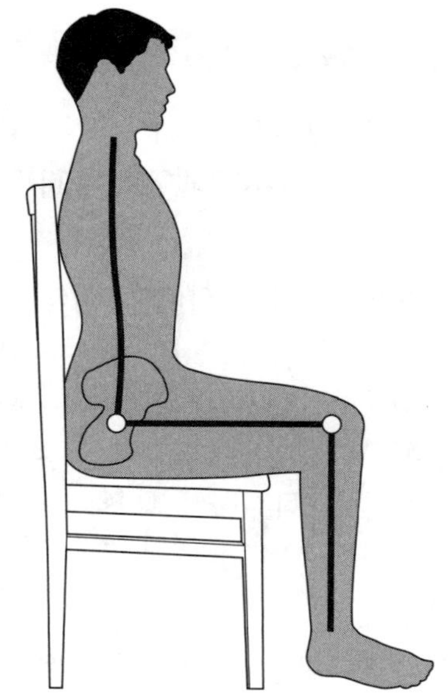

Good sitting posture is characterized by the following:

- Ears over shoulders
- Shoulders relaxed but not elevated
- Upper back relaxed and over hips
- Hips bent 90 degrees
- Knees bent 90 degrees
- Buttocks flat on seat with even weight on both hips
- Feet flat on floor or foot rest

Figure 8.3 **Sitting Posture**

If you have upper back or shoulder pain, even when you have not assisted your care partner, think about what else might be causing it. For example, many people experience pain that stems from poor posture while using a computer (see Figure 8.4). If you identify a cause, take note of your posture and do what you can to improve it.

Using Recommended Transfer Postures

Helping your care partner change positions can put strain on your back and limbs. There are many ways to practice and use safe and steady transfers. Encourage your care partner to actively participate, even if having your care partner involved takes more time. Use the tips discussed in the previous section to protect your

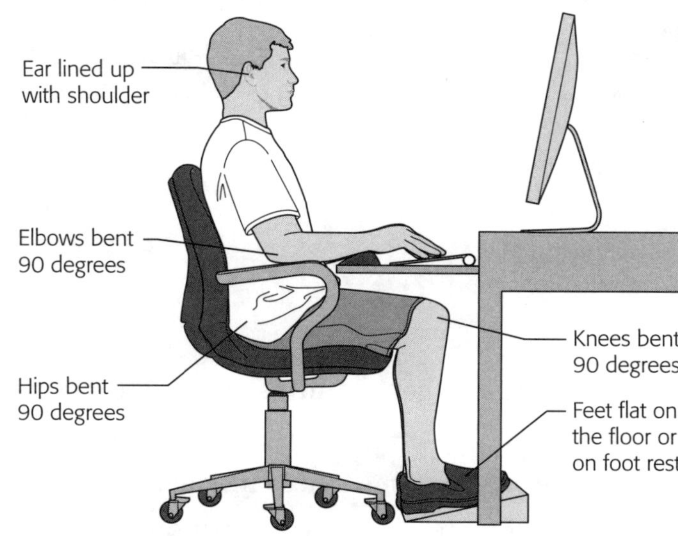

Figure 8.4 **Good Sitting Posture for Computer Use**

Body Mechanics for Daily Caregiving Activities

Good body mechanics involve using good posture when helping your care partner with activities such as getting dressed, taking a shower, or changing position. The following tips can protect your back and limbs:

- Bend your knees and hinge at the hips if you need to lean forward. Do not bend at the waist as it strains your spine.

Incorrect

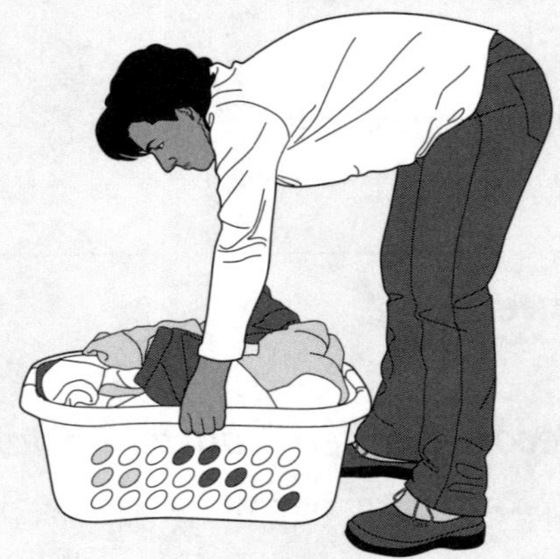

Do not bend at the waist.

Correct

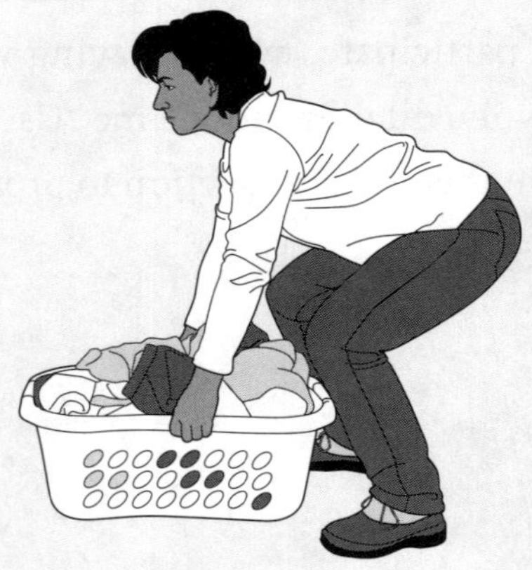

Protect your back by bending your knees or hinging at your hips.

- Use equipment or change your position to avoid awkward body posture. For example, consider sitting on a low stool to help your care partner put on shoes or socks. Use a long-handled sponge to reduce bending and twisting while helping your care partner shower.
- Reduce twisting, especially bending forward and twisting. One helpful trick is to imagine you are wearing a belt buckle; keep your imaginary belt buckle and your feet pointing in the same direction.
- Avoid assisting your care partner with your arms outstretched. Make sure that you are close to the bed when you assist your care partner with transfers.
- Make sure you feel steady and your care partner feels steady. Place your legs about hip distance apart and one foot in front of the other.
- Gently tighten and lift your stomach muscles to support your spine.
- Use a gait belt (see Table 8.3 on page 132) to increase safety as needed.

back and limbs. If a total assist is needed, get help or use equipment.

In this section, we illustrate a few types of transfers. Carefully review the complete instructions before practicing with your care partner. Adjust the instructions so that you and your care partner feel safe, steady, and balanced. If these instructions do not work for you, consult an occupational or physical therapist.

Moving from Sitting in an Arm Chair to Standing

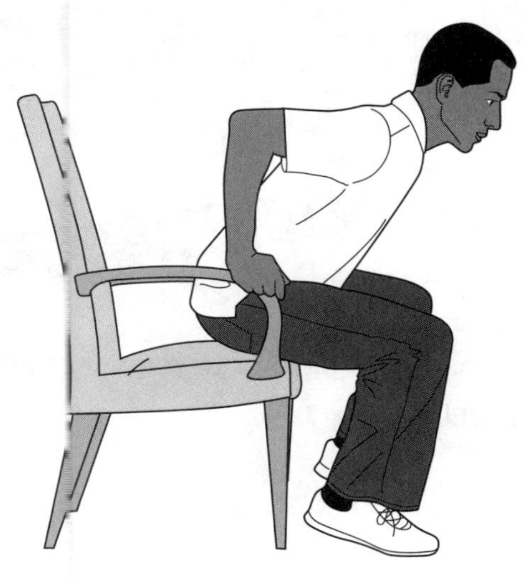

1. Have care partner slide hips forward to sit near the front half of the chair.
2. Make sure care partner's feet are on floor (making 90-degree angle with knees).
3. Have care partner lean forward (nose over toes).
4. Have care partner push from chair arms to come to a standing position (if assistance is needed, consider using a gait belt; see Table 8.3 on page 132).

Getting into Bed

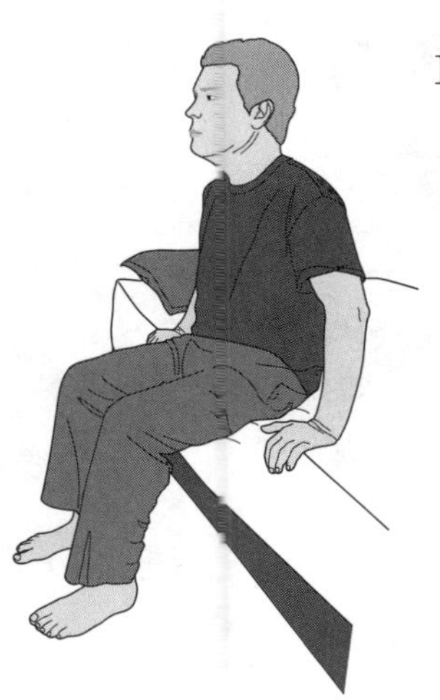

1. Have care partner sit on the bed about a foot from the pillow.

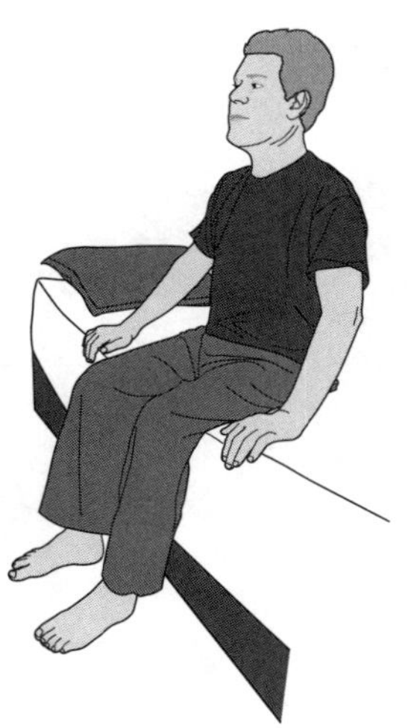

2. Ask care partner to scoot back so not sitting on very edge of bed. The backs of the knees should be touching the mattress (or assist care partner to move from edge).

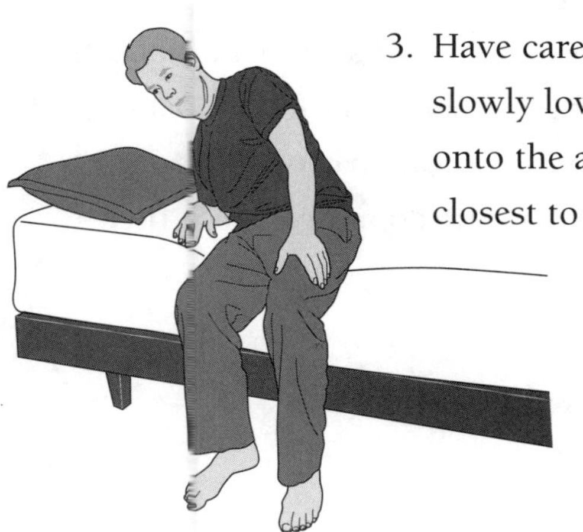

3. Have care partner slowly lower body onto the arm that is closest to the pillow.

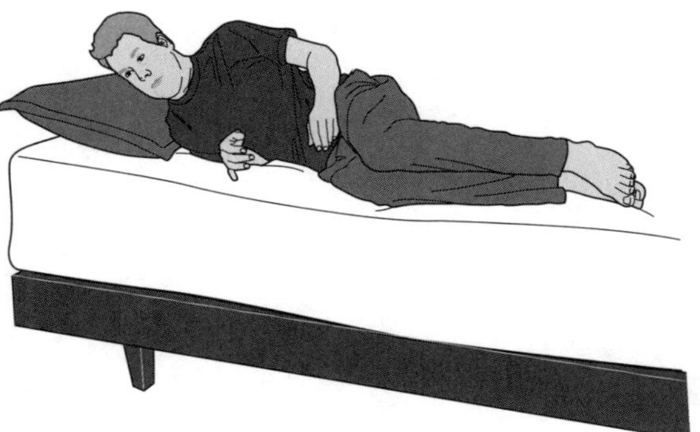

4. Ideally, at the same time, have care partner bend knees and pull them onto the bed. (If assistance is needed, guide your care partner's legs into the bed, keeping knees bent.)

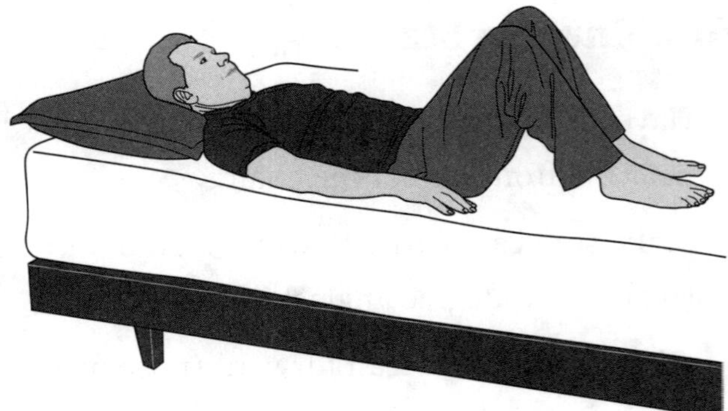

5. Have care partner roll onto back.

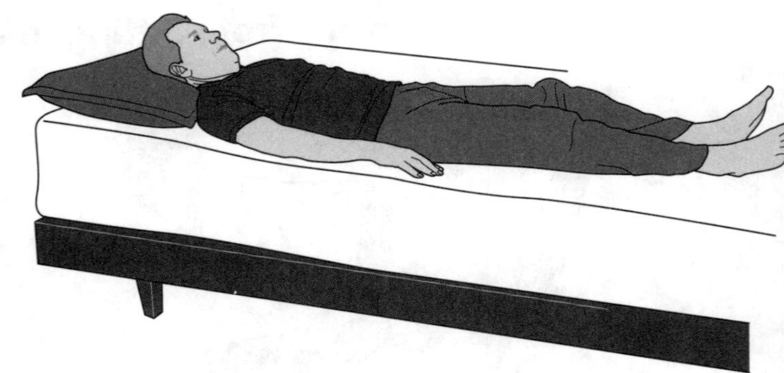

6. Encourage care partner to relax legs and get comfortable.

Getting out of Bed

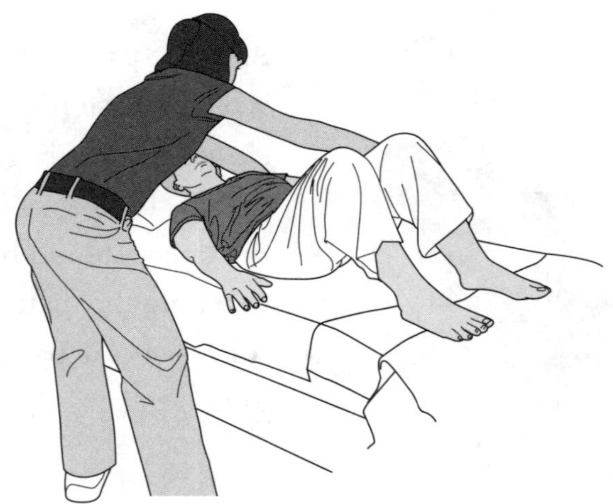

1. Have care partner bend knees while lying on back (or bend knees for them).

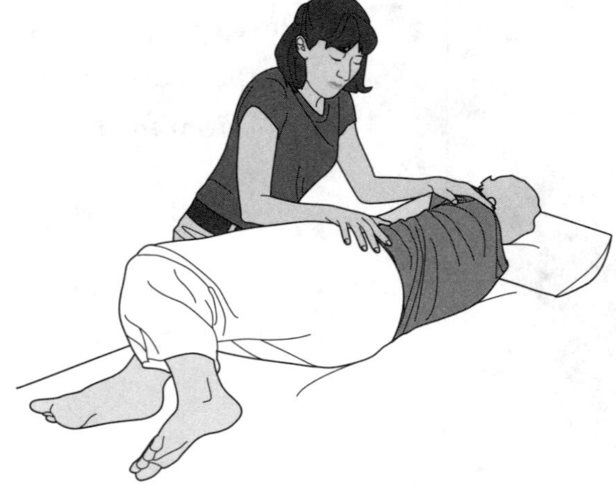

2. Ask care partner to roll toward you as you stand at side of bed. (If assistance is needed, get as close to the bed as possible and gently guide with one hand on care partner's shoulder and other on care partner's hip. Make sure care partners do not roll onto their hands.)

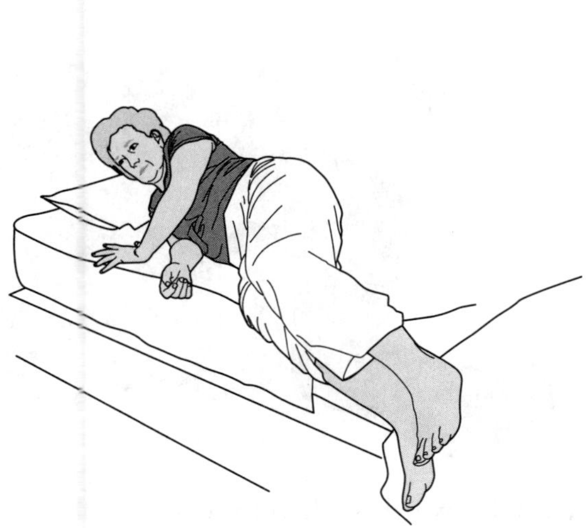

3. Ask your care partner to move feet over the edge of the bed while pushing up onto one elbow. (If assistance needed, guide care partner's feet over the edge.)

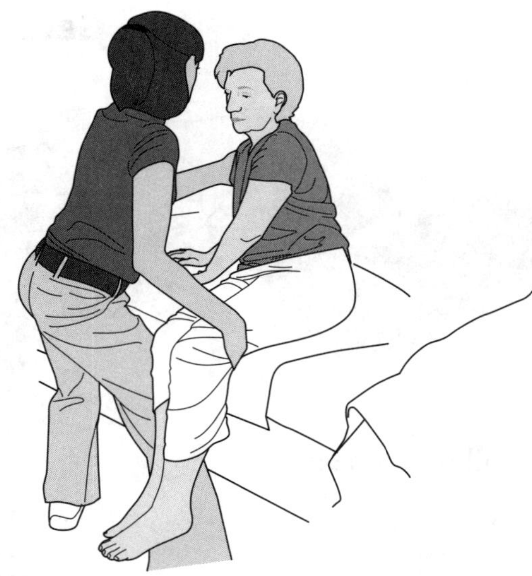

4. Ask care partner to move to sitting position. (If assistance is needed and you are able, cradle care partner's shoulders in one hand and place your other hand under your care partner's knees to guide care partner up to sitting position.)

Troubleshooting Tip for Transfers

- Sometimes one side of the bed is easier than the other.
- Consider installing a safety rail on the side of the bed to help with pushing up.
- If using an assistive device (for example, a walker or a cane), push up from a steady, permanent surface rather than the device, as it is safer.
- **DO NOT LIFT** care partners even if they are small enough to make this possible.

Getting up from the Floor

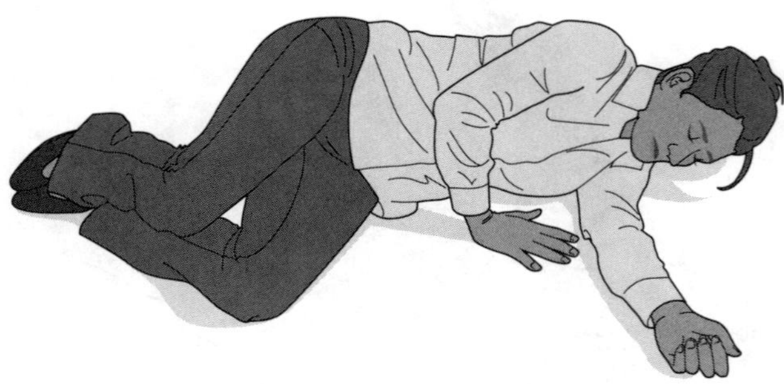

1. Roll onto one side.

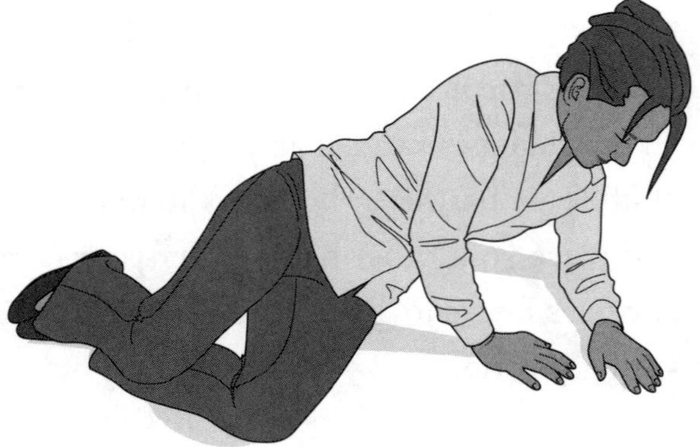

2. Push up with upper hand enough to get lower elbow under the body.

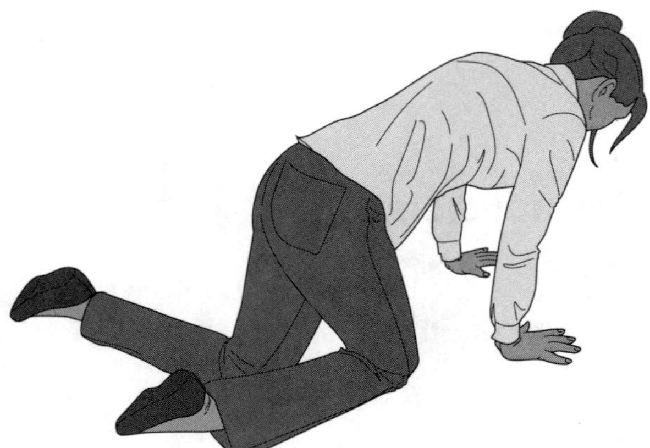

3. Tuck knees under the body and roll to all fours.

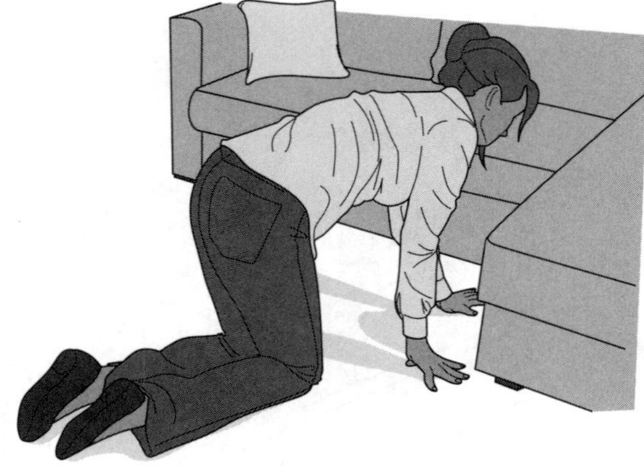

4. Crawl toward the bed or a sturdy chair.

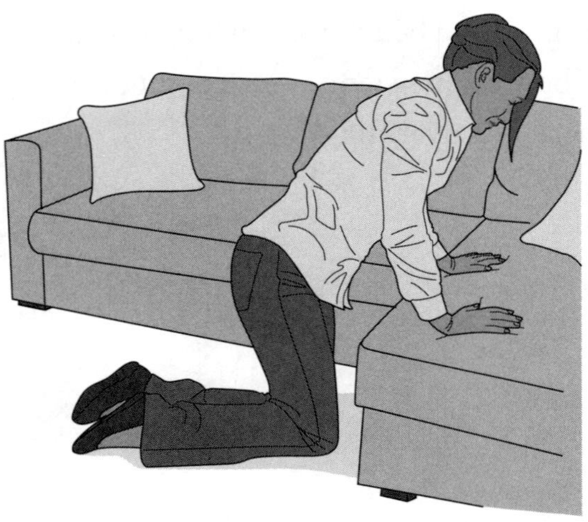

5. Place hands on sturdy surface (chair or bed).

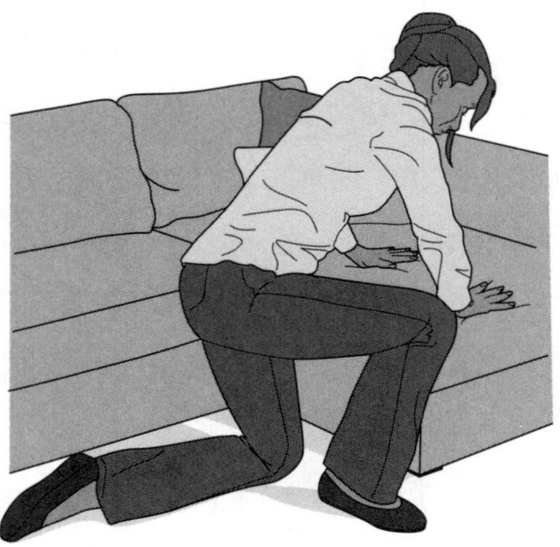

6. Bend stronger leg and put the foot of that leg flat on the floor.

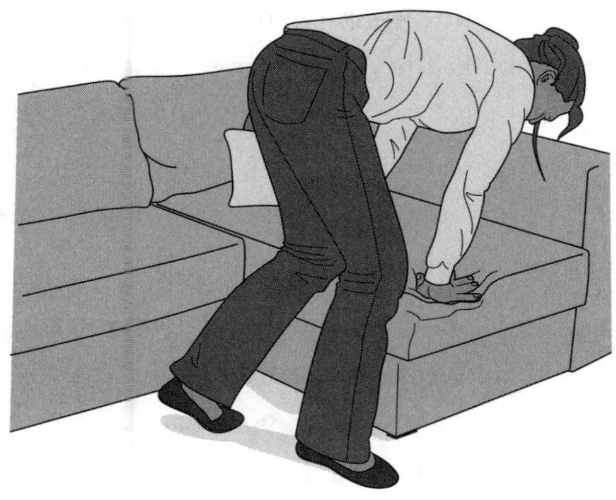

7. Push up to standing position.

Staying Safe during Transfers and Daily Activities

Preparation, communication, and moving with teamwork is a three-step approach to organize common tips and strategies for assisting your care partner with transfers. This process can be applied to other difficult daily tasks, such as dressing or bathing.

Step 1. Preparing

- *Stress assessment.* What is your and your care partner's state of mind? Consider using the quieting reflex by taking a few breaths prior to each transfer or use another cue to "check in" with yourself. Ask your care partner to also take a few deep breaths.
- *Assistance assessment.* How much help do you and your care partner need? If it has been a bad day due to illness or mood, you or your care partner may need more assistance. If two people are required for the transfer, have a plan so that neither person is injured. Think ahead about the task and have a clear picture of what your care partner can do and what assistance you need to provide.
- *Equipment assessment.* What equipment will you need today? We discuss gait belts, transfer boards, and mobility aids later in this chapter (see Tables 8.2 and 8.3 on pages 129–134); one or all of these could enhance your safety during the activity.
- *Safety assessment.* What can you do to make your environment safer? If your care partner uses a wheelchair, make sure to lock it and swing away or remove the legs before you start. Safe transfers start and end with a stable surface.

Safely Swinging away Wheelchair Leg Rests

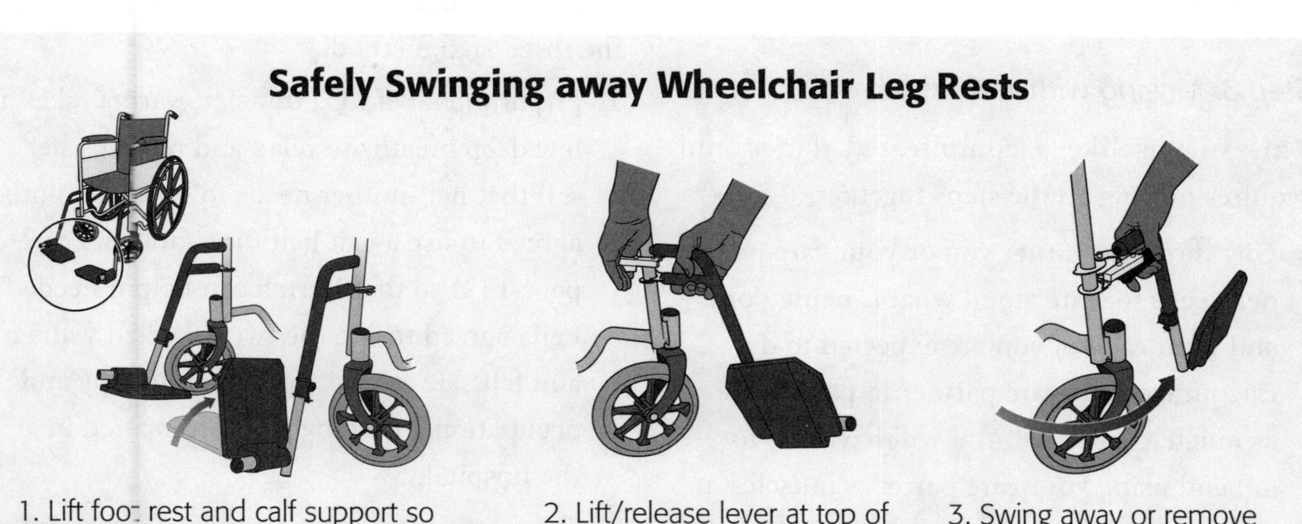

1. Lift foot rest and calf support so they fold toward the leg rest.
2. Lift/release lever at top of leg rest.
3. Swing away or remove leg rest.

Step 2. Communicating and Creating Calm

There is no single correct way to communicate with your care partner. The person giving assistance and the person receiving assistance must work together. It is a dance. Communicating clearly and calmly is always helpful in a partnership.

- If possible, *be sure your care partner helps.* Talk about your ideas and your care partner's ideas. Decide who will give the cues and what each of you will do. You might need to have this discussion only once, or you might go over this several times a day. Remember, in most cases, your care partner is trying to do it right.
- *Decide on commands.* Give quick clear simple commands that the two of you have agreed on. Keep them the same every time and make sure all caregivers use them. Too many words and repetition tend to result in confusion and frustration. Consider cues such as "take a breath," "push," "up," or "turn." If you like the recommended transfer postures, consider using shortened versions of those cues.

Step 3. Moving with Teamwork

This step is like a complicated dance and requires putting all the steps together.

- *Give direction.* Either you or your care partner needs to state aloud what is being done and what each of you are expected to do. Encourage your care partner to participate as much as possible. You will have less to do, and using your care partner's muscles, it will help maintain muscle strength. Even if you are strong enough to get the job done, repeatedly lifting your care partner increases your risk of injury and your care partner's dependence. Try to work out consistent ways of moving so that both of you know what to expect. This will decrease frustration and increase efficiency.
- *Tune into your body.* You could do a quick body scan to tune into pain or soreness. Small twinges of pain in your back and arms are easily overlooked, but pain can add up. If you have aches or pain, try some stretches or some ice (not more than 20 minutes at a time). You may find a few deep breaths help.

The following two examples show the three-step process in action:

Situation 1: Leila, the care partner, is a widow, and her daughter, Karina, is the caregiver. Karina became so afraid her mother would fall again that she and her husband restricted Leila's movement and even picked her up for transfers. Leila became so weak as a result of not helping herself with daily tasks that she fell and was admitted to the hospital. Following this accident, Karina committed to helping her mother to do more and regain her strength. They used the three-step method.

1. *Preparation:* Before a transfer, Karina takes a few deep breaths to relax and reminds herself that her mother needs to do more. Both agreed to use a gait belt (see Table 8.3 on page 132) so that Karina can help if needed. Leila agreed to use the two-wheeled walker and felt safe after the physical therapy and occupational therapy she participated in at the hospital.
2. *Communication:* Karina expressed her worry, and her mother expressed her desire to

regain her independence. Together they decided that Karina can stay nearby during transfers, and Leila will use her walker all the time. Both agreed to use the gait belt. Karina agreed to remain quiet unless a command is needed.

3. *Moving together:* Leila needs assistance for shower transfers and dressing. Karina stands by and remains calm and quiet during transfers to a shower chair. Karina pays attention to maintain her posture and Leila does too. Leila requests assistance during dressing but does most of it herself. This helps her feel more independent as well as strengthens her body.

Situation 2: Alex, the care partner, is a 41-year old-combat veteran. He recently fell at the grocery store. He went home after the emergency room visit. Since then, he has gotten progressively weaker. His wife, Elena, hurt her back while getting him out of bed. She hired a caregiver to help. Alex and Elena asked the doctor for physical therapy. Participating in therapy helped Alex build up his strength. The physical therapist also taught Alex and Elena to work together for transfers.

1. *Preparation:* Before a transfer, Elena asks Alex how he is doing today. When he says he is feeling tired, she puts on the gait belt (see Table 8.3 on page 132) so she can help him. Alex always keeps his walker near his chair or bed. Elena takes a couple of deep breaths as a cue to remind herself to use good body mechanics. Alex is using a walker now and keeps it close during a transfer.
2. *Communication:* The physical therapist taught Elena to break the transfer into steps because Alex is forgetful at times. Alex is very agreeable to Elena using cues for each step of the transfer. He reminds her to pay attention to her posture because he doesn't want her to injure her back again.
3. *Moving together:* Elena puts on a gait belt when Alex feels he needs it. She says: "Slide hips forward," "Feet under knees," "Nose over toes," and "Push up." She is careful to use the body posture position shown in Figure 8.2 on page 116 as it takes strain off her back. After the transfer, she does a quick body scan, and if her back is at all sore, she does a few stretches.

Emphasizing Your Self-Care Needs

Because of lack of time and increased responsibility, you might not be meeting your own needs or making time for yourself. You might be edgy or short tempered. Think about your own basic needs and set priorities. What are the current activities that cause you the most frustration and fatigue? Which activities bring you satisfaction or calm you down? Explore the advice and suggestions offered in this book. Consider testing out one or two suggestions in Chapter 5, Using Your Mind to Manage Stress, that could make your habits healthier and lessen your stress level. Some of the activities to build positive connections and calming experiences described in the following sections may help you meet your own needs while helping your care partner. One caregiver we know has made the time to do a daily 15-minute mindful meditation for the past two years. She finds that setting aside this short time period is possible on most days. The meditation leaves her more refreshed and energized to deal with the many requirements of caregiving. She reports that she is less likely to lose her temper with her care partner and more optimistic about the future.

Building Calm and Positive Connections and Experiences

You may get frustrated because your care partner's personality is so different than it was in the past, because it's a struggle to get tasks done, because you feel at risk for an injury working with your care partner, or for any number of good reasons. You might become frustrated by unexpected demands, such as picky eating or bowel and bladder accidents. When you dwell on frustration, the focus on negative thoughts can make daily tasks more challenging. It is not unusual to experience tension. And tension could put you into a negative state before there is real difficulty. Tension between you and your care partner can increase the risk of an injury. Increasing calm interactions between you and your care partner can reduce frustration during transfers and other challenging daily tasks.

If your care partner has difficulties with moods, making the mood calmer can be especially helpful in reducing unexpected episodes of upset or agitation. Being calm and connected can help reduce the risk of another source of injury, physical combativeness. If the suggestions offered here don't fit your situation, use them as a starting place to do your own brainstorming. Changing the atmosphere may be a work in progress rather than a simple fix.

Remaining calm and connected while still managing the changes life has dealt you and your care partner is not always easy. Sometimes activities you enjoyed in your former life aren't feasible and too much time is spent watching TV and managing daily living basics. Listed below are some options that allow you to relate to your care partner and provide pleasure for both of you:

- **Music creates a mood.** Choose music you both enjoy. Play music that is calming to reduce agitation, or upbeat to promote participation. You could use a favorite radio station or internet site. Some people load favorite music onto an MP3 player or cell phone, add speakers, and then listen with their care partner. If your care partner has memory issues, music is organizing and might enhance positive mood and increase participation in daily activities. Just a note, not everyone likes calming music. If your care partner likes Gilbert and Sullivan, marches, or jazz, it is alright to play these.
- **Enjoy nature.** Observing nature does not require memory or physical ability. Taking your care partner for a wheelchair walk in the park is an opportunity to be outside and notice nature. It is both stimulating and calming to many. Similarly, there are botanic gardens and greenhouses you can visit. Focus on natural beauty; many find it calming. Even a care partner with limited memory can participate and enjoy the experience in the moment. If you are confined indoors, the action around a bird feeder viewed through a window can offer simple entertainment. Sitting and watching the birds with your care partner for even 10 minutes can be a source of stimulation and calm. It might even bring joy.

- **Shared activities.** Games offer an opportunity to relate. If your care partner was a game player in the past, those are the best games. If games of the past, such as bridge, are too hard, try simple game such as Go Fish or Parcheesi. Consider your care partner's abilities and interests in choosing games. The current trend toward adult coloring books is another option for an activity you might be able to do together.
- **Laugh together.** It is easy to get wrapped up in required activity or the frustrations of the day. Make some time to laugh. Maybe you have funny memories you share. Maybe you can read each other jokes from an online source. Sometimes you can just laugh about everyday things. Humor is a wonderful outlet for frustration. Many argue that laughter is good medicine.

Practicing Mindful Movement

Do you find yourself rushing through tasks or notice that you are sometimes hasty or preoccupied? Rushing might mean speeding to a doctor's appointment because getting ready took longer than expected, running to answer the phone, or hurrying through your care partner's shower. Rushing can lead to accidents and problems. Rushing focuses on a future task and makes it easy to lose sight of the task you are doing. If rushing becomes a habit, you might not notice your care partner's faltering balance or bumping into furniture until it's too late. You may overlook fall hazards on the floor and trip over something. Rushing can also create a silent tension between you and your care partner.

It is easy to get caught up in thinking about the next thing on your to-do list. Rushing and worrying distracts us and increases risk of injury. Being mindful is the opposite of being rushed or preoccupied. Recall from Chapter 5, Using Your Mind to Manage Stress, that mindfulness is a way of calmly and consciously observing and accepting whatever is happening in that moment of your life. When you are mindful, you can be more present and pay closer attention while doing your daily tasks. Sometimes caregiving is unpredictable, but there are times you can change things to gain more control. To practice being more mindful, consider the following suggestions.

- **Reduce rushing.** One way to reduce rushing is to gain control of predictable tasks and allow extra time to complete them. Start breakfast early if you have to get to an appointment. Schedule planned appointments at your care partner's best time of day or a time of day that won't require a mad dash for you to "make it." If you aren't successful all the time, you can at least disrupt the rushing cycle.
- **Reduce worrying.** To reduce worry and preoccupation, start by thinking about what worries you the most and brainstorm your own ideas for addressing those topics. Would calling a friend to talk or attending a support group help? Would having more physical assistance with care giving tasks reduce your worry? Is there some other action you can take that would reduce your worry?
- **Cue yourself to pay attention in the present moment.** There are many ways to cue yourself to pay attention during caregiving activities. One common way is the quieting reflex. You can use the quieting reflex at

any time, but before and after transfers and challenging daily tasks are excellent times to tune into your body. We provide an example to create a habit of tuning into your body and emotions in the steps to safer movement later in this chapter.

Making Activities Easier and Safer with Special Equipment

Making daily activities easier and safer reduces caregiver fatigue and stress. Adaptive equipment or mobility aids can compensate for your or your care partner's limitations. Special equipment provides additional support to your care partner so your job will require less effort. The important questions to ask are: "What devices are available?" "How do I choose the right one?" and "How do I use the device properly?" Be sure to get the answers you need.

Using Mobility Aids

Mobility aids such as walkers, canes, and wheelchairs are common. If you or your care partner are experiencing any of the following, think about using a mobility aid:

- You or your care partner are touching furniture or steady surfaces to get around the house.
- One leg is weaker than the other.
- You or your care partner are unsteady outside of house or when walking on uneven surfaces.
- You or your care partner are falling due to poor balance, weakness, or slow reaction times.

Falls of almost any type could signal the need for mobility aids. Unfortunately, not using a mobility aid correctly or using the wrong or improperly fitted aid can also lead to falls and injury. Sometimes mobility changes and thus there is a need to change aids. If you have any questions about which aid is right for you or how to use it, seek guidance from health care professionals such as a physical therapist and get proper training. You might even want to take a short video with your cell phone during the training so that you remember how to use it correctly when you get home.

Table 8.2 lists commonly used mobility aids and tips to prevent injuries. While you should seek a professional's help, you can use the information from the table to get started and know what questions to ask.

Reducing Caregiver Strain and Effort with Adaptive Devices

Adaptive devices can decrease caregiver effort. For example, if your care partner can stand up by holding onto a grab bar, less effort is required from you.

Table 8.3, Special Equipment, lists and describes devices that reduce the effort you need to put forth to physically support your care partner. You will likely not need all of these devices and it is not a goal to own all of these devices. Instead, you want to select the devices that can provide an answer to a problem that you cannot solve with other strategies, techniques, or tools. In addition to the devices listed in Table 8.3, there are many other types of equipment that have the potential to improve your care partner's independence in daily living tasks and

Table 8.2 **Mobility Aids and Injury Prevention Tips**

Mobility Aids	Qualities	Injury Prevention Tips
Walking sticks	◆ Often longer than a conventional cane ◆ Can use one or two ◆ Use two walking sticks on uneven or rough terrain ◆ Two sticks provide a standing rest break ◆ Designed for people who have adequate balance on flat ground ◆ Tends to hold less stigma than a cane	◆ Use of two sticks is helpful when hiking or on uneven terrain. ◆ Choose cork or molded rubber hand grips; plastic grips tend to get sweaty.
Single-point cane or straight cane	◆ Good for people who need some stability while walking ◆ Increases safety and balance compared with no assistive device ◆ Helps to maintain mobility when there is pain or weakness on one side of the body	◆ Hold vertical with upright posture. ◆ Keep the cane close to your body. ◆ Don't drag the cane. ◆ Is not useful if held in air and not touching ground. ◆ Hold in hand opposite weak or injured leg; step out with injured or weak leg and cane at same time.
Quad cane	◆ Good for people who need more stability than a single-point cane ◆ Can stand upright ◆ Larger base than standard cane	◆ Hold vertical with upright posture. ◆ Keep the cane close to your body. ◆ Don't drag the cane. ◆ Is not useful if held in air and not touching ground. ◆ Hold in hand opposite weak or injured leg; step out with injured or weak leg and cane at same time. ◆ All four feet at cane base must touch surface to be safe.

Continued ▶

Table 8.2 **Mobility Aids and Injury Prevention Tips** (*continued*)

Mobility Aids	Qualities	Injury Prevention Tips
Hemi walker	• Good for people who have had a stroke and/or need more support than a cane • Most stable device for people with use of one arm • Large base of support • Folds for storage • Bulky/heavy	• Advance the walker as you advance the affected side, then take a small step to bring it in line with other foot. • Have someone close by for balance if concerned about falling.
Rollator with 4 wheels	• Good for people who have more balance but reduced endurance • Fastest walking speed • Offers seat for rest break and basket to carry items	• Stand tall. • Stay close to walker. • Handles of walker should be at user's wrist height (arms hanging straight at side). • Lock the brakes before you sit down or go from chair to standing. • Can tip if you put full weight on the hand rests.
Rolling walker with 2 wheels	• Good for people with some balance issues who need some support to walk • Moves faster than standard walker • Glides forward only	• Stand tall. • Stay close to walker. • Handles of walker should be at user's wrist height (when arms are hanging straight at side). • Consider attached tennis balls or glides to back legs to allow back legs to slide.

Table 8.2 **Mobility Aids and Injury Prevention Tips** (*continued*)

Mobility Aids	Qualities	Injury Prevention Tips
Standard walker	◆ Good for people with limited balance who need a lot of support to walk ◆ Slow to move ◆ No wheels ◆ Need to pick up	◆ Stay close to walker. ◆ Handles of walker should be at user's wrist height (when arms are hanging straight at side). ◆ Keep all four legs in contact with the ground when walking. ◆ Stand tall.
Manual wheelchair	◆ Good for people with enough upper body strength to propel the wheelchair ◆ Good for people who lack the endurance to use a walker or cane for outings (museums and outdoor gardens often have wheelchairs available if you call ahead) ◆ Good for people who have someone to push them	◆ Always lock the brakes before getting in and out of the wheelchair. ◆ Swing away the wheelchair legs for a safer transfer (see box content on p. 123). ◆ Avoid putting heavy loads on the back of a wheelchair. ◆ Avoid going up or down steep inclines. ◆ If there are no curb cuts, consider backing up wheelchair to go up/down to/from a curb.
Scooter	◆ Good for people who don't require a power wheelchair full time.	◆ Always ride solo. ◆ Wear seat belt. ◆ Keep track of battery charge indicator so battery is fully charged. Consider carrying an extra battery.
Power wheelchair	◆ Good for people who cannot push a wheelchair with their own arm strength ◆ Power wheelchairs with standing options are available that allow people with paraplegia to stand independently	◆ Turn the power off before transferring. ◆ Avoid riding in the rain. ◆ Avoid going up or down steep inclines. ◆ Keep track of battery charge indicator so battery is fully charged.

Table 8.3 **Special Equipment**

Device	Purpose	Tips
Gait belt	• Assists with transfers and unstable walking • Allows you to grasp the belt in order to assist in transferring or moving a person	• Place the gait belt low around your care partner's waist. • Fasten the belt tight enough so it does not slide but loose enough so you can slip a finger under the belt. • When you put the belt on your partner who is sitting, fasten tighter than you might think is necessary as it will loosen up when you partner becomes more upright.
Mobility bed rail	• Helps with sitting up or getting out of bed • Prevents falls from bed • Allows you to exert less effort to sit your care partner up in bed if the care partner has strength in upper extremity	• Place on your care partner's stronger side. • Test that the rail is secure before your care partner grasps it. • May need more than rail if care partner puts excessive weight on the rail. • The rail is not designed to keep people in bed, rather to help them sit up and to prevent them from falling out of bed accidentally.
Hoyer lift	• Assists with getting out of bed or chair • Useful in reducing injury if your care partner needs full assistance and/or is too heavy for you to lift	• Seek professional guidance from your health care team before purchasing. • Proper use is critical and requires special training.
Chair lift up	• Assists with safely standing from a seated position • Best if used in a rigid chair, not for use on a soft chair or couch. • It is safest used in a chair with arms.	• Test the seat yourself before your care partner uses to make sure that the seat is stable and not sliding.

Table 8.3 **Special Equipment** (*continued*)

Device	Purpose	Tips
Raised toilet seat/ uplift commode assist	◆ Assists with safely standing from a seated position ◆ Assists with safely sitting from standing position ◆ Allows one to follow precautions needed after hip replacement ◆ There are many different models; some types are easier to remove if there is only one bathroom and commode must be used by others	◆ Make sure the seat fits securely. ◆ Test for stability before your care partner uses.
Toilet safety rails	◆ Assist with safely standing from a seated position ◆ Assist with safely sitting from standing position. ◆ This is a good alternative (to the raised toilet seat/uplift commode assist described above) if your care partner only needs the armrest but not the raised toilet seat	◆ Test to make sure this is sturdy enough to hold your care partner's weight when pushing up. ◆ Measure your toilet (width and height) to make sure the rails will fit before purchasing.
Grab bars	◆ Assist with getting out of tub/shower ◆ Assist with slowly and safely assuming a seating position from a standing position ◆ Provides stability and supports longer standing time (for example, so caregiver can wash entire body)	◆ Can be used to enter the shower, to get up from the toilet seat, or get over a step or a few stairs in a hall, not just in a bathroom. ◆ See the box "Tips for Installing Grab Bars" in the Bathroom on p. 136. ◆ Have grab bars professionally installed so they will not pull out of the wall. ◆ Request assistance and a home visit with an occupational therapist to learn where to place and install bars. ◆ Avoid suction grab bars options; these must be tested every time they are used to ensure that they don't pull away from wall. ◆ Use professionally installed grab bars, NOT towel bars; a towel bar is not a grab bar and with repeated pressure, it will unexpectedly pull out of the wall.

Continued ▶

Table 8.3 **Special Equipment** (*continued*)

Device	Purpose	Tips
Shower chairs/bench 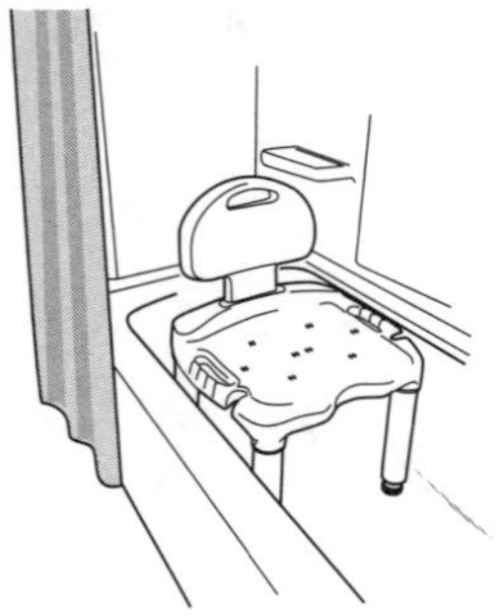	◆ Provides stability and prevents falls in shower/tub ◆ A shower stool or folding shower seat is adequate if your care partner only needs place to rest ◆ Choose a shower chair with armrest/back if your care partner needs more support ◆ Choose a shower chair without armrest if you are using transfer board (described below) ◆ Choose a tub transfer bench if your care partner cannot safely step over the tub edge ◆ Portable chairs are available for travel	◆ Measure your tub/shower to make sure the chair fits before purchasing. ◆ Install a hand showerhead to increase the care partner's independence and control over water flow.
Handy bar 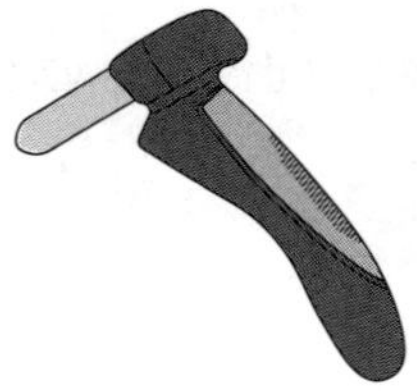	◆ Assists with getting in and out of car 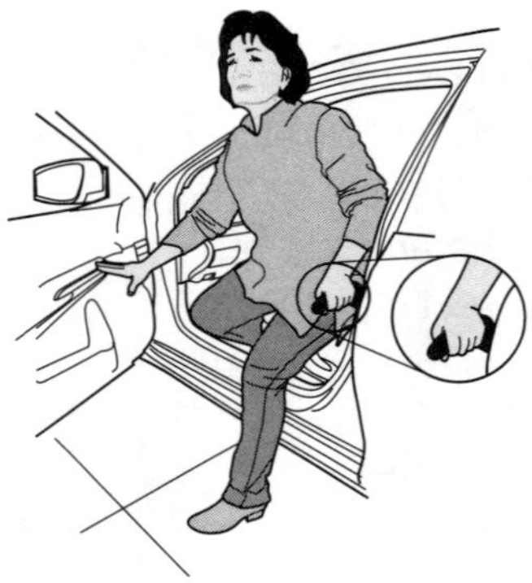	◆ Before your care partner uses the handy bar, make sure to test its sturdiness.
Swivel cushion 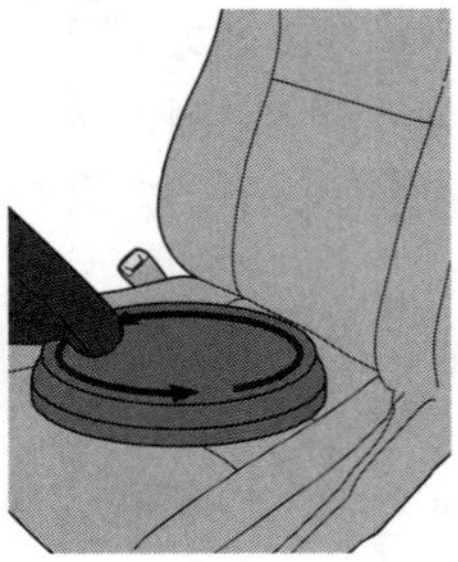	◆ Assists with getting in and out of cars ◆ Helps with swiveling around when one is in a chair or car seat	◆ Test the cushion yourself before your care partner uses.
Transfer board 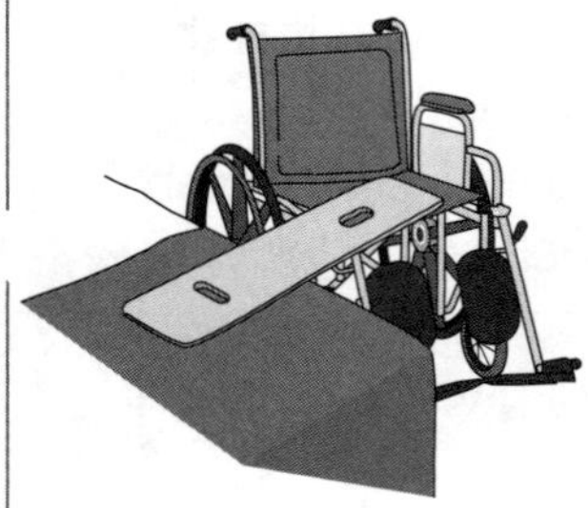	◆ Assist chair-to-chair transfer (wheelchair-to-car, -tub bench, -bed, -chair) ◆ Allow your care partner to slide over the board instead of lifting him/her	◆ Make sure your care partner has good arm and trunk strength before using transfer board. ◆ Before using with your care partner, try the transfer board yourself and seek instruction from a healthcare professional to make sure you understand how it works.

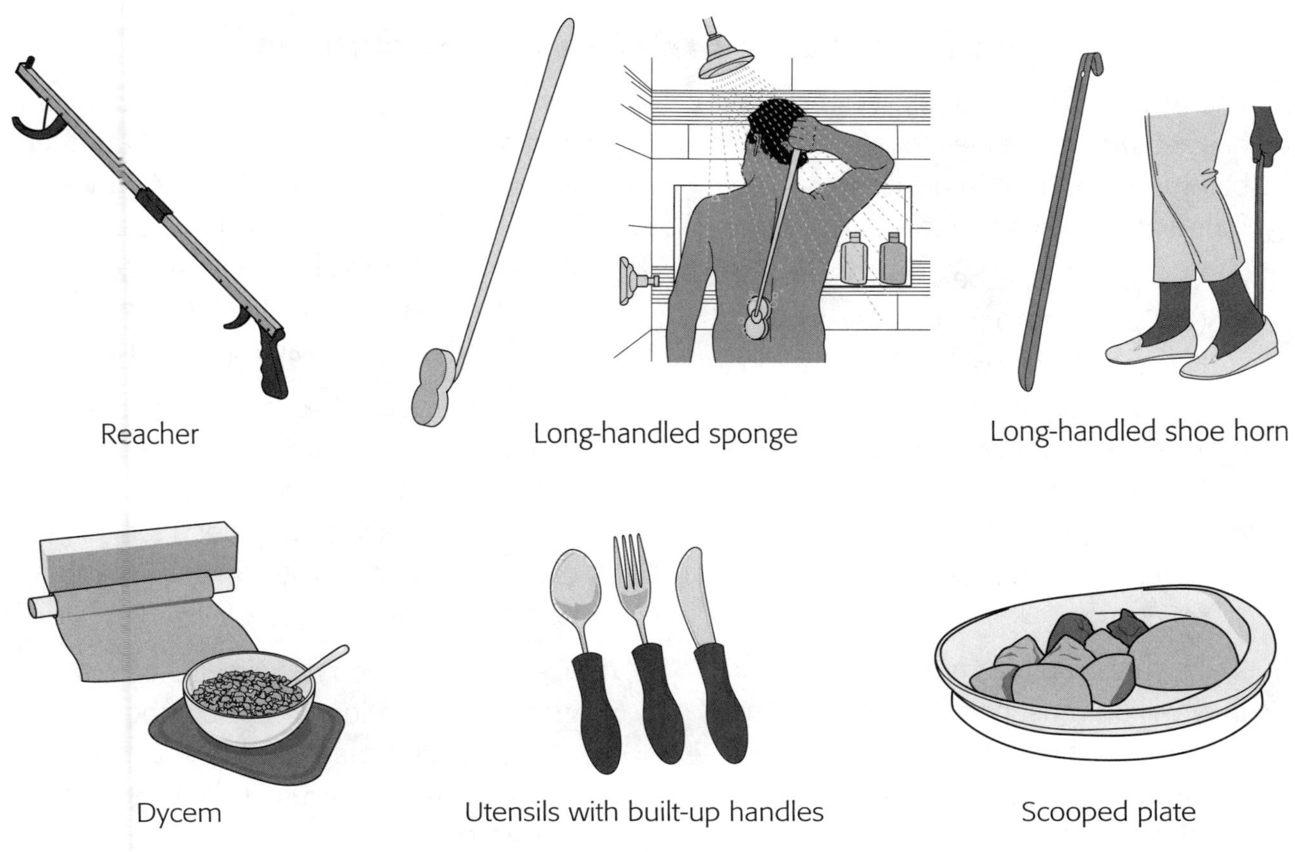

Figure 8.5 **Tools to Make Tasks Easier**

thus to reduce caregiver effort. Equipment specifically made for people with impairments is called adaptive equipment, but sometimes you can also find commercially available items that can make tasks easier. Sometimes, just a small change makes a task less frustrating and safer. If your care partner struggles to get on clothes or shoes, you can consider buying new items a size bigger and look for clothes with larger neck openings. You can also add Velcro closures to clothing or shoes, or use elastic shoelaces. If your care partner has reduced balance or mobility, have them use a long-handled shoe horn while sitting. For bathing, your care partner can use a long-handled sponge to address reduced balance, motion limitations, and motion restrictions. Installing a hand-held shower head or using a pump dispenser for shampoo or body wash can make bathing easier. For eating, use Dycem, which is a non-slippery substance you can purchase to keep plates from moving. Utensils with built-up handles or other special utensils, such as a rocker knife, can also increase your care partner's independence during eating. A scooped plate can prevent food spills. Some of these items are pictured in Figure 8.5.

To find these devices, check a local medical supply store, drug store, or online (see the Other Resources section at end of the chapter). Often the easiest way to purchase them is online. You can do an online search of the names of the devices listed in Table 8.3 and Figure 8.5 to find equipment, devices, or tools that meet your safety needs. If you are not sure whether

Tips for Installing Grab Bars in the Bathroom

1. The Americans with Disabilities Act (ADA) has set forth guidelines for an accessible bathroom. Detailed information can be found at http://www.adabathroom.com.
   a. Mount grab bars between 33–36" high (840–915 mm) for best leverage.
   b. Horizontal side-wall grab bars need to be 42" (1,065 mm) minimum length.
   c. There are currently no ADA guidelines for vertical grab bars.
   d. The guidelines on the website provide pictures of common grab bar placement.
2. Make sure grab bars are installed where they will be most helpful. Try a "dry run" without water in the shower or tub to figure out where you and your care partner need a grab bar for maintaining balance. When you are in the bathroom, notice where you and your care partner reach out for support. This usually indicates a good location for a grab bar. If you find that either of you put weight on towel bars, then replace towel bars with grab bars. If you are unsure, consult with an occupational therapist or physical therapist to receive help with the decision. Look for one that is a certified aging in place specialist (CAPS).
3. Consider a vertical bar to help you and your care partner safely enter the tub or shower. If there is a big difference between your heights, consider a longer bar so that both of you can grab at your natural heights.
4. Hire someone who has experience with grab bar installation. Make sure the installer uses anchors or attaches the grab bar to studs so that it is secure. Following the installation, pull the grab bar with all your strength to test its holding power. Have someone stand by in case the bar comes loose.

the device is the right choice or you know that you will only need it temporarily, you might be able to borrow a used item. Look for a lending closet, senior center, or community organization in your area that rents or loans out equipment.

Adapting Your Home and Surroundings

You may not have noticed the injury hazards in your home and surroundings. There are many small changes that can make your home safer and help you worry less. Increased awareness can help you manage risks outside your home, such as uneven surfaces, damaged sidewalks, or streets without curb cuts. In this section, we introduce various ways you can make your surroundings safer. Most of them are general tips that can help both you and your care partner. Walk around your house and see how these tips apply.

Rearranging the Layout and Setup of Your Home

You can make your home safer by reducing hazards and rearranging furniture and daily items.

Your goal is to make sure you establish a clear pathway to areas where you and/or your caregiver frequently walk to, such as the bathroom, bedroom, and kitchen. Rearrange furniture and remove clutter. Clearing a straight path minimizes the need to navigate hazards or step over obstacles. A wide path way means you and your care partner don't need to twist to go through a narrow space. Twisting can increase fall risks. Take the following steps to clear the high-traffic areas in your home:

- **Remove or organize cables or cords.** Cables on the floor are major tripping hazards. Use cable or cord covers to hide cords.
- **Remove or secure throw rugs.** Throw rugs tend to slip, slide, or bunch up and are easy to trip over. The best option is to not use them, but if you want to keep one, secure it with nonslip under-padding or rug anchors.
- **Rearrange the layout of furniture.** While you clear clutter to establish a clear pathway, you can also strategically place furniture so it can be used as support. For example, place a sturdy cabinet at waist height on the path to the bathroom so there is something to grab when losing balance. Make sure low coffee tables are not near or in pathways. These are tripping hazards. Place sturdy chairs throughout the house. A chair in the bedroom can be used for dressing and one in kitchen can be used to rest while waiting for the water to boil.
- To prevent repetitive movement in an awkward position, **re-organize items in your cabinets** Put the most frequently used items in the front of the cabinet and store them between shoulder and hip height. This prevents bending over or reaching every time you use the items.
- **Keep frequently used items in each room or on each floor** if you live in a multi-story house. Keep canes, phones, reading glasses, or other important things in areas you often use it. Rushing to answer an inconveniently placed phone often results in a fall. Placing a phone in every room or keeping a cell phone nearby will prevent you and/or your care partner from hurrying to answer it. At the same time, you will have a phone close at hand in emergencies. Check each day that cell phones are charged and landline phones are on their chargers.

Changing the Lighting in Your Home

- **Improve lighting.** You need to see where you are walking. If your home is dimly lit, it is more likely that you or your care partner might trip over something. Check the lighting in all areas in your home and change the bulbs to brighter ones or add more lighting as needed. Do the same for entrances to your home.
- **Install nightlights.** Light is particularly important at night. People often fall when they go to the bathroom. Install nightlights or motion-sensitive lights throughout your home, particularly around the path to the bathroom. You may want to purchase lights that are light sensitive and will turn on when it is dark. These types of light don't require that you turn them off and on; you do not even have to think about them.

Choosing Furniture to Help Reduce Strain

The type of furniture in your home can increase or reduce the amount of assistance your care partner needs. Choose chairs and beds carefully. These pieces of furniture are especially important because if you help your partner with transfers, you will transfer them from chairs and beds frequently.

- **Choose sturdy, firm chairs with arms.** Unstable chairs are likely to cause falls. It is far more difficult to bring up your care partner from a recliner or sofa than from a kitchen chair with arm support.

- **Use beds and chairs at the right height.** Chairs or beds that are too low can be difficult to exit without help. At the same time, chairs that are too high with limited support, such as stools, are not safe. While a high bed might make it easier to stand up, you may consider purchasing a bed that is height adjustable. If your care partner is suddenly having difficulty getting out of a bed or a chair, consider getting a consult from a rehabilitation professional, such as an occupational therapist or physical therapist.

Providing Environmental Cues for Your Care Partner

You can use the environment to create reminders for yourself and your care partner that can help keep both of you safe. These cues are particularly helpful if your care partner has visual or cognitive impairments. However, a cue can help anyone in the household especially in a busy environment where it is easy to lose track of things or become careless.

- **Apply brightly colored, non-slip tape on stairs** to prevent tripping or sliding. Stairs are common fall hazards. You and your care partner can trip over steps or slip because of weakness, balance issues, visual impairment, or carelessness. If you wear slippers at home, the risk of falling increases when walking on surfaces and stairs that are slippery (such as wooden floors and staircases). To prevent tripping, slipping, or missing steps, mark the edge of each step (or the last step only) with non-slip, brightly colored tape (for example,

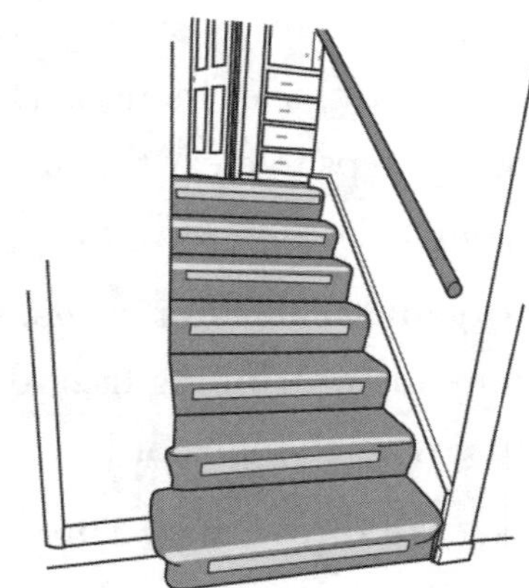

colored duct tape). There are also glow-in-the-dark tapes that are useful in darker areas such as stairs to the basement.

- **Use high contrasting colors** to make it easy to locate items or spaces. If your care partner has dementia, it helps to clearly mark frequently used areas. Often, injuries occur at night as care partners wander around to find the bathroom. Paint the doors of the bathroom or bedroom with a bright color. Post signs on the doors. Or use glow-in-the-dark tape to mark the path from the bed to the bathrooms. High-contrast colors also help when locating items. In a white bathroom, install or use special equipment or bathing items that do not blend in. For example, in the illustration below, the bathtub bench is dark so it stands out in the all-white bathroom environment. Wise use of contrasting

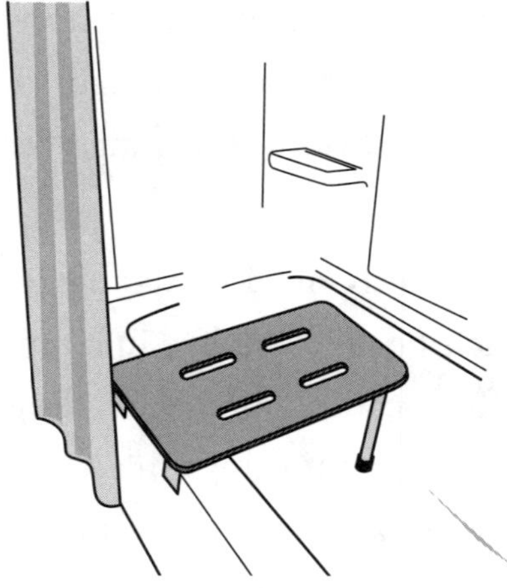

What Can You Do to Prevent Falls?

Below are specific ways you can reduce fall risk. These strategies are supported by research. You can also address the fall risk of your care partner. If your care partner is safer, you will be too.

- Exercise to improve leg strength and balance.
- Ask your doctor or pharmacist to review your medications.
- Ask to have your balance and hearing checked if you are feeling dizzy.
- Check your vision and wear eyeglasses with your current prescription.
- Wear sturdy footwear with a back—do not wear flip flops or slippers.
- Make your home safer.
  - Install and maintain good lighting.
  - Remove trip hazards and clutter.
  - Install strong railings on all stairs.
  - Install and maintain safety equipment and grab bars in the bathroom.

colors can improve your care partner's independence.

- **Post signs to prevent dangerous situations.** Care partners with cognitive or visual impairments are also at risk of injuring themselves by eating spoiled food or inedible materials. Lock and put up "stop" or "no" signs on cabinets where you store cleaning materials to ease your mind about dangerous situations. Explore available safety aids designed to protect young children and see what might work for you.

Advocating for Accessibility in Your Neighborhood or Community

As we mentioned before, fall and injury hazards are not just problems at home. Curbs or uneven pavements are common dangerous fall hazards. Being mindful about your surroundings can help you to avoid dangerous situations when you are out in the community. However, in the long run, you want to make changes so those barriers do not get in your and your care partner's way every time you get out in your neighborhood. Under the Americans with Disabilities

What Can You Do to Reduce Body Pain and Injury?

- Exercise regularly.
- Make good posture and good body mechanics a habit in your everyday life.
- Ask healthcare professionals for training and feedback on safe position changes and ways to modify activities to protect yourself and your care partner from body pain and injury.
- Use mindful movement practices to reduce rushing, worrying and inattention.

Act, you and your care partner have the right to request evenly paved sidewalks and curb cuts at inaccessible sidewalks. You can contact your city hall or alderman's office to request changes in your neighborhood. If you live in a large city, there might be a phone number to call to issue complaints about inaccessible areas. Sometimes it takes a long time to get these fixed. Be assertive and regularly check on the progress so the job gets done to your advantage. In addition to working with your local government, you can work with your neighbors to help make the neighborhood more accessible for all. For example, if you have a neighbor with foliage that extends onto the walk, kindly ask them to cut it. They are probably unaware of the problem and will be happy to help.

Seeking Guidance from Health Professionals

Self-management is always a good strategy, but you do not have to do everything alone. Both your doctor and your care partner's doctor should have access to a range of health professionals to support safety and well-being. It is best if you approach a doctor with a specific problem and some possible solutions. For example, if your partner falls, you might say, "Sam keeps falling and I think he needs a walking aid. Can you refer us to someone who can give us advice on this?" Request a medication review to make sure none of the prescribed medications increase fall risk. This can be done by your physician or a clinical pharmacist. Many retail pharmacists can also review your or your care partner's medications for fall risk. If there are equipment needs, find out if the equipment is covered by your insurance and if it can be ordered by your doctor's office. Sometimes a nurse or care coordinator can assist you. If not, call the number on the back of your insurance card.

If you or your care partner needs rehabilitation services such as occupational therapy, physical therapy, or speech therapy, ask the doctor's office or insurance company if a referral is needed. All therapy services begin with an evaluation. The following are some services you can expect from various therapists:

- Speech therapy focuses on enhancing communication and understanding and safe eating. Common services offered by speech and language pathologists include: sustaining attention, enhancing problem solving and understanding, speech training, and swallowing assessment and safe eating practices (to reduce choking risk).
- Physical therapy focuses on restoring normal and safe movement. Common services offered by physical therapists include: instruction in exercise and proper gait; home exercise programming to increase flexibility, strength, balance, and endurance post-fall or post-injury; transfer training for you and your care partner; selection of mobility aids and training in their proper use; and manual therapy procedures for pain management.
- Occupational therapy focuses on helping people to regain independence and active participation in everyday activities. Common services offered by an occupational therapist include: home safety assessment, transfer training, self-care training with an emphasis on proper body mechanics, problem solving related to reduction of safety

risks, modifying home and surroundings, modifying tasks to make them safer, and guidance with selecting and using special equipment.

Therapists can provide visits in a hospital, clinic, skilled nursing home, or home setting.

One last note: The Veterans Administration has caregiving coordinators in most facilities. Some insurance plans also offer care coordinators. Find out if you are eligible for these services and make sure to talk to these people as you may be entitled to many services.

Putting It All Together: Utilizing Your Tools to Avoid Risks

In this chapter, we identified risks that contribute to unintentional accidents and injury and we described tools to reduce injury risks. These tools can make your caregiving experience easier and more positive. In this chapter, we discussed the tools individually, but you can put them together to reduce your risk of falls and body pain.

Suggested Further Reading

Curtis, Jason. *Fix your posture: Over 70 Effective Exercises to Fix Posture and Stop Back Pain*. S.l.: Fundamental Changes, 2017. A simple guide to posture-correcting exercises and techniques. http://amzn.to/2ERFf6g

Reynolds, Roxanne. *A Senior's Guide to Fall Prevention and Healthy Living*. Bloomington, IN: Balboa Press, 2011. An outline of causes of falls, diseases affiliated with falls, home safety, foot health, diet, nutrition, and activities that promote balanced movement. http://amzn.to/2EDgHyr

Scott, Vicky. *Fall Prevention Programming: Designing, Implementing, and Evaluating Fall Prevention Programs for Older Adults*. S.l.: Vicky Scott, 2012. A unique approach to fall prevention for health care professionals and community support providers who work with older persons in community, residential, and acute care settings. http://amzn.to/2sDVAX9

Smith, William, and Jo Brielyn. *Exercises for Better Balance: The Stand Strong Workout for Fall Prevention and Longevity*. S.l.: Hatherleigh Press, 2015. Instruction on how to build balance through resistance exercises, flexibility, and cardiovascular activities. http://amzn.to/2FfdphM

Teater, Martha, and John W. Ludgate. *Overcoming Compassion Fatigue: A Practical Resilience Workbook*. Eau Claire, WI: Pesi Publishing & Media, 2014.

A workbook approach for compassion fatigue, providing tools for burnout and stress. http://amzn.to/2C6LjGS

Other Resources

AgingCare.com provides information on mobility and preventing falls. https://www.agingcare.com/mobility-falls

Centers for Disease Control and Prevention (CDC) gives fall prevention and educational materials for patients on their site. https://www.cdc.gov/steadi. On the CDC site, **Check for Safety** is a brochure offering aa home gall prevention checklist to see if you have any fall hazards at home. https://www.cdc.gov/steadi/pdf/check_for_safety_brochure-a.pdf

Websites for balance programs

The Evidence-Based Leadership Council provides information on evidence-based health. http://www.eblcprograms.org

A Matter of Balance addresses fear of falling and emphasizes practical coping strategies to reduce fear of falling in an eight-session program. https://mainehealth.org/healthy-communities/healthy-aging/matter-of-balance

The Otago Exercise Program is an individualized program often taught by a physical therapist that consists of 17 leg muscle strengthening and balance exercises to prevent falls. Walking and flexibility exercises are part of the program. http://www.med.unc.edu/aging/cgec/exercise-program

Stepping On is a seven-week program for adults who do not use a mobility aid. https://www.ncoa.org/resources/program-summary-stepping-on

Stay Active and Independent for Life (SAIL) is a strength, balance, and group fitness program taught three times per week on an ongoing basis. http://www.wellnessplacewenatchee.org/sail-home

Tai Chi for Arthritis is a 16-session program held once or twice weekly for people with arthritis or pain to reduce fall risk. http://taichiforhealthinstitute.org/programs/tai-chi-for-arthritis

Tai Ji Quan: Moving for Better Balance is a 24-week program held twice weekly. A DVD is available for home practice. https://tjqmbb.org

Websites for managing caregiver emotion supports and safety

The Family Caregiver Alliance website gives you caregiving tips and strategies including condition specific information. https://www.caregiver.org

The VA Caregiver Support website provides caregiver support toolbox to help manage emotion and physical burden. https://www.caregiver.va.gov

Websites for home safety tips:

The National Association of Area Agencies on Aging and the Administration on Aging provide checklists to make your home safer. Contact the Elder Locator and Rebuilding Together affiliate to find local community resources including assistance for low-income adults to modify their living space. https://www.n4a.org/files/PreventingFalls.pdf

The National Council on Aging offers this website to check eligibility for benefits including deductible home modifications to support environment modification. https://www.economiccheckup.org

The Partnership for Healthy Aging created by MaineHealth offers a guidebook for caregivers. This guidebook includes a home environment evaluation tool (page 31). https://mainehealth.org/healthcare-professionals/clinical-resources-guidelines-protocols/elder-care-services/partnership-for-healthy-aging

Websites on daily living equipment and medical alert systems:

Medical alert

American Association of Retired Persons (AARP) offers specific tips for choosing the right medical alert system. Search for "Medical Alert" using the search box in the upper right-hand corner on the home page. https://www.aarp.org/caregiving/home-care/info-2017/medic-alert-systems-options.html

Adaptive equipment

You can find many medical supplies and adaptive equipment at local medical supply stores. Here are two online sources of supplies and special equipment:

https://www.amazon.com A number of products from a range of companies are available when you type "adaptive equipment" in the search box. You can be more specific in your search to locate specific items such as "adaptive equipment seniors."

http://www.adaptivespecialties.com This website offers a variety of adaptive devices and tools to assist caregiving activities.

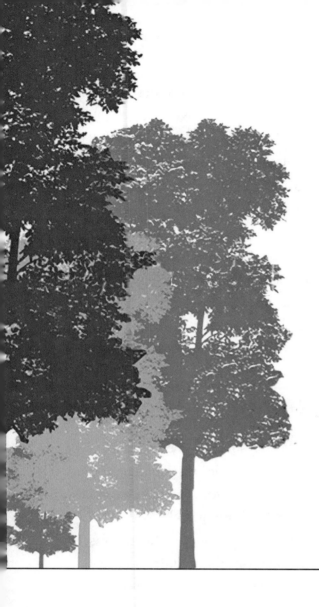

Chapter 9

Exercising for Health and Wellness

You probably already know that regular exercise is important for both you and your care partner, but if your life includes caring for another person or you have a chronic health problem, you might feel that you are already too busy or to tired to add anything else to your day. You may want to exercise but don't want to do anything that could cause injury. You might wonder what you could possibly do to make a difference in your health and wellness. You might be worried about your current health and capacity, your limited skills, or natural ability. These are common thoughts, but you (and often your care partner) can learn and do many activities that can make you feel better, increase your energy, and reduce your risk of injuries as you care for another person. The information in this chapter will help you get started and be successful.

When you are physically active and exercise, you improve your strength, flexibility, and endurance. You also reduce your risk of injuries from strained muscles, overstressed joints, fatigue, and poor balance. Regular exercise improves self-confidence and lessens feelings of stress, anxiety, and depression. In addition, regular exercise can help you sleep better and feel more relaxed and happy. Exercise can help you maintain a good weight, which takes stress off your back and legs. Exercise is also part of keeping bones strong. Published research, medical recommendations, and public health guidelines from many countries point to the effectiveness and importance of regular physical activity to maintain health and improve fitness.

The good news is that it doesn't take hours of painful, sweat-soaked exercise to achieve health benefits. Even short periods of moderate physical activity can improve health and fitness, reduce disease and injury risks, and boost your mood. Being active also helps you feel more in control of your life and capable of carrying out your daily tasks. If you can exercise with your care partner, both of you can achieve physical, emotional, and relationship benefits!

What Exercise Can Do for You

In the same way that different types of food (such as vitamins, protein, fats, and fiber) provide different benefits for your body, different kinds of exercises have different positive effects. Exercise can provide specific and important benefits to improve and maintain health and reduce risk of injury. In this chapter, we outline four types of exercise: those make you more flexible, those that boost strength, those that improve your endurance, and those that improve your balance.

- **Flexibility.** Being flexible helps you move comfortably and safely. Limited flexibility can cause pain, lead to injury, and make muscles work harder and tire more quickly. You lose flexibility when you are inactive or your daily movement is limited. Certain illnesses and diseases can also result in a loss of flexibility. However, you can improve flexibility by doing gentle stretching exercises such as the ones described in this chapter.
- **Strength.** Muscles need to be exercised to be strong. Inactive muscles weaken and atrophy (shrink). When your muscles get weak, you feel weak and tire quickly. Much disability and lack of mobility is due to muscle weakness. Exercises that require muscles to do more work (such as lifting a weight) strengthens muscles.
- **Endurance (aerobics).** Endurance depends on the fitness of your heart, lungs, and muscles. The heart and lungs must work efficiently to send enough oxygen-rich blood to the muscles. The muscles must be fit enough to use the oxygen. Aerobic ("with oxygen") exercise is exercise that uses the large muscles of your body in continuous activity, such as walking, swimming, dancing, mowing the lawn, or riding a bike. Numerous studies have proven that aerobic exercise promotes a sense of well-being, eases depression and anxiety, promotes restful sleep, and improves mood and energy levels.

- **Balance.** Strong and coordinated muscles in your trunk and legs are a key part of good balance. Flexibility, strength, and endurance also contribute to balance. Of course, there are many causes of falls (poor vision, poor lighting, obstacles such as rugs on the floor, dizziness, or being tired or distracted), but being strong and coordinated are very important and can help prevent falls from these other causes. Certain exercises described in this chapter are especially good for improving balance.

The descriptions and illustrations in this chapter include all these kinds of exercise. You can select what you want to do depending on what you want to accomplish. The exercises illustrated in the following sections are arranged in groups of flexibility, strength, and balance. Suggestions and examples of endurance exercise are described later in this chapter. In Chapter 8, Preventing Injuries, there are more details of how exercise can help you protect yourself and your care partner from getting hurt. In that chapter, you will also find Table 8.1, Exercises to Reduce Injury Risk, which references the exercises in this chapter.

Flexibility Exercises

1. The Whole-Body Stretcher

This exercise is a whole-body stretch to be done lying on your back. You can do it in bed first thing in the morning and last thing at night. Start the motion at your ankles as explained here (or you can reverse the process if you want to start with your arms first).

- Point your toes, and then pull your toes toward your nose. Relax.
- Bend your knees. Then, straighten your knees and let them relax.
- Arch your back. Do the pelvic tilt (Exercise 6 on page 149). Relax.
- Breathe in and stretch your arms above your head. Make gentle fists and then straighten your fingers and spread them apart. Breathe out and lower your arms. Relax.
- Stretch your right arm above your head, and at the same time stretch your left leg by pushing down with your heel. Hold for a count of 10. Switch to the other side and repeat.

Neck and Back Exercises

2. Heads Up

This exercise relieves jaw, neck, and upper back tension or pain. It also helps promote good posture. You can do it while driving, sitting at a desk, sewing, reading, or exercising. Just sit or stand straight and gently slide your chin back. Keep looking forward as your chin moves backward. You'll feel the back of your neck lengthen and straighten. To help, put your finger on your nose and then draw your nose straight back from your finger. (Don't worry about a little double chin—you really look much better with your neck straight!)

The following are clues for finding the correct position when doing the Heads Up exercise:

- Ears over shoulders, not out in front
- Head balanced over neck and trunk, not in the lead
- Neck vertical, not leaning forward
- Bit of double chin

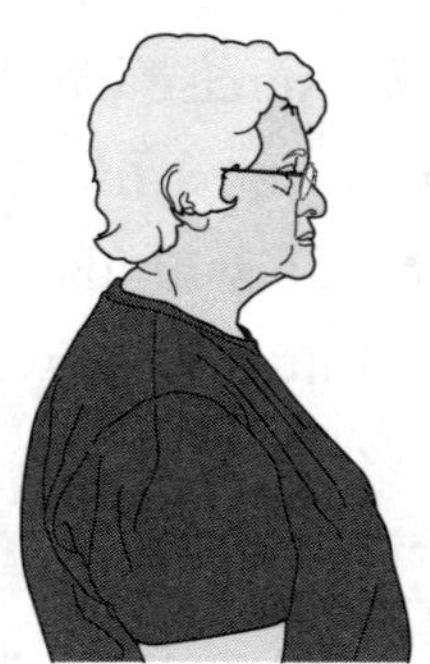

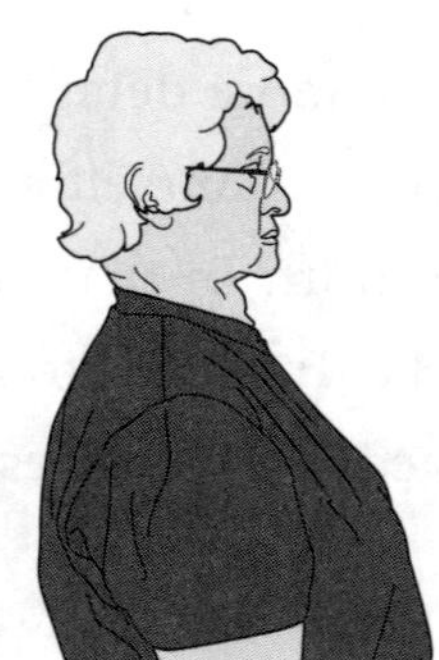

3. Neck Stretch

In heads-up position (Flexibility Exercise 2) with your shoulders relaxed, turn slowly to look over your right shoulder. Then, turn slowly to look over your left shoulder. Next, tilt your head to the right and then to the left. Move your left ear toward your left shoulder and your right ear toward your right shoulder. Do not lift your shoulder up to your ear.

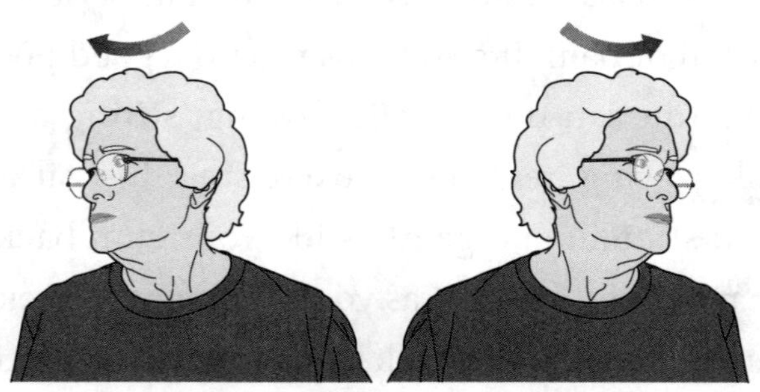

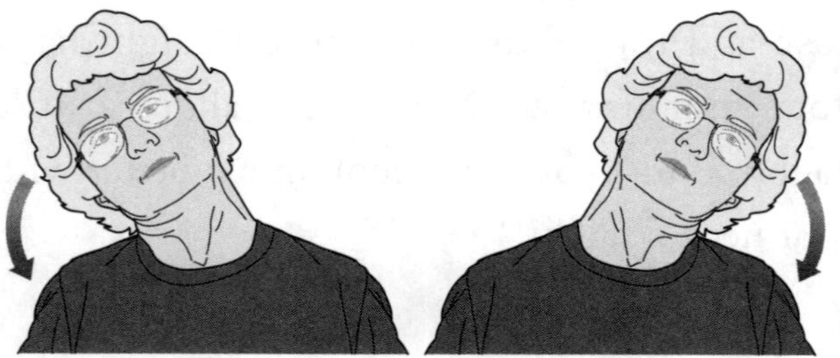

4. Cat and Cow Pose in Seated Position

This two-part exercise stretches and improves flexibility in the entire spine and opens the chest. It is a yoga exercise that can reduce tension and calm the mind. At first, keep your movements small so that you do not strain your lower back. If you have neck problems, make sure to keep your neck in line with your body, not letting your neck go too far back or too far forward.

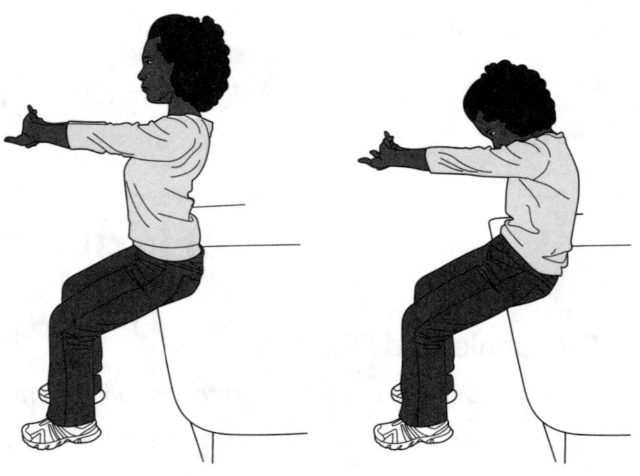

Sit in a straight-backed chair so that your back is not against the back of the chair. Sit with your head over your shoulders and shoulders over your hips. Place your feet flat on the floor with your knees over your heels and your hands rested gently on your thighs.

Imagine a string attached to the top of your head lifting your body to its full length. Start the "cat" by exhaling slowly as you bring your belly toward your spine and your back toward the back of the chair. Allow your back and shoulders to round and your head to come forward. Then, move into the "cow" by inhaling and bringing the chest forward and up as you let the shoulders come up and back. As you do this, your head raises and gently looks up as far as is comfortable. This puts the back in a gentle back bend. Repeat the cat and cow several times at your own pace.

5. Knee-to-Chest Stretch

For a low back stretch, lie on the floor with knees bent and feet flat. Bring one knee toward your chest, using your hands to help. Hold your knee near your chest for 10 seconds, and then lower the leg slowly. Repeat with the other knee. You can also bring both legs to your chest at the same time if you wish. Relax and enjoy the stretch.

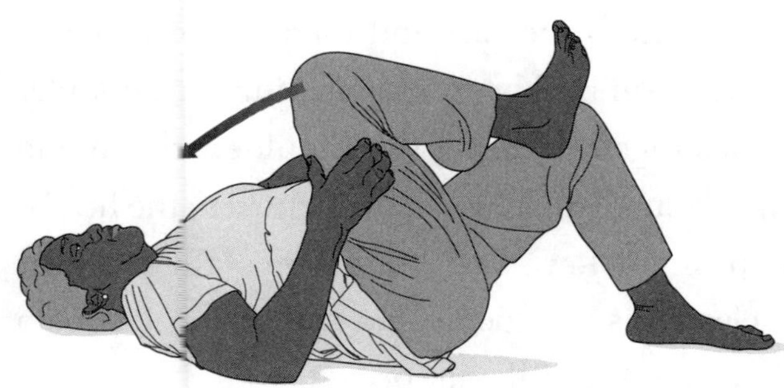

6. Pelvic Tilt

This is an excellent exercise for the low back and can help relieve low back pain. Lie on your back with knees bent, feet flat on the floor. Place your hands on your abdomen. Flatten the small of your back against the floor by tightening your stomach muscles and your buttocks. When you do this exercise, you will be tilting your tailbone forward and pulling your stomach back. Think about trying to pull your stomach in enough to zip a tight pair of trousers. Hold the tilt for five to 10 seconds. Relax. Arch your back slightly. Relax and repeat the pelvic tilt. Keep breathing. Count the seconds out loud. Once you've mastered the pelvic tilt lying down, practice it sitting, standing, and walking.

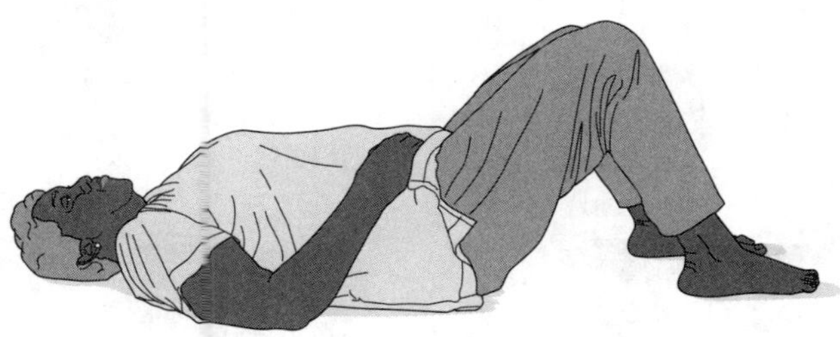

7. Back Lift

This exercise improves flexibility along your spine and helps you lift your chest for easier breathing. Lie on your stomach, and raise your upper body up onto your forearms. Keep your back relaxed, and keep your stomach and hips down. If this is comfortable, straighten your elbows so that your upper trunk is raised higher. Breathe naturally and relax for at least 10 seconds. If you have moderate to severe low back pain, do not do this exercise unless it has been specifically prescribed for you.

To strengthen back muscles, lie on your stomach with your arms at your side or extended overhead. Lift your head, shoulders, and arms off the floor. Do not look up. Keep looking down with your chin tucked into that double-chin position. Count out loud as you hold for a count of 10. Relax. You can also lift your legs, instead of your head and shoulders, off the floor.

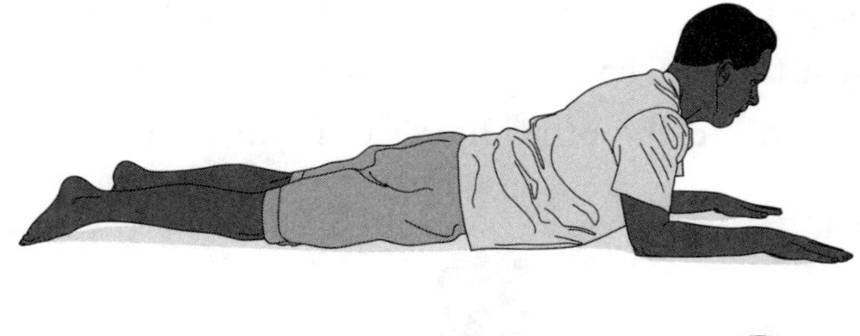

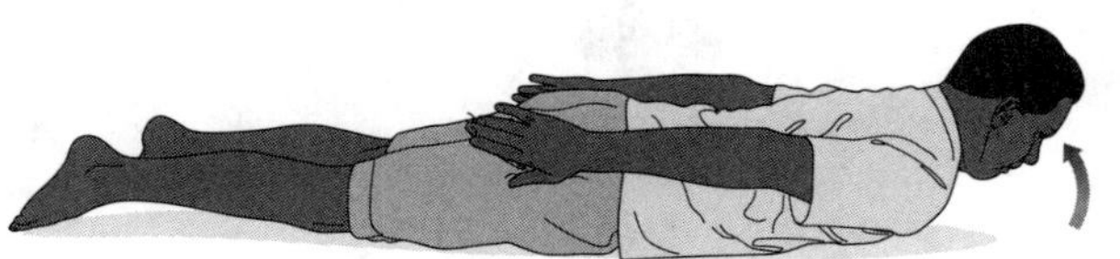

Note that lifting both ends of your body at once is a fairly strenuous exercise. It might not be helpful for a person with back pain.

8. Low-Back Rock and Roll

Lie on your back and pull your knees up to your chest. You can keep holding on to your legs with your hands on your shins or stretch your arms out to your sides to lie on the floor at shoulder level. Rest in this position for 10 seconds, and then gently roll your hips and knees to one side and then the other. Rest and relax as you roll to each side. Keep your upper back and shoulders flat on the ground.

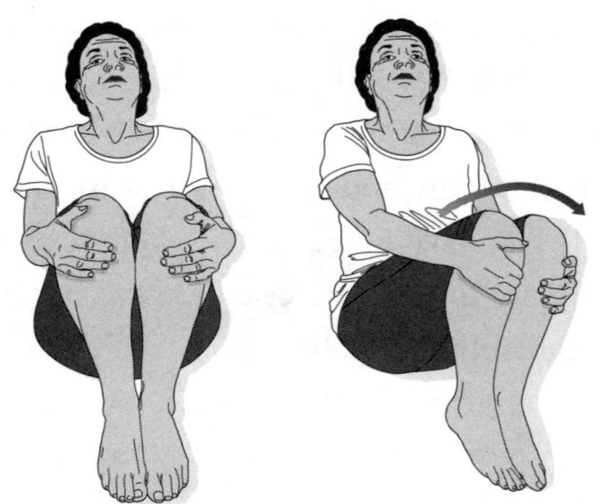

Arm and Leg Exercises

9. Pat and Reach

This double-duty exercise helps increase both flexibility and strength for shoulders. Raise one arm up over your head, and bend your elbow to pat yourself on the back. Move your other arm to your back, bend your elbow, and reach up toward the other hand. Can your fingertips touch? Relax and switch arm positions. Can you touch on that side? For most people, one position will work better than the other. Do not worry if you cannot touch. Many people cannot touch, but you will improve as you practice. If you wish, you can use a towel as if you were drying your back; this can provide you with feedback and assist in the motion.

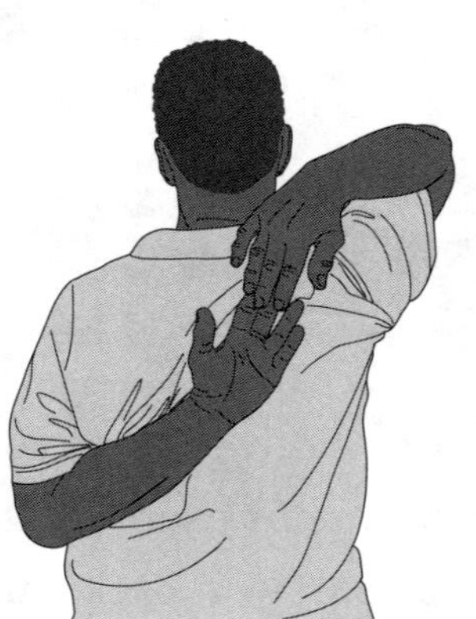

10. Shoulder Shape-Up

In heads-up position (Exercise 2), slowly raise the shoulders to the ears; hold the position and then drop your shoulders. Next, raise the shoulders again to the ears and then begin to slowly rotate them backward by pinching the shoulder blades together; bring the shoulders down and forward to complete a circle. Return to the heads-up position. Reverse the direction of the shoulder circles. This is a good exercise if the neck stretch (Exercise 3) is difficult for you.

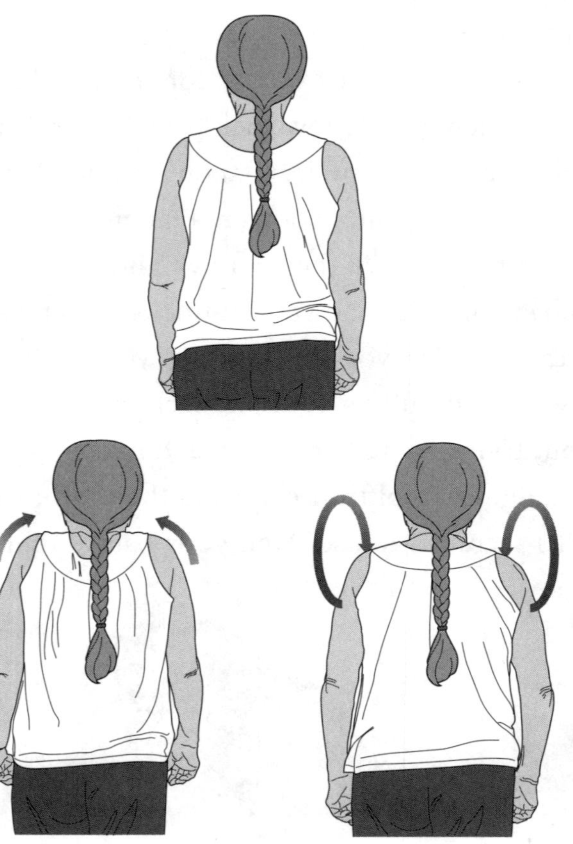

11. Good Morning

This exercise can be done seated or standing. Start with hands in gentle fists, palms down, and wrists crossed. Breathe in and stretch out your fingers while you uncross your arms and reach up for the sky. Straighten your elbows as much as you can as you reach up. Bend your elbows to touch your fingers to your shoulders and then reach up to the ceiling again. Breathe out as you stretch your arms and relax.

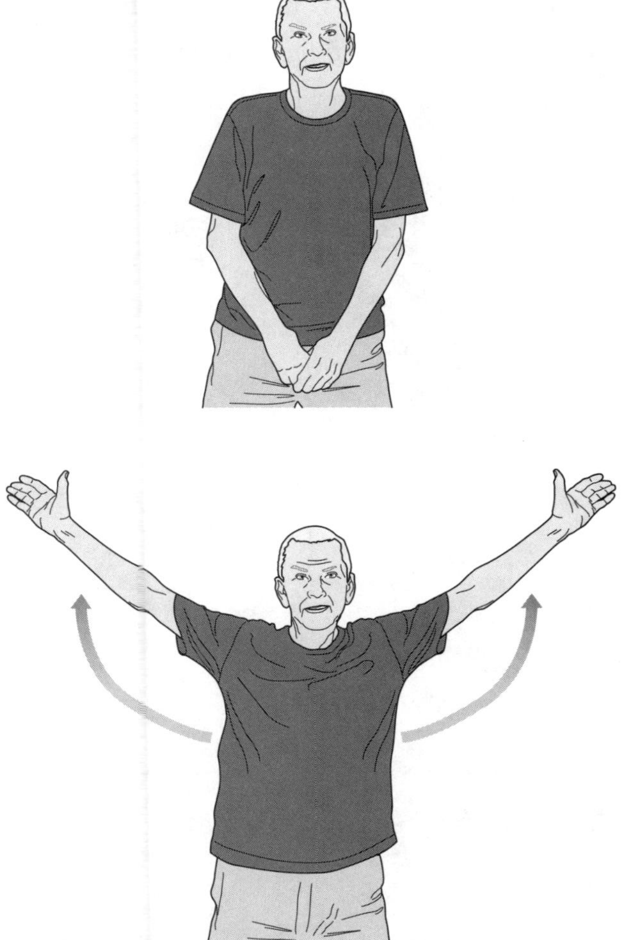

Maintaining the same position, stretch your wrists as described in the following instructions. The purpose of the wrist stretches is to fully extend the muscles that attach to the elbow on the top and the bottom of your forearm. Repetitive tasks can make these muscles stay in a tight and shortened position resulting in forearm or elbow pain. Stretching them often helps prevent this.

Wrist Stretch Down

Start with your elbow straight and palm facing down toward the floor. Make a fist with your hand and bend at the wrist to lower your knuckles down until you feel a stretch in your forearm or elbow. Hold for five seconds. Repeat several times.

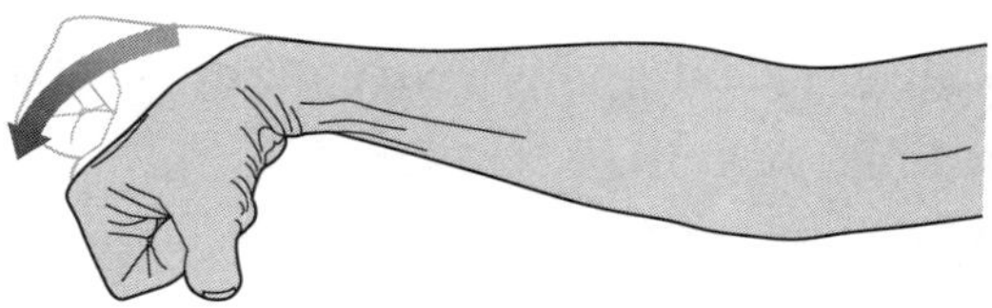

Wrist Stretch Up

Start with your elbow straight and palm facing away from you. Put your opposite hand over the away-facing palm. Gently stretch your palm toward you until you feel a stretch on the underside of your forearm near the elbow. Hold for five seconds. Repeat several times.

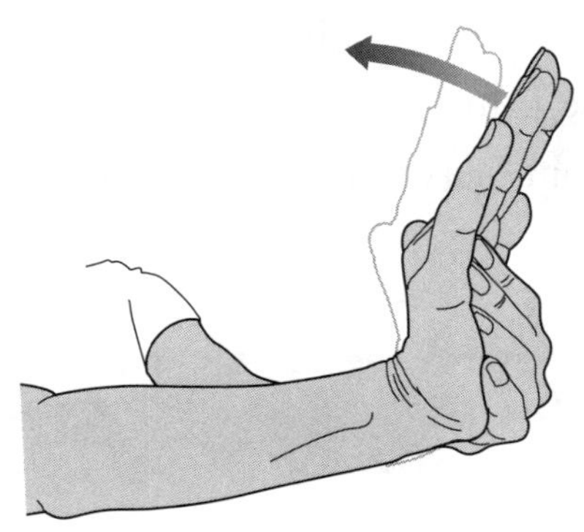

12. Hamstring Stretch

Lie on your back, knees bent, feet flat on the floor. Grasp one leg at a time behind the thigh. Holding the leg out at arm's length, slowly straighten the knee and extend the leg. Hold the

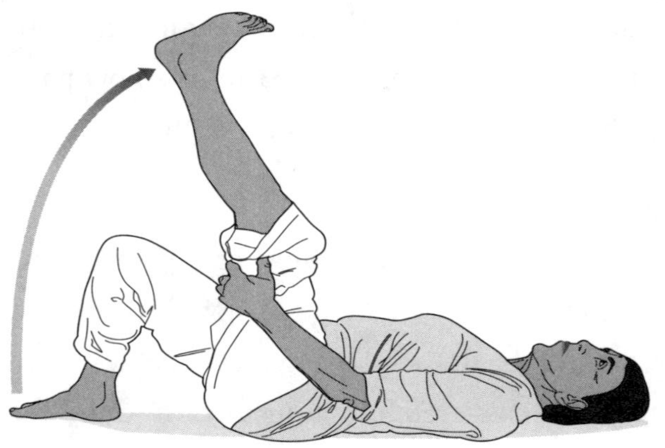

leg as straight as you can as you count to 10. You should feel a slight stretch at the back of your knee and thigh.

Be careful with this exercise. It's easy to overstretch and end up sore.

13. Achilles Stretch

Stand at a counter or against a wall. Place one foot in front of the other, toes pointing forward and heels on the ground. Lean forward, bend the knee of the forward leg, and keep the back knee straight, heel down. You will feel a good stretch in the calf. Hold the stretch for 10 seconds. Do not bounce. You can adjust this exercise to also stretch the other large calf muscle by slightly bending your back knee while you stretch.

This exercise helps maintain flexibility in the Achilles tendon, the large tendon at the back of your ankle. Good flexibility helps reduce the risk of injury, calf discomfort, and heel pain. The Achilles stretch is especially helpful for cooling down after walking or cycling and for people who get cramps in the calf muscles. If you have trouble with standing, balance or spasticity (muscle jerks), you can do a seated version of this exercise. Sit in a chair with feet flat on the floor. Keep your heel on the floor and slowly slide your foot (one foot at a time) back to bend your ankle and feel some tension on the back of your calf (lower leg).

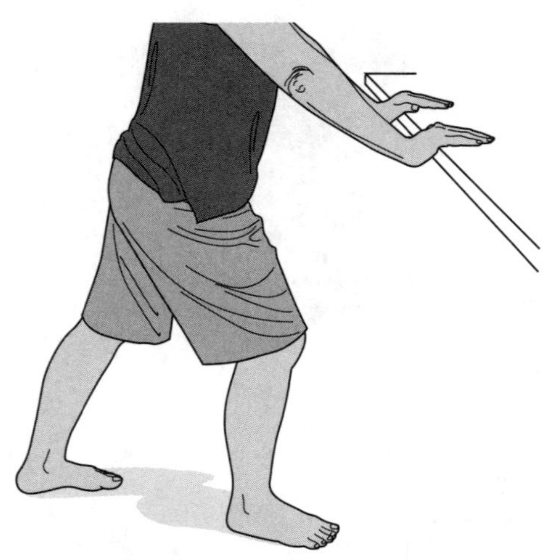

Strength Exercises

Strength for Better Posture

14. Shoulder-Blade Pinch

This is a good exercise to strengthen the middle and upper back and to stretch the chest; it can be an especially good exercise if you have breathing problems. Sit or stand with your head in heads-up position (Exercise 2) and your shoulders relaxed. Raise your arms out to the sides at shoulder height with elbows bent and forearms up. Pinch your shoulder blades together by moving your elbows as far back as you can. Hold briefly, and then slowly move your arms

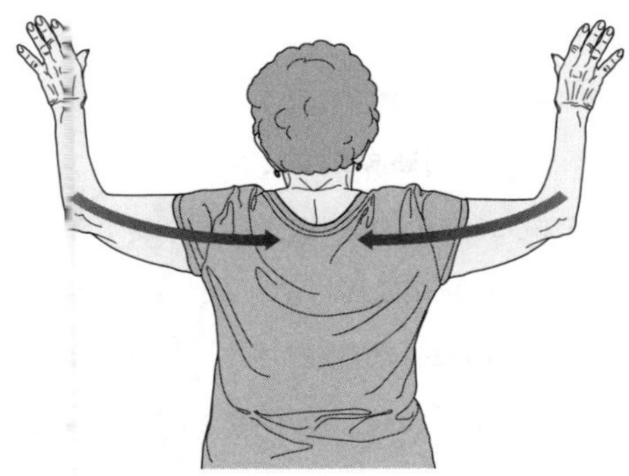

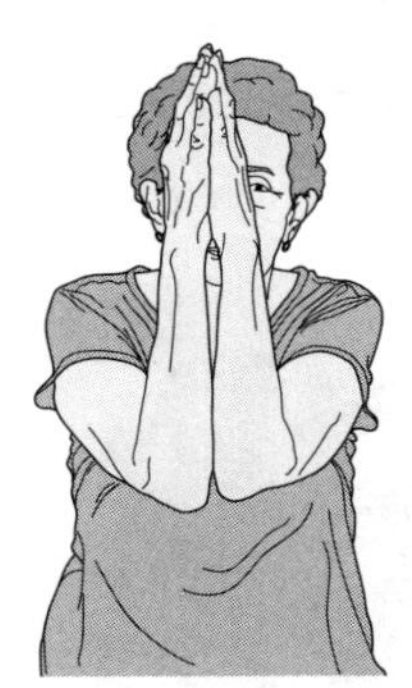

forward to touch your elbows together. If this position is uncomfortable, lower your arms or rest your hands on your shoulders.

15. Curl-Up

A curl-up is a good way to strengthen stomach muscles. Lie on your back, knees bent, feet flat. Do the pelvic tilt (Exercise 6). Slowly curl up in segments. Tuck your chin as you roll your head up and begin to lift your shoulders off the floor. Slowly uncurl back down, or hold for 10 seconds and slowly lower. Breathe out as you curl up, and breathe in as uncurl back down. Do not hold your breath. If you have neck problems or

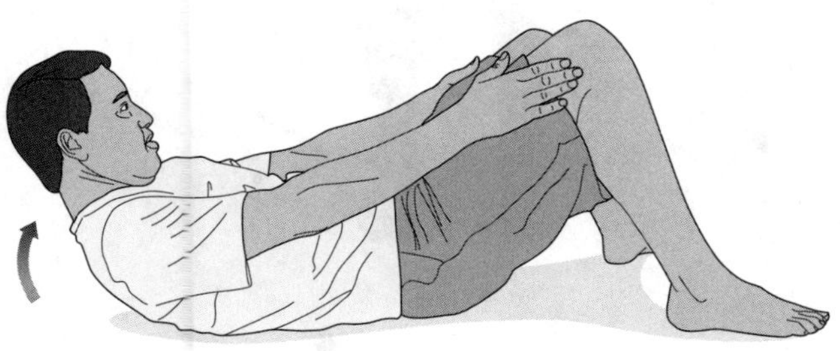

if your neck hurts when you do this exercise, try the roll-out (Exercise 16) instead. Never tuck your feet under a chair or have someone hold your feet!

16. Roll-Out

This is another good stomach strengthener, and it is easy on the neck. Use it instead of the curl-up (Exercise 15). If neck pain is not a problem, do both exercises.

Lie on your back with knees bent and feet flat. Do the pelvic tilt (Exercise 6), and hold your lower back firmly against the floor.

Slowly and carefully, move one leg away from your chest as you straighten your knee. Move your leg out until you feel your lower back start to arch. When this happens, tuck your knee back to your chest. Reset your pelvic tilt and roll your leg out again. Breathe out as your leg rolls out. Do not hold your breath. Repeat with the other leg.

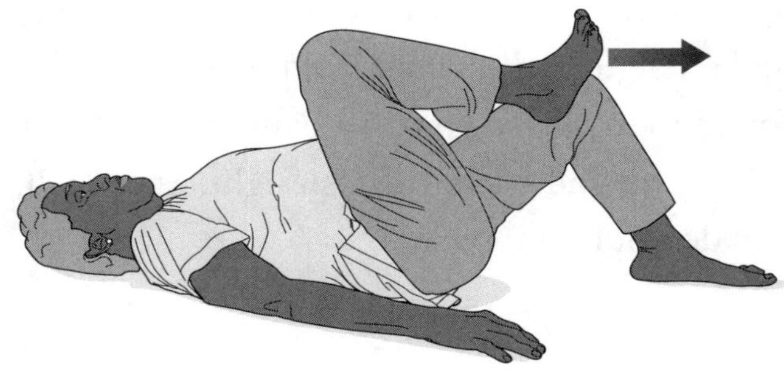

You are strengthening your abdominal muscles by holding your pelvic tilt against the weight of your leg. As you get stronger, you'll be able to straighten your legs out farther and move both legs together.

Leg Strength

17. Straight-Leg Raises

This exercise strengthens the muscles that bend the hip and straighten the knee. Lie on your back, knees bent, feet flat on the floor. Straighten one leg. Tighten the muscle on the upper surface of that thigh, and straighten the knee as much as possible. Keeping the knee straight, raise your leg a foot or two (up to 20 inches or 50 centimeters) off the ground. Do not arch your back. Hold your leg up, and count out loud for 10 seconds. Relax. Repeat with the other leg.

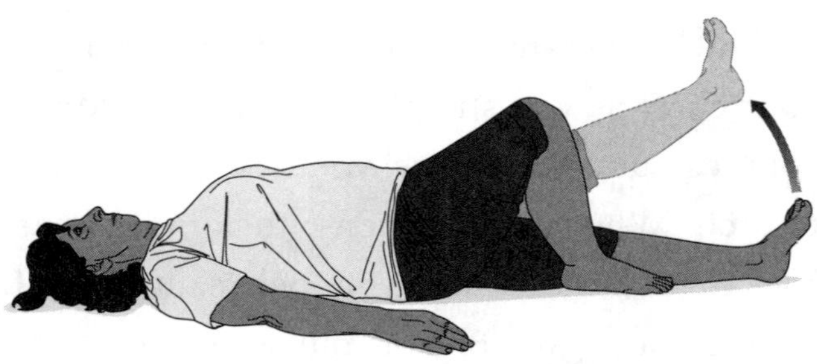

18. Back Kick

This exercise increases the backward mobility and strength of your hip. Hold on to a counter for support. Raise your leg behind you. Move the leg up and back, knee straight. Stand tall, and do not lean forward.

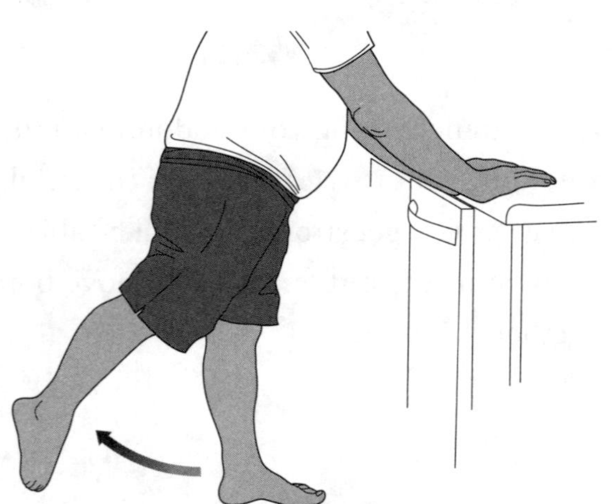

19. Hip Hooray

This exercise can be done standing or lying on your back. If you lie down, spread your legs as far apart as possible. Roll your legs and feet out like a duck, then in to be pigeon-toed. Then, move your legs back together. If you are standing, move one leg out to your side as far as you can. Lead out with the heel and in with the toes. Hold on to a counter for support. You can make the muscles work harder while you are standing by adding a weight to your ankle.

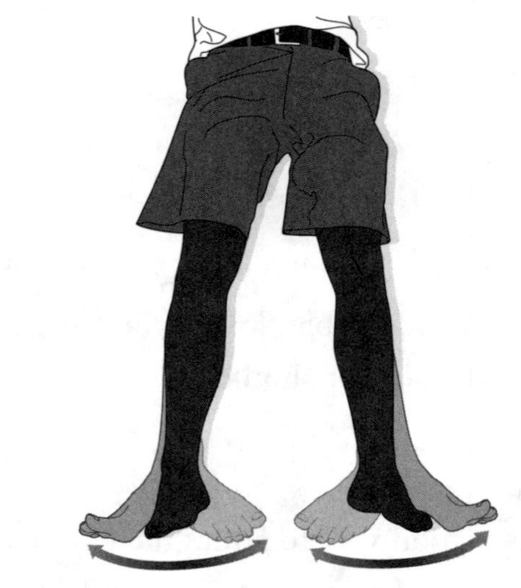

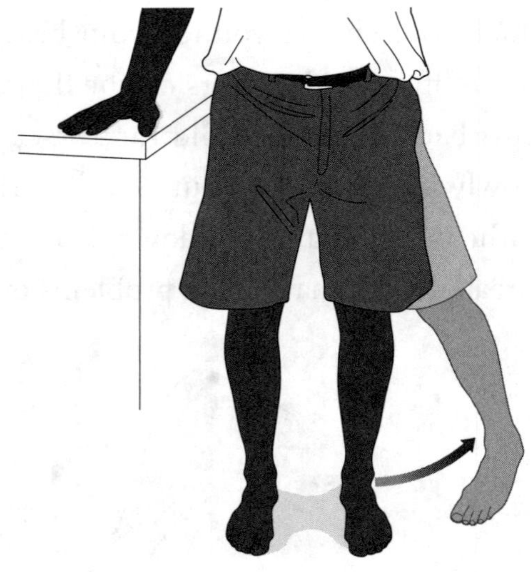

20. Knee Strengthener

Strong knees are important for walking and standing comfortably. Sitting in a chair, extend your leg and straighten your knee by tightening up the muscle on the upper surface of your thigh. Place your hand on your thigh and feel the muscle work. If you wish, make circles with your toes. As your knees strengthen, see if you can build up to holding each leg out for 30 seconds. Count out loud. Do not hold your breath.

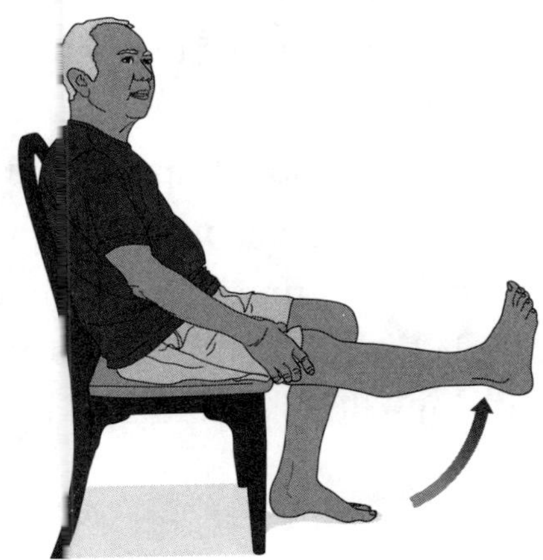

21. Power Knees

This exercise strengthens the muscles that bend and straighten your knees. Sit in a chair and cross your legs at the ankles. You can bend your knees as much as you like but keep your feet touching the floor. Try several positions to find one that works for you. Push forward with your back leg, and press backward with your front leg. Exert pressure evenly so that your legs do not move. Hold and count out loud for 10 seconds. Relax. Switch leg positions. Be sure to keep breathing. Repeat.

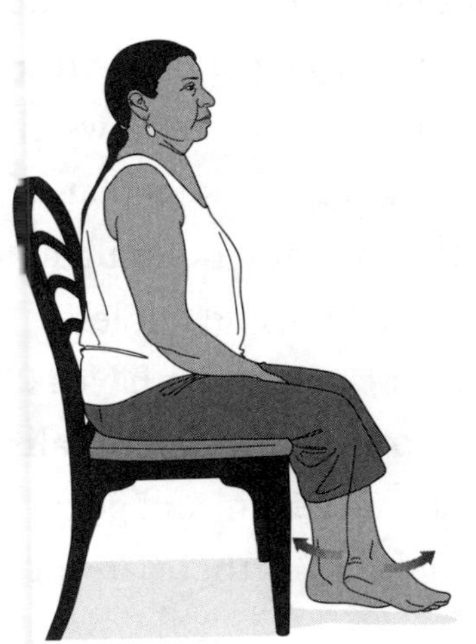

22. Ready-Go

Stand with one leg slightly in front of the other with the heel (of the front leg) on the floor, as if ready to take a step with the front foot. Now tighten the muscles on the front of the thigh on your front leg, making your front knee firm and straight. Hold to a count of 10. Relax. Switch positions and repeat with the other leg.

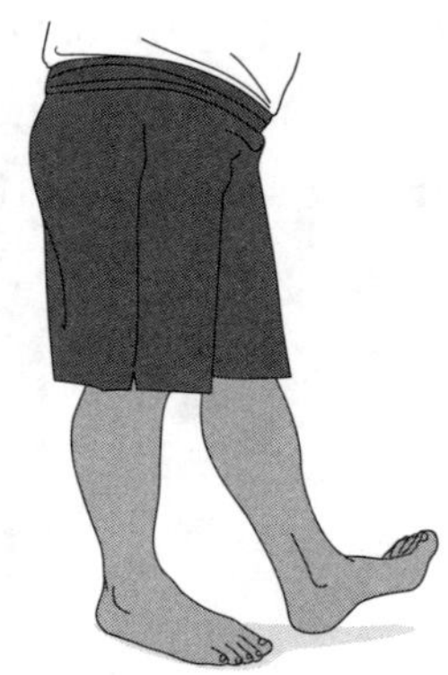

23. Tiptoes

This exercise will help strengthen your calf (lower leg) muscles and make walking, climbing stairs, and standing less tiring. It might also improve your balance. Hold on to a counter or table for support and rise up on your tiptoes. Hold for 10 seconds. Lower slowly. How high you go is not as important as keeping your balance and controlling your ankles. It is easier to do both legs at the same time. If your feet are too sore to do this standing, start doing it while sitting. If this exercise makes your ankle jerk,

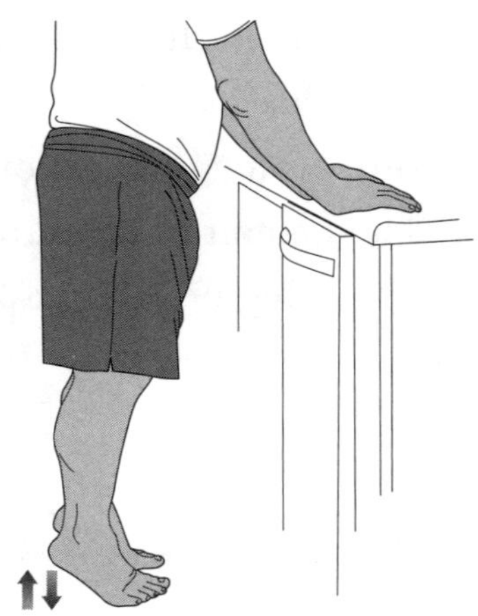

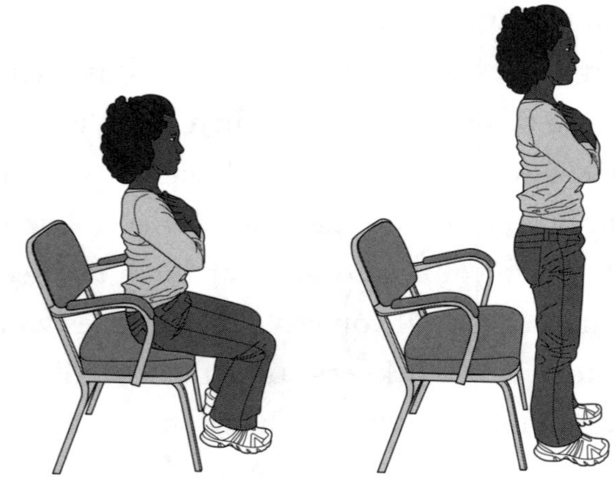

stop doing it and talk to your therapist about other ways to strengthen these calf muscles if needed.

24. Sit-to-Stand

Sit toward the front edge of a straight-backed chair with arms and a firm seat. Bend your knees so that your feet are flat on the floor and behind your knees. Lean a bit forward and stand up. Practice going from sitting to standing using your arms as little as possible. The exercise is to work on being able to stand up without using your arms. At first you may need your arms to push up. Stand up five times. Rest a bit and do five more. Little by little, as your hips and legs get stronger, you will be able to stand without using your arms.

Balance Exercises

Sometimes people decide that the best way not to fall is to spend more time sitting. At first you might think that if you and your care partner are not up walking around, you won't be at risk for falling. However, inactivity causes weakness, stiffness, slower reflexes, slower muscles, and even social isolation and depression. All of these harm balance and increase the risk of falling. Once you or your care partner are weaker, even simple things such as getting up or sitting down in a chair, going to the bathroom, or going down a step can cause problems.

Physical conditions such as weakness, dizziness, stiffness, poor eyesight, loss of feeling in feet, or inner ear problems can put you at risk for falls, as can the side effects of medications. Falls can also happen because of your personal environment: poor lighting, uneven ground, rugs, and cluttered floors. To avoid falls, reduce all these risks and keep yourself strong, flexible, and coordinated. Research shows that people who have strong legs, ankles that are flexible, and who do things that require them to balance have less fear of falling and fall less.

If you or your care partner have fallen or you are afraid that one of you might fall, talk with your health care providers and get your balance checked to make sure there are no vision or inner ear problems or medication problems that need to be fixed. Make sure your home is safe. (You can learn more about keeping your home safe for you and your care partner in Chapter 8, Preventing Injuries.) Exercising to keep yourself strong, flexible, and active also helps protect you from falling.

The exercises in this section are designed to let you or your care partner practice balance activities in a safe and progressive way. The exercises are presented in order of difficulty. Start with the first exercises and work up to the more difficult ones as your strength and balance improve. If you feel that your balance is particularly poor, exercise with someone else close by who can give you a supporting hand if needed. Always practice by a counter or stable chair that you can hold on to if necessary. Signs of improving balance are being able to hold a position longer or without extra support or being able to do the exercise or hold the position with your eyes closed.

There might be some balance exercise classes in your community to help continue your progress. Tai chi is a wonderful program to help you work on balance and strength. It is low-impact and gentle on your joints. The A Matter of Balance program is a excellent program and is offered widely. The National Institute on Aging offers an exercise video and guide, as well as a list of available exercise programs, but you can use the exercises we include here to get started. You can find links to many of these at the end of chapter 8

25. Beginning Balance

Stand quietly with your feet comfortably apart. Place your hands on your hips, and turn your head and trunk as far to the left as possible and then to the right. Repeat five to 10 times. To increase the difficulty, do the same thing with your eyes closed.

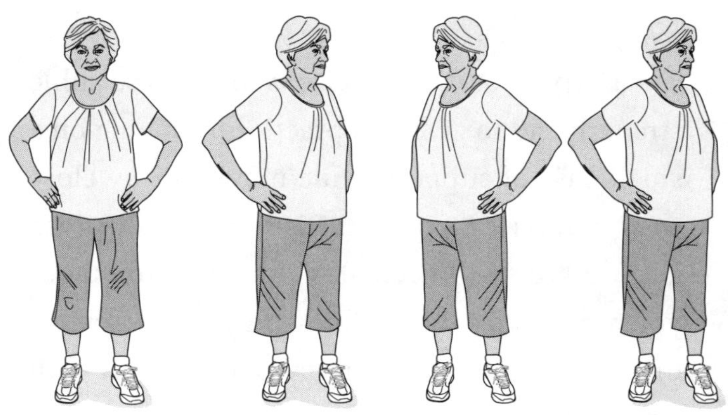

26. Swing and Sway

Using a counter or the back of a stable chair for support, do each of the following five to 10 times: Rock back on your heels and then rise up on your toes.

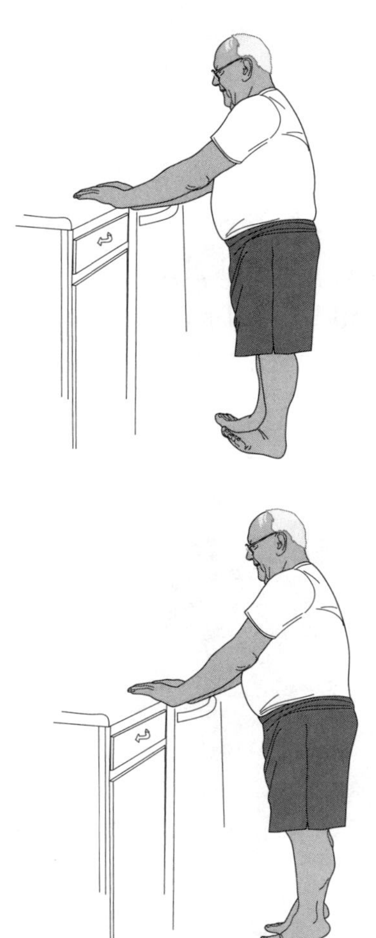

27. Toe Walk

The purpose of this exercise is to increase ankle strength and to give you practice balancing on a small base of support while moving. Stay close to a counter or support. Rise up on your toes and walk up and back along the counter. Once you are comfortable walking on your toes without support and with your eyes open, try it with your eyes closed.

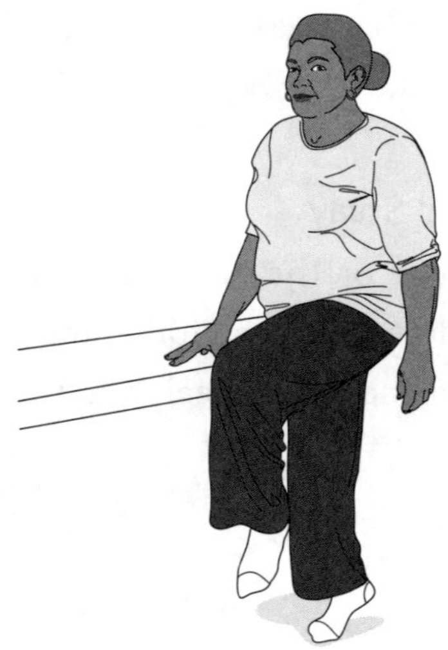

28. Heel Walk

The purpose of this exercise is to increase your lower leg strength and give you practice moving on a small base of support. Stay close to a counter for support. Raise your toes and forefoot and walk up and back along the counter on your heels. Once you are comfortable walking on your heels without support and with your eyes open, try it with your eyes closed.

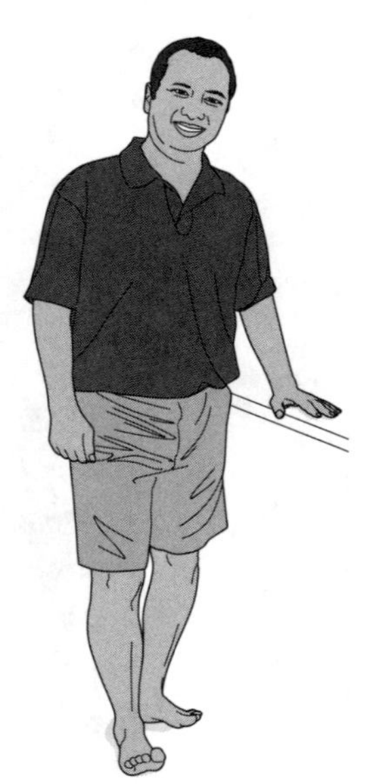

If you are not ready to walk, you can modify the heel walk with a heel stand and practice in place.

29. One-Legged Stand

Holding on to a counter or chair, lift one foot completely off the ground. Once you are balanced, lift the hand that is not holding on to the support. The goal is to hold the position for 10 seconds. Once you can do this for 10 seconds without holding on, practice it with your eyes closed. Repeat for the other leg.

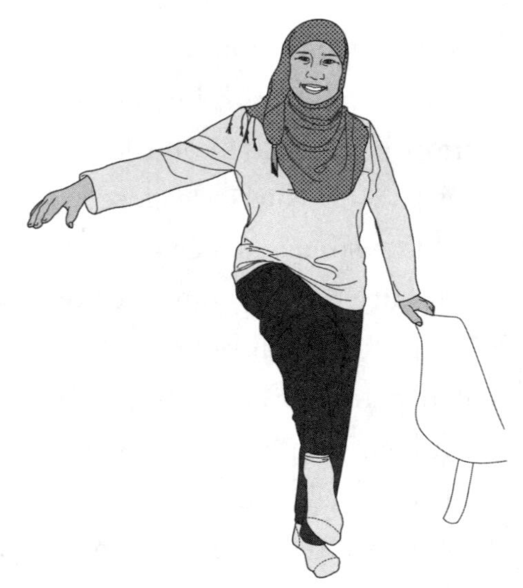

30. Walk-the-Line

Find a place to walk a few steps next to a kitchen counter or in a hallway with hand rails so you have support if you need it. Practice walking heel-to-toe (also called tandem walking). At first you will probably watch your feet, but with practice you will be able to look straight ahead.

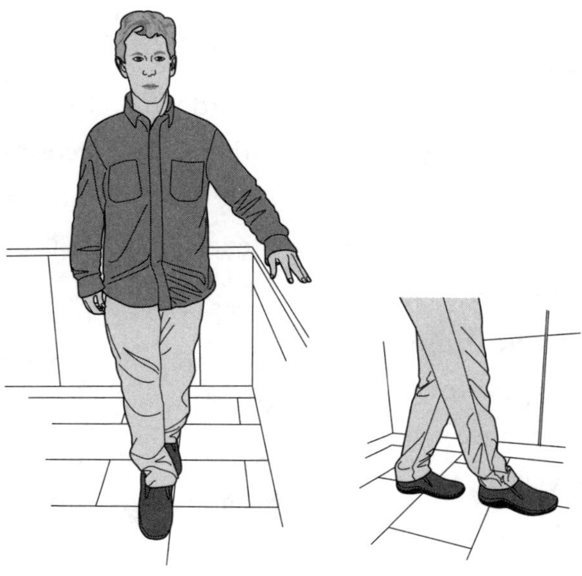

Endurance Exercises

Having good endurance means you can do your daily tasks without feeling tired or "worn out" all the time. It can also be an opportunity to include your care partner in an activity that can help you both. Aerobic (endurance) exercise can increase your energy and make it so you don't tire as quickly. Health guidelines recommend that adults exercise at a moderate intensity for at least 150 minutes each week in activities spread throughout the week. There are many ways to work exercise into your day. The most important thing to remember is that some activity is better than none. If you start off doing what is comfortable and increase your efforts gradually, it is likely that you will build a healthy, lifelong habit. You will learn how to stay active and how to return to being active even when changes in your life or responsibilities may slow you down or derail your exercise efforts for a while. Remember, it is better to begin your program by underdoing rather than overdoing and to add more activity at a comfortable pace.

Flexibility and strengthening exercises are described by how many you do at a time and how often you do them. Endurance exercise is described by how often you do it (frequency), how long you exercise at a time (duration), and how hard you work (intensity).

- **Frequency (how often).** Most guidelines suggest doing at least some exercise most days of the week. Exercising three to five times a week is a good choice.
- **Duration (how much time).** According to the guidelines, it is best if you can exercise at least 10 minutes at a time. You can add up your 10-minute exercise periods all week to work to meet the 150-minute recommended amount. For example, taking three 10-minute walks each day for five days gets you to 150 minutes for the week. If 10 minutes is too much at first, start with what you can do and work toward 10 minutes.

- **Intensity (how hard you work).** Aerobic or endurance exercise is safe and effective at a moderate intensity. When you exercise at moderate intensity, you'll feel somewhat warmer, you'll breathe more deeply and faster than usual, and your heart will beat faster than normal. Exercise intensity is relative to your fitness. For an athlete, running a mile in 10 minutes is probably low-intensity exercise. For a person who hasn't exercised in a long time, a 10-minute walk at a constant pace may be moderate to high intensity. For someone with severe physical limitations, a slow walk might be high intensity.

The trick, of course, is to figure out what is moderate intensity for you. There are a couple easy ways to do this.

- **Talk Test.** When exercising, talk to another person or yourself, or recite poems out loud. Moderate-intensity exercise allows you to speak comfortably. If you can't carry on a conversation because you are breathing too hard or are short of breath, you're working at a high intensity. Slow down. The talk test is an easy and quick way to recognize your effort and regulate intensity. If you exercise with your care partner, the talk test is an easy way to keep track of your care partner's intensity and make adjustments if needed. If you or your care partner have lung disease, the talk test might not work for you. If that is the case, try using the perceived-exertion scale.
- **Perceived Exertion.** Another way to monitor intensity is to rate how hard you're working on a scale of perceived exertion. On a 0-to-10 scale, 0, at the low end of the scale, is lying down, doing no work at all, and 10 is equivalent to working as hard as possible—very hard work that you couldn't do for more than a few seconds. A good level for moderate aerobic exercise on the 0-to-10 perceived-exertion scale is between 4 and 5.

There are several kinds of exercise that you can use to improve your endurance. Walking, bicycling, swimming, or low-impact aerobics classes are good choices and let you start comfortably and at your own pace.

Walking

Walking is easy, inexpensive, safe, something you might be able to do with your care partner, and it can be done almost anywhere. You can walk inside or outside, by yourself or with company. Walking is safer than jogging or running and puts less stress on the body. It's an especially good choice if you have been sedentary or have joint or balance problems.

If you walk to shop, visit friends, and do household chores, then you can probably walk for exercise. Using a cane or walker need not stop you from getting into a walking routine. Be cautious the first two weeks of walking. If you haven't been doing much for a while, five or 10 minutes might be enough. Alternate brisk walks and slow walks to build up your endurance. Each week increase the brisk walking interval by no more than five minutes until you are up to 20 or 30 minutes.

Remember that your goal is to walk most days of the week at moderate intensity and to build your time to get up to at least 10 minutes each time you walk. Don't forget that you are in charge of your walking. You control the frequency, duration, and intensity. The following walking tips can help you be safe and successful:

- **Choose your ground.** Walk on a flat, level surface. Walking on hills, uneven ground, soft earth, sand, or gravel is hard work and often leads to hip, knee, or foot pain. Fitness trails, shopping malls, school tracks, streets with sidewalks, and quiet neighborhoods are good places.
- **Always warm up and cool down with a stroll.** Walk slowly for five minutes to prepare your circulation and muscles for a brisker walk. Finish up with the same slow walk to let your body calm down gradually. Experienced walkers know they can avoid shin and foot discomfort if they begin and end with a stroll.
- **Set your own pace.** It takes practice to find the right walking speed. To find your speed, start walking slowly for a few minutes, then increase your speed to a pace that is slightly faster than normal for you. After five minutes, check your exercise intensity with the perceived-exertion or talk test. If you are working too hard or feel out of breath, slow down. If your exertion is below your desired intensity, try walking a little faster. Walk another five minutes and check your intensity again. If you are still below your target intensity, keep walking at a comfortable speed and simply check your intensity in the middle and at the end of each walk.
- **Use a walking or hiking stick.** You can learn more about walking sticks in Table 8.2, Mobility Aids and Injury Prevention Tips, in Chapter 8, Preventing Injuries.

Choosing Shoes

Choose shoes of the correct length and width with shock-absorbing soles and insoles. Make sure they're big enough in the toe area. The rule of thumb is there should be a thumb width between the end of your longest toe and the end of the shoe. You shouldn't feel pressure on the sides or tops of your toes. The heel counter (the back of the shoe) should hold your heel firmly in the shoe when you walk. Be sure your shoes are in good repair.

Wear shoes with a continuous composite sole. Avoid shoes that have very thick, rubbery, or sticky soles that may create a tripping hazard. Shoes with laces or Velcro let you adjust width as needed and give more support than slip-ons. If you have problems tying laces, consider Velcro closures or elastic shoelaces. Shoes with leather soles and a separate heel don't absorb shock as well as athletic and casual shoes. Good shoes do not need to be expensive; any shoes that meet the criteria we have just described will serve your purposes.

Many people like shoes with removable insoles that can be exchanged for more shock-absorbing ones. You can find insoles in sporting goods stores and shoe stores. When you shop for insoles, take your walking shoes with you. Try on the shoe with the insole inserted to make sure there's enough room for your foot to be comfortable with the insoles in place. Insoles come in different sizes and can be trimmed with scissors for a custom fit. If your toes take up extra room, try the three-quarter insoles that stop just short of your toes. If you have prescribed inserts in your shoes already, ask your doctor about insoles.

Preventing Possible Problems

If you have pain around your shins or leg cramps when you walk, you might not be spending enough time warming up or you could be walking too fast. Start your walk at a slow pace for at least five minutes. Keep your feet and toes relaxed. Sore knees are another common problem. Take care of your knees by starting with a slower warm-up walk and walk on smooth and even surfaces (for example, on a sidewalk, mall trail, or track). If you are exercising with your care partner, you should be watching out for these problems for both of you.

Swimming

When you swim, the buoyancy of the water lets you move your joints through their full range of motion and strengthen your muscles and cardiovascular system with less stress than on land. For most people, swimming is excellent exercise. It uses the whole body. If you haven't been swimming for a while, consider a refresher course. To make swimming an aerobic exercise, you eventually need to swim continuously for 10 minutes. Try different strokes, changing strokes after each lap or two. This lets you exercise all joints and muscles without overtiring any one area. Although swimming is an excellent aerobic exercise, you also will need to do other standing and walking exercise to improve balance and bone strength.

Stationary Bicycling

Stationary bicycles offer the fitness benefits of bicycling without the outdoor hazards. Stationary bicycling also allows you to exercise without leaving home when you need to be present. Indoor use of a stationary bicycle may also be preferable to outdoor bicycling for people who live in a cold or hilly area or in an area with lots of car traffic or limited bike lanes or paths. You can choose between the traditional upright or recumbent bicycle style. Make sure the bike is steady and you can get on and off safely.

The most common complaint about riding a stationary bike is that it's boring. Watching television, reading, or listening to music helps the time go by faster. Penny keeps her indoor cycling interesting by mapping out tours of places she would like to visit and then charts her progress on a map as she rolls off the miles. Other people set their bicycle time for the half hour of a favorite television or radio program. There are also videocassettes and DVDs of exotic bike tours. Book racks that clip onto the handlebars make reading easy.

The following cycling tips can help you be safe and successful:

- **Remember that stationary bicycling uses different muscles than walking.** Until your leg muscles get used to pedaling, you might be able to ride for only a few minutes. Start off with no resistance. Increase resistance slightly as riding gets easier. Increasing resistance has the same effect as bicycling up hills.
- **Pedal at a comfortable speed.** For most people, 50 to 70 revolutions per minute (rpm) is a good starting pace. As you get used to bicycling, you can increase your speed. However, faster is not necessarily better. Listening to music at the right tempo makes it easier to pedal at an enjoyable and consistent speed.

Experience will tell you the best combination of speed and resistance.

- **A good target goal is 20 to 30 minutes of pedaling at a comfortable speed.** Build up your time by alternating intervals of brisk pedaling with periods of less exertion. If you get out of breath, slow down.
- **Keep a record of the times and distances of your bike trips.** You'll be amazed at how much you can do.

Exercise Classes

For many people, an exercise class is a good choice for building endurance. One advantage of an exercise class is that you benefit from the experience and knowledge of a teacher and class members. You can take an exercise class in your community or find a class on television or a DVD. A TV show or DVD lets you exercise at home, choose your time, and stop and start when you want, as well as to do it with your care partner. A community class adds social time and a change of scenery to your daily routine. There are many types of classes, including aerobic dance, ballroom and square dance, yoga, tai chi, and water exercise—all with different benefits.

Your local Y, senior center, or community recreation center are also good places to look for classes. Talk to friends and family about what they do. Visit and observe classes. Choose a place, time, and class that feels comfortable and works for your needs and schedule. Talk with the instructor and "sample" a class before signing up for a long-term commitment. Look for an instructor who encourages everyone to go at their own pace and a class where people are friendly and having fun. There are some suggestions for classes listed in the Other Resources section at the end of the chapter including programs that may be available in your community and others that are available online, on DVD, or on television.

Exercising with Your Care Partner

Many exercises and activities can be adapted in ways to let people with different needs take part. If your care partner is physically limited, for example, there are exercises that can be used sitting or lying down instead of standing. The good morning exercise (Exercise 11) and the shoulder-blade pinch (Exercise 14) can be done standing, sitting or lying down. The toe walk and the heel walk (Exercises 27 and 28,) are described as standing and moving exercises, but also they can be done seated. The exercises shown lying down are best done on the floor or a firm mat, but could be done in bed too.

As you choose exercises for yourself, discuss the exercises with care partners and explore what they might want to do. Try a couple exercises. Try to find an exercise time during the day to exercise together. You don't need to do the same things, just be active together. You might also ask your care partner to count or keep time for you as you exercise, like a coach or cheerleader. When you are active together, you are encouraging and supporting each other in a healthy habit, and it is a pleasant way to spend time together.

Anuj and Leila do stretches and balance exercises for 10 minutes each morning after breakfast and before it is time to get Anuj dressed for the day. Anuj's favorite exercise is good morning. When the weather permits, on Monday, Wednesday, and Friday afternoons, they walk to the park, which is 20 minutes away. Leila takes a beginning adaptive yoga class at the local Y that meets three times a week while Anuj's sister visits with Anuj.

Overcoming Exercise Barriers

Health and fitness make sense. Yet when faced with being more physically active, people often come up with many excuses, concerns, and worries. These barriers can prevent you from taking the first step. Here are some common barriers and possible solutions:

- **"I don't have enough time."** When you are a caregiver, you have many tasks to complete every day that require time and energy. Think how becoming stronger and more energetic can make the rest of your day better. Exercise doesn't take a lot of time. Ten minutes at a time two or three times a day can make a big difference in how you feel. Try adding some exercise on to what you do already. Do some stretching while you watch TV. Make a morning stretch or several short walks part of your daily routine.
- **"I'm too tired."** When you're a full-time caregiver, stressed out, out of shape, or depressed, you might feel tired. You have to break out of the "too tired" cycle. Try an experiment: Next time you are too tired, do a few stretches or take a short walk (five minutes or even just two!). You may be surprised how this changes your outlook and gives you energy. As you become more active, you will recognize the difference between feeling listless and feeling physically tired.
- **"I'm too old."** You're never too old for physical activity. No matter what your level of fitness or your age, you can always find ways to increase your activity, energy, and sense of well-being. Fitness is especially important as we age.
- **"I get enough exercise."** This might be true, but for most people, their jobs and daily activities do not provide enough sustained exercise at a moderate level to keep them fit and energetic. An interesting and often surprising way to really find out how active you are is to use a step counter. There are a variety of choices—some that you can wear on your wrist and some that hang on a belt or you carry in a pocket. There are also apps for smartphones and smart watches that will count and record steps.

- **"Exercise is boring."** You can make exercise interesting and fun. Exercise with other people. Entertain yourself with a headset and musical tapes, or listen to the radio. Vary your activities and your walking routes. You might find exercise time a good opportunity to think and problem solve.
- **"Exercise is painful."** The old saying "no pain, no gain" is simply wrong. Health benefits come from regular moderate-intensity physical activity. Choose exercises that are comfortable and do not cause pain.
- **"I'm afraid I might fall."** Check where you will exercise to make sure it is safe (good lighting, well-maintained parking lots and walkways, handrails, and uncluttered floors). Choose exercises that feel safe—chair exercise, water exercise, or recumbent bicycling provide a lot of support as you get started. Remember, having good posture and balance and staying active reduces the risks of falls.
- **"I'm afraid I'll have a heart attack."** In most cases, the risk of a heart attack is greater for people who are not physically active than for those who exercise regularly. But if you are worried about this, check with your doctor.
- **"I'm afraid I won't be able to do it right or won't be successful."** Many people don't start a new project because they are afraid they will fail. If you feel this way, remember two things. First, whatever activities you are able to do—no matter how short or "easy"—will be much better than doing nothing. Be proud of what you have done, not guilty about what you haven't done. Second, new projects often seem overwhelming—until we get started and learn to enjoy each day's adventures and successes.

Perhaps you have some other barriers. Be honest with yourself about your worries. Talk to yourself and others to develop positive thoughts about exercise. If you get stuck, ask others for suggestions, or try some of the positive thinking suggestions in Chapter 5, Using Your Mind to Manage Stress.

Getting in the Habit of Healthy Exercise and Keeping It Up

If you haven't exercised recently, you'll probably experience some new feelings and frustrations when you first start exercising. Don't be surprised by setbacks. There will be interruptions. You might get off track for a while. Don't be discouraged. You may need a rest, a different schedule, or different activities. If you get derailed, take a short break and when you are ready, start again. Begin at a lower, gentler level. It can take you the same amount of time to get back into shape as you were out. For instance, if you missed three weeks, it might take at least that long to get back to your previous level. Go slowly. Be kind to yourself. You're in this for the long haul.

With exercise experience, you develop a sense of control over yourself and your schedule. You learn how to choose your activity to fit your needs. You know when to do less and when to do more. When there are interruptions, you know it isn't a disaster. You know you have the tools to get back on track. Give yourself a chance to succeed. Sticking with it and doing it your way makes you a sure winner.

For most people who are not already active, starting an exercise routine means getting into a new habit. This means making time on most days of the week to exercise. Exercise is part of good self-care and relaxation. Think of your head as the coach and your body as your team. For success, all parts of the team need attention. Be a good coach. Encourage and praise yourself. Design "plays" you feel your team will like. Choose places that you like and are safe. Good coaches know their teams, set good goals, and help the team succeed and get more confident. A good coach is loyal. A good coach does not belittle, nag, or make anyone feel guilty. Be a good coach to yourself.

Besides a good coach, everyone needs a good cheerleader or two. Of course, you can be your own cheerleader, but being both coach and cheerleader is a lot to do. Successful exercisers usually have at least one family member or friend who encourages them. Sometimes cheerleaders pop up by themselves, but don't be bashful about asking for a hand. Your cheerleader can exercise with you, help you get other chores done so you can exercise, praise you, or just consider your exercise time when making plans. Your care partner can be a good cheerleader and participate in exercise with you, remind you and encourage you to take time for yourself to exercise.

We hope this chapter helps you learn to use exercise to feel better and stay healthy. Start by knowing your own needs and limits and respect your body. Talk to other people like you who exercise. Talk with your doctor and other health professionals. Always pay attention to your own experience. That helps you know your body and make wise choices.

Suggested Further Reading

Hammarstrom, Gwen Wendy. *Circles of Healing: The Complete Guide to Healing with Massage and Yoga: For Caregivers, Practitioners, Students and Clients*. Ama Press, 2012. Outlines self-care techniques, such as conscious breathing, exercise, and giving and receiving healing touch. http://amzn.to/2o3CbdC

Kisner, Carolyn, Lynn Allen Colby, and John Borstad. *Therapeutic Exercise: Foundations and Techniques*. Philadelphia: F.A. Davis Company, 2018. A guide to customize interventions for individuals with movement dysfunction with a balance of theory and clinical techniques. http://amzn.to/2Glyyq1 Videos also available at www.Davis*Plus*.com (redeem code from purchased book).

Kozak, Joshua. *Stay Fit for Life: More Than 60 Exercises to Restore Your Strength and Future-proof Your Body*. Indianapolis: DK, 2017. A training program to restore strength and balance to your everyday movement with 62 functional exercises, targeted workout routines, and three four-week fitness programs. http://amzn.to/2HlBTH3

Liebman, Hollis Lance. *1,500 Stretches: The Complete Guide to Flexibility and Movement*. New York: Black Dog & Leventhal Publishers, 2017. A collection of stretches organized by body part demonstrated in photographs, with additional chapters on yoga and partner stretches. http://amzn.to/2ENitMH

Otto, Michael W., and Jasper A. J. Smits. *Exercise for Mood and Anxiety: Proven Strategies for Overcoming Depression and Enhancing Well-Being*. New York: Oxford University Press, 2011. Examples and practical advice on using exercise to relieve stress, anxiety, and depression. http://amzn.to/2CqBlvH

Plahay, Tania. *Yoga for Dementia: A Guide for People with Dementia, Their Families and Caregivers*. London: Jessica Kingsley Publishers, 2018. A program to enhance well-being, posture, breathing, and sleep and to reduce anxiety and agitation. http://amzn.to/2Bxyp3w

Quarta, Cynthia. *Seated Taiji and Qigong: Guided Therapeutic Exercises to Manage Stress and Balance Mind, Body and Spirit*. Philadelphia: Singing Dragon, 2012. Provides simple techniques for anyone working with people with physical disabilities to make big improvements on their physical and mental well-being. http://amzn.to/2EyQRYm

Stephens, Mark. *Yoga Sequencing Designing Transformative Yoga Classes*. Berkeley, CA: North Atlantic Books, 2012. Offers 67 model sequences of yoga poses (*asanas*) for beginners, intermediates, and advanced students; yoga for kids, teens, and seniors; and classes to relieve depression and anxiety. http://amzn.to/2obKEdW

Other Resources

Try some of these resources to help you and your care partner build an enjoyable exercise routine. The websites will help you find the options for home use and where the classes are taught locally. You will find television shows, streaming programs, CDs and DVDs, and community classes.

AgingCare.com provides information on elderly activities, outing ideas and animal therapy. https://www.agingcare.com/activities-recreation

Enhanced Fitness is a group exercise program for older people and those with limitations. It is offered in many places with trained instructors. http://www.projectenhance.org/enhancefitness.aspx

Moving Easy and Exercises for Chronic Conditions audio CDs talk you through gentle exercise sessions. https://www.bullpub.com/catalog/exercises-for-chronic-conditions-cd

Silver Sneakers is a program taught in many communities by trained leaders. Some insurance plans provide it as a benefit. https://www.silversneakers.com

Sit and Be Fit offers the classes through public television, streaming, YouTube, and DVDs. https://sitandbefit.org

Special thanks to Bonnie Bruce, DrPH, MPH, RD, and Cindy Tran, MPH for their help with this chapter.

Chapter 10

Healthy Eating

We all have very personal preferences about eating. These are shaped by our families, our cultures, our religion, our health, the media, and society. What was considered healthy when we were children may no longer be considered healthy. As we learn more, this will continue to change. This chapter was written based on recent information from the United States Department of Agriculture. We present this information to help you make your own decisions.

Healthy eating is one of your best personal investments. Eating healthy means making good and healthful food choices most of the time. It does not mean being rigid or perfect. It can mean finding new or different ways to prepare your meals to make them tasty and appealing. If you or your care partner have certain health conditions, it may mean that you must be choosier. Eating well does not usually mean you can never indulge in your favorite food.

Unfortunately, due to the internet, books, other media, friends, and relatives, we can get overloaded with information about what we should and should not eat. No matter what the media or your friends say, there is no one best way of eating for everyone. There is no perfect food. There is no perfect way to eat. Many eating patterns can contribute to health and wellness but the whole eating thing can be confusing.

In this chapter, we give you basic science-based nutrition and diet information. We are not going to tell you what to eat or how to eat. That is your decision. We do, however, share basic, clear information about adult nutrition and some ways to help you integrate that information with your and your care partner's specific likes and needs. On pages 183–188 we give information for individuals with the most common long-term health conditions. We know that eating can be a source of joy or a source of stress, especially when you must navigate the choices of your care partner as well for as yourself. We hope this chapter will help make eating a joy and not another cause of stress.

Why Is Healthy Eating So Important?

The human body is a marvelous machine, sort of like an automobile. Cars need the proper mix of fuel to run right. Without it, they may run rough and may even stop working. The human body is similar. It needs the proper mix of good food (fuel) to keep it running well. It does not run right on the wrong fuel or on empty.

Healthy eating cuts across every part of your life. It is linked to your body and your mind's well-being, including how your body responds to some illnesses. Of course, the same is true for your care partner. When you give your body the right nourishment, here's what happens:

- You have more energy and feel less tired.
- You increase your chances of preventing or lessening further problems from health conditions, such as heart disease, diabetes, high blood pressure, and cancer.
- You feed your brain, which can help you handle life's challenges as well as its emotional ups and downs.

What Is Healthy Eating?

At the heart of healthy eating are our daily choices. For some of us, healthy eating means having to be somewhat choosy about the foods we eat. For example, people with diabetes need to watch their carbohydrate intake to manage blood sugar levels. They do best by planning which and how much of carbohydrate foods, such as milk, fruit, breads, beans, cereals, and rice, that they will eat daily. Others, with heart disease or who are at risk for heart disease, find that watching the amount and kinds of fat they eat can help control their blood cholesterol levels. Those with high blood pressure can help lower their blood pressure by eating lots of fruits, vegetables, low-fat dairy foods (and, for some people, by cutting back on salt). Anyone who wants to lose or gain weight needs to pay attention to how many calories they eat.

The real issue for most of us is not the healthy foods we choose but the less healthy ones. Healthy eating is being flexible and allowing yourself to occasionally enjoy small amounts of foods that may not be so healthful. Being overly strict or rigid and not allowing yourself ever to have a treat will likely cause your best efforts to fail.

However, one-third of the American diet is made up of foods that can damage health—these are foods are high in added sugars (e.g., candy and other sweets), solid fats (e.g., butter, stick margarine, shortening, and fat from beef, pork, and chicken), and sodium (e.g., salt). Added sugars, fats, and sodium can contribute to health problems such as high blood pressure, diabetes, and obesity. People in the United States also tend to eat a lot of food made from white flour and other refined grains (e.g., white rice and bread and baked goods), that have been stripped of the original nutrients.

Trade-offs are a big part of healthy eating. This means learning how food affects you and making good decisions about when to treat and when not to treat yourself. For instance, it might be important for you to have a very special meal on your birthday. If this is the case, as a trade-off, you can make healthier choices when you are out for a casual lunch. Trading off is a tool that can help you stay on the path of healthy eating. As you get better at making trade-offs to keep yourself from over-doing it too often, you will find it gets easier and even becomes a natural habit in your everyday life. Another important tool is being aware of how much you eat. Many of us eat more than we need to eat, even if the foods we eat are mostly healthy choices.

Most dietary guidelines suggest that a good starting place is to move toward eating more plant foods including whole grains, fruits, vegetables, cooked dry beans and peas, lentils, nuts, and seeds. This does not mean giving up meats and other foods high in sugar, fat, or sodium, but rather eating them in smaller amounts or less often. Many current dietary guidelines recommend moderate amounts of lean meats, poultry, and eggs. We have come a long way since meat and potatoes were thought of as the foundation for a great diet. Today, we know that vegetables, fruits, whole grains, low-fat dairy products, lean meats, poultry, and fish are at the core of a healthy diet. There is still a place for meat and potatoes; it is just not the most important place.

A Special Note for Caregivers

It may be that your care partner is nearing the end of life or that eating is one of his or her few pleasurable activities. While healthy eating is important, making perfect food choices might not be as important during this time. For example, it could be fine for your care partner to have dessert first, not eat all their greens, or have ice cream every night. If you are concerned about your care partner's nutrition, talk with a health care professional.

Key Principles of Healthy Eating

Balancing the kinds of food you eat and how much you eat are the primary elements of a healthy diet. (We'll have more to say about this later in this chapter.) This all sounds simple, but every day we are faced with hundreds of food choices. It is often easier and quicker to grab something less healthful than to think about what we will eat, much less cooking it. So, how do we put together meals that are tasty and enjoyable yet healthful? The following key principles can help make this task as simple as possible:

- **Choose foods as nature originally made them.** This means the less processed the better. By *processed* we mean foods that have been changed from their original state by having ingredients added (often sugar or fat) or removed (often fiber or nutrients) to make them tastier or more appealing. Examples include whole grains made into white flour for baked products, such as cookies, or animal foods made into luncheon or deli meats. Choices that are less processed include a grilled chicken breast instead of fried breaded chicken nuggets, a baked potato (with skin) rather than French fries, and whole grains, or whole-grain bread and pasta and brown rice instead of refined grains, such as white bread and white rice.
- **Get your nutrients from food, not supplements.** For most people, the nutrients from vitamin, mineral, and other dietary supplements cannot take the place of nutrients from real food. Foods as nature made them contain nutrients and other healthy compounds, such as fiber, in the right combinations and amounts to help our bodies work properly. When we remove naturally existing nutrients from food, those nutrients may not work the way they should. They might have harmful side effects.
  - For instance, beta carotene is an important source of vitamin A, found in plant foods, such as carrots and winter squash. It helps our vision and enhances our immune system. However, artificial beta-carotene supplements have been shown in some people to increase some cancer risks. There is no such risk when beta carotene is eaten as it is naturally found in food, such as carrots.
  - Another reason to get your nutrition from food rather than supplements is that real foods contain a host of nutrients as well as other healthful compounds. When you take a supplement such as a vitamin pill, you are missing out on other helpful substances that are naturally partnered within a food.
  - In most of the world, including the United States, diet and nutrition supplement manufacturers do not have to follow government regulations for quality or goodness. Unlike over-the-counter medications, with supplements there is no guarantee that you are getting what is on the label or that you are not getting harmful substances.
  - Is there ever a place for dietary supplements? Yes, sometimes we cannot get enough of one or more of the nutrients we need. For example, older men and

women often need a large amount of calcium to help prevent or slow osteoporosis. Although we get calcium from milk and milk products such as yogurt or cheese, consuming the amount needed can be difficult. If you are thinking of taking a supplement, first talk to your health care professional or a registered dietitian.

- **Eat a wide variety of colorful foods in their original forms.** "Eat the rainbow" is an easy way to remember this. Choose foods that are as close as possible to how they come from the garden, field, or farm. The more variety in your diet, the better; the more colors on your plate, the better; and the closer foods are to their original form, the better.
    - By following these three simple rules, your body has a great chance of getting all the good things it needs. This means a plate containing lean, simply prepared meat, fish, or poultry and a lot of colorful fruits and vegetables—think red, blue and purple grapes and blueberries; yellow and orange pineapple, oranges, winter squash, and carrots; red tomatoes, strawberries, and watermelon; and green leafy greens and beans—along with the white and warm brown tones from mushrooms, onions, and cauliflower and whole grains, such as brown rice.
- **Eat foods high in phytochemicals.** Phytochemicals are health-promoting and disease-fighting compounds found only in plant foods (*phyto* means "plant"), such as fruits, vegetables, whole grains, nuts, and seeds. Phytochemicals include the compounds that give fruits and vegetables their bright colors. Whenever a food is refined or processed, as when whole wheat is made into white flour, phytochemicals are lost. The more often you choose foods that are not refined, and as close as possible to how nature made them, the better.
- **Eat regularly.** A gas-fueled machine will not run without the gas, and a fire eventually burns out without more wood. Your body is much the same. It needs regular refueling to work at its best. Eating something, even a little bit, at regular intervals helps keep your "fire" burning.
    - Eating at regular times during the day, preferably evenly spaced over the day, helps maintain and balance your blood sugar level. Blood sugar is a key player in supplying the organs in your body, especially the brain, with energy. If you do not eat regularly, your blood sugar drops, and depending on how low it gets, you may feel weak, shaky, sweaty, and nauseous. You may also experience mood changes (e.g., irritability, anxiety, or anger), headaches, or poor coordination. Low blood sugar (hypoglycemia) can be a dangerous condition.
    - Eating regularly helps you get the nutrients you need and helps your body use those nutrients. Of course, not skipping meals or not letting too many hours go between meals also helps keep you from getting overly hungry. Being overly hungry often leads to overeating. This can in turn lead to problems such as indigestion, heartburn, and weight gain.

- Eating regularly does not mean that you must stick to the same daily routine. Nor does it mean that you must follow the "normal" pattern of eating three meals a day. Allow yourself room for flexibility.
- If you have certain health conditions, such as cancer, you might find that at times several small meals over the day are best for you, while at other times fewer, bigger meals work best. If you are diabetic, spacing meals regularly and balancing what you eat is key, but this could mean several small meals a day, three meals mixed with a snack, or just three meals. Whatever is best for you.

- **Eat what your body needs (not more or less).** How much you should eat depends on the following:
  - Your age (we need fewer calories as we get older)
  - If you are a man or woman (men usually need more calories than women)
  - Your body size and shape (in general, if you are taller or have more muscle, you can eat more)
  - Your health needs (some conditions affect how your body uses calories)
  - Your activity level (the more physically active you are, the more calories you can eat)

Managing How Much You Eat

It is easy to say that you should eat the amount (not more or less) that your body needs, but more difficult to put that plan into action. The following tips can help you manage how much you eat:

- **Stop eating when you first feel full.** This helps keep you from overeating. Pay attention to your body to learn what this feels like. Like all new skills, it takes some practice. If it is hard to stop eating when you begin to feel full, remove your plate or, if you can, get up from the table.
- **Eat slowly.** Eating slowly gives you more enjoyment from food and helps keep you

A Note about Breakfast

Breakfast is just that: "breaking the fast." It refuels your body after going without eating for many hours and helps you resist the urge to eat extra snacks or overeat the rest of the day. Increasing scientific evidence backs up that eating breakfast can help promote health and links skipping breakfast to higher risk of obesity and poorer glucose (blood sugar) control and diabetes.

We know that you might not want to eat breakfast, not only because you don't have the time or aren't hungry or perhaps you do not like the usual breakfast foods. There are no rules about what you should eat for breakfast. It can be anything that appeals to you—fruit, beans, rice, bread, broccoli, even leftovers. The important thing is to kick-start your body each day by refueling it.

from overeating. Make your meals or snacks last at least 15 to 20 minutes. It takes this much time for the brain to catch up and tell your stomach that it is getting full. If you finish quickly, wait at least 15 minutes before getting more food.

- **Pay attention to what you eat.** Be mindful when you eat. If you are not paying attention, it is easy to eat an entire bag of chips or cookies or eat too much food without even knowing it. This can happen easily when we are sharing food and socializing with friends, reading, using the computer, or watching television. In these situations, try measuring the portion you want to eat before you sit down, or keep food out of reach or out of sight. What you eat is called a portion.
- **Know a serving size looks like.** A serving is the recommended portion to be eaten. What you eat, a portion, may be more or less than a serving. It is good to know what a serving looks like. A 1/2-cup serving is about the size of a tennis ball or a closed fist. A 3–4 ounce serving of cooked meat, fish, or poultry is about the size of a deck of playing cards or the palm of your hand. The end of your thumb to the first joint is about 1 teaspoon: three times that is a tablespoon. (*Tip:* Using a measuring cup is a great way to learn what a serving size looks like and very helpful in determining how well you are estimating your portions.) In addition, there is a Nutrition Facts label on most packaged foods which, among other things, tells you the serving size for that food (see p. 184).
- **Watch out for supersizing.** In recent years, portion sizes have literally "beefed up." The typical adult cheeseburger used to be about 330 calories; now it is about 590 calories! Twenty years ago, an average cookie was about 1½ inches wide and had 55 calories; now it is 3½ inches wide and has 275 calories—*five times* the calories! Sodas typically came in 6½–8-ounce bottles with 85 calories; today it's 20 ounces in a bottle with 250 calories.

  It takes an extra 3,500 calories more than we need to gain a pound of body fat. This means that over a year's time, it takes only an extra 100 calories a day to put on 10 pounds; 100 calories are equal to eating only an extra third of a bagel each day! Recommended serving sizes vary for different foods.
- **When practical, select foods that come in a single-serving.** Foods that come prepackaged as single servings can help you see what a suggested serving looks like. If a prepackaged serving size seems too small compared to what you would usually eat, start to adjust slowly by cutting how much you now eat by just a small amount at a time. For example, if you usually eat 1 cup of rice, try eating a 1/2 or 3/4 cup instead.
- **Make your food attractive.** We really do eat with our eyes! Compare a monotone plate with white fish, white rice, and white cauliflower with the colorful mouth-watering appeal one of golden brown chicken, grilled sweet potato, and bright green spinach. Which of these two meals seems more appetizing?

A Map for Healthy Eating

A map helps you along your journey and get you to where you want to go. Put your meal together so that a little less than one-fourth of the plate is covered with colorful fruit; a little more than one-fourth with vegetables; one-fourth with a protein source (lean meat, fish, or poultry, or better yet, plant-based protein) and one-fourth with grains (aiming for at least half from whole grains) or other starches, such as potatoes, rice, yams, or winter squash. Finish off your plate with calcium-rich foods. These could be milk or foods made from milk (preferably fat-free or low-fat), such as cheese, yogurt, frozen yogurt, puddings, or, for variety, calcium-fortified soy foods such as soy milk. Of course, your food choices and amounts will depend on what you like and need. For more information about this way of eating, check out the U.S. Department of Agriculture's MyPlate website at http://www.chooseMyPlate.gov and see Figure 10.1.

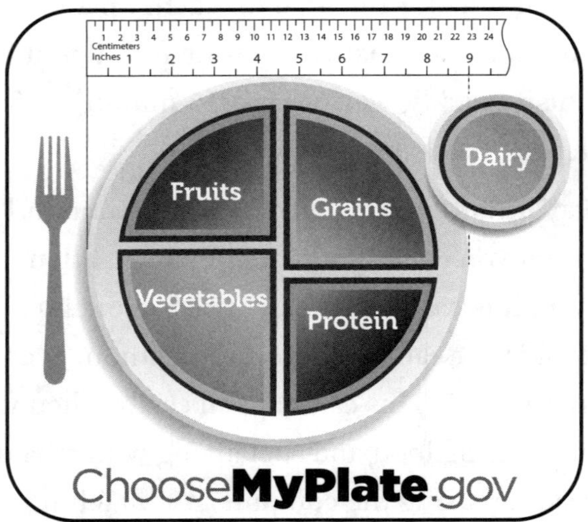

Figure 10.1 **MyPlate: Map for Healthy Eating**

For people with diabetes, the American Diabetes Association recommends a similar plate. See Figure 10.2, Create Your Plate from the American Diabetes Association, on page 186.

Even with this map, calories and portion sizes are important. Plate sizes are now typically bigger, making it easier to get more calories than you want or need. The plates referenced in Choose MyPlate and the Create Your Plate for diabetes are nine inches in diameter. Many dinner plates, on the other hand, are 10–11 inches in diameter. The box "Guidelines for Healthy Eating" on page 182 can help you plan meals that fit your situation. It lists examples of serving sizes based on Choose MyPlate. If you have questions about how much you should eat, check with your healthcare provider or a registered dietitian.

Note, too, that on the internet there are many people who claim to be nutrition experts but may not be. If you want a real expert, look for a registered dietitian (R.D.). These health professionals are specially trained and are the best sources for diet and nutrition advice and information.

Feeding Your Body the Nutrients It Needs

Earlier, we emphasized the need to get nutrients from food. In the following sections, we focus on carbohydrates, fats, protein, water, and a few vitamins and minerals. We also discuss fiber, although technically this is not a nutrient. Fortunately, it is not difficult to get the nutrients that we need from healthy eating.

Carbohydrates and Fiber

Carbohydrates are your body's go-to fuel for the brain, central nervous system, and red blood cells. Carbohydrates largely determine your blood glucose (sugar) level—more so than protein or fat. But carbohydrates do a great deal more. They provide basic materials to help our bodies make vital parts for the body. Nearly every part of your body, from your toenails to the top of your head, uses some part of a carbohydrate in its construction.

Carbohydrates are found mostly in plant foods. Milk and yogurt are about the only animal foods rich in carbohydrates. Foods with carbohydrates can be categorized by whether they are high in sugar or high in starch. Foods that are high in sugar usually break down faster, get into your blood faster, and give you energy faster than high-starch foods.

Sugary carbohydrates are found in fruit and juice, milk, yogurt, table sugar, honey, jellies, syrups, and sugar-sweetened drinks. Starchy carbohydrates are found in vegetables such as corn, green peas, potatoes, winter squash, dried beans and peas, lentils, and grains such as rice. Pasta, tortillas, and bread are also high in carbohydrates. The amount of carbohydrate in whole grains, brown rice, and whole wheat bread is like that in refined grains, such as white bread and white rice. The big difference between these two sources of carbohydrates is that the refined grains have been stripped of nutrients, phytochemicals, and fiber during processing.

Many minimally processed plant foods that contain carbohydrates also contain fiber. Most fiber is not absorbed into the body and does not have calories. Fiber is found only in plant foods with "skins, seeds, and strings." For example, whole grains, dried beans, peas, lentils, fruits, vegetables, nuts, and seeds all have some fiber. Some foods have added fiber (as when pulp is added to juice). Animal foods and refined and processed foods (white flour, bread, many baked and snack foods, such as cookies and chips) have little or no fiber unless it was added by the manufacturer.

Different types of fiber help your body in different ways. Wheat bran, some fruits and vegetables, and whole grains act as "nature's broom"; they keep your digestive system moving and help prevent constipation. The fiber in oat bran, barley, nuts, seeds, beans, apples, citrus fruits, carrots, and psyllium seed can help manage your blood sugar because they help slow the amount of time it takes for sugar to get into the bloodstream. These fiber sources can also help lower blood cholesterol. High fiber diets are also thought to help reduce the risk of rectal and colon cancers.

Oils and Solid Fats: The Good, the Bad, and the Deadly

Many of us think that all fat is bad. But we need some fat for survival and for our bodies to work properly. The body needs about a tablespoon of fat a day. Fat can also be used almost without limit, to store energy as body fat.

Although all fats for the same serving size have the same number of calories, some fats are more healthful than others (we call these good fats), and some can be harmful when we eat too much (bad fats).

Good fats (also called unsaturated fats) are usually liquid at room temperature. These good unsaturated fats help keep our cells healthy, and some can help reduce blood cholesterol. Good fats include soybean, safflower, corn, peanut, sunflower, canola, and olive oils. Nuts, seeds, and olives (and their oils), as well as avocados, are rich in good fats.

There is another group of good fats, the omega-3s, which can be helpful for some people in reducing the risk of heart disease and may help with rheumatoid arthritis symptoms. These fats are found in fatty deep-water fish, such as salmon, mackerel, trout, and tuna. Other sources of omega-3s include wheat germ, flaxseed, and walnuts, although the body might not be able to use omega-3s from plants as readily as it does the omega-3s from fish.

The bad fats (also called saturated fats) are usually solid at room temperature. Consuming these bad saturated fats can increase blood cholesterol and the risk of heart disease. Most bad fats are found in animal foods such as butter, beef fat (tallow, suet), chicken fat, and pork fat (lard). Other foods high in bad fats include stick margarines, red meat, ground meat, processed and cured meats (sausage, bacon, luncheon and deli meats), poultry skin, whole- and low-fat milk and milk products (hard cheese, yogurt, cottage cheese) including cream cheese and sour cream. Palm oil, palm kernel oil, coconut oil, and cocoa butter are also high in saturated fat.

The worst fats that we can eat are the trans fats. These deadly fats have more harmful effects on our blood cholesterol and risk of heart disease than the bad fats. The best advice is to eat as little trans fat as possible, and avoid them if possible. Trans fats are found mostly in processed foods, including pastries, cakes, cookies, crackers, icing, margarine, and most microwave popcorn. They are listed on food labels as "partially hydrogenated" or "hydrogenated" oils.

Tips for Choosing Healthier Carbohydrates and Increasing Fiber

- Fill at least half of your plate with different kinds of vegetables and whole fruits (versus juice).
- Make at least half of the grains you eat each day whole grains (brown rice, whole-grain breads, whole-grain pasta, and tortillas.
- Choose foods with whole wheat or a whole grain, such as oats, listed first on the ingredients list on the food label.
- Choose dried beans and peas, lentils, or whole-grain pasta instead of meat or as side dishes at least a few times a week.
- Choose whole fruit rather than fruit juice. Whole fruit contains fiber, takes longer to eat, fills you up better than juice, and can help keep you from overeating.
- Choose higher-fiber breakfast cereals, such as oatmeal, shredded wheat, Grape-Nuts, or raisin bran.
- Eat higher-fiber crackers, such as whole-rye or multigrain crackers and whole-grain flatbread.
- Snack mostly on whole-grain crackers or breads, whole fruit, or nonfat yogurt rather than sweets, pastries, or ice cream.
- When you add fiber to your diet, do it gradually over a period of a few weeks. Drink plenty of water to help process the fiber and prevent constipation.

Tips for Choosing Good Fats and Healthier Fats

The following tips will help you eat less bad fat and more good fat. Just be sure that if you decide to choose more good fats, that you are not increasing the amount of fat you eat and that you are eating less bad fat.

When Choosing Foods

- Serve and eat cooked portions of meat, fish, and poultry that are 2–3 ounces. This is about the size of a deck of cards or the palm of your hand.
- Eat poultry without skin.
- Eat more deep-water fish, such as salmon, tuna, and mackerel.
- Choose leaner cuts of beef (round, sirloin, or flank).
- Use low-fat or fat-free milk and dairy foods (cheese, sour cream, cottage cheese, yogurt, and ice cream).

When Preparing Foods

- For cooking and baking, use oil, such as olive or canola oil, and soft (tub) margarines (not the reduced fat or diet kinds) instead of solid fats, such as shortening, lard, butter, or stick margarine.
- Trim off all the fat from meat before cooking.
- Use a nonstick pan or a pan with small amounts of cooking oil spray.
- Broil, barbecue, or grill meats.
- Do not fry or deep-fry foods.
- Skim the fat from stews and soups during cooking. (If you refrigerate them overnight, the solid fat lifts off easily.)
- Use less butter, margarine, gravies, meat-based and cream sauces, spreads, and creamy salad dressings.

Be warned! Food companies can legally claim "no" or "0" trans fats on the label even when the food has up to half a gram (0.5 g) per serving.

Most people get more than enough fat. The best recommendation is to eat very little bad and deadly fats and to replace them with the good fats, without increasing the amount of fat you eat.

There is one more thing you should know about fat. All fats contain twice the number of calories per teaspoon as proteins or carbohydrates. Calories from fat add up quickly. For instance, 1 teaspoon of sugar has about 20 calories, but 1 teaspoon of any fat has about 35 calories. When we eat more calories than we need—no matter where they come from—the extra calories get stored as body fat, which leads to weight gain.

Protein

Protein is vital for hundreds of activities that keep you alive and healthy. Protein is part of your red blood cells and the enzymes and hormones that help regulate your body as well as your muscles. It helps your immune system fight infection and builds and repairs damaged tissues. Protein can also give you some energy. But like fat, protein is not as good a source of energy as carbohydrate.

We divide proteins into two types: complete proteins and incomplete proteins. Complete proteins have all the right components in the right amounts. Your body uses complete proteins just as they are. Complete proteins are found in animal foods—meat, fish, poultry, eggs, milk and other dairy products—as well as in soy foods, such as soybeans, tofu, and tempeh. Incomplete proteins are low in one or more key components. Incomplete proteins are found in plant foods, such as grains, dried beans and peas, lentils, nuts, and seeds. Most fruits and vegetables contain little, if any, protein.

For your body to be able to use incomplete proteins best, you need to eat them with at least one other incomplete protein or along with a complete protein. Over centuries, people have learned to survive by eating protein combinations when complete protein sources are not available. Two of the most plentiful and commonly eaten incomplete protein pairs are beans and rice and peanut butter and bread. Although nearly all plant proteins are incomplete proteins, they are still the heart of eating healthy. By eating a small amount of animal protein, such as chicken, with a plant food, such as lentils or black beans, you get all the benefits of a complete protein. In addition, some plant foods, such as nuts and seeds in particular, are great sources of good fats, and many plants foods are good sources of fiber. Plant foods have no cholesterol and little to no trans fats.

The good news is that most people get more than enough protein in their diet. Unless you have a special medical condition, there is no need to be concerned. Unfortunately, many people get most of their protein from meat, which tends to be high in the bad fats. The best sources of protein are plant foods along with small amounts of lean meat, poultry, or fish.

Vitamins and Minerals

Vitamins help regulate the body's inner workings. Minerals are part of many cells and cause important reactions to happen in the body. All vitamins and minerals are essential for survival and health, and most of us can get what we need from healthy eating. But the minerals, sodium, potassium, and calcium stand out because they are related to current health problems, and many of us eat either too much or too little of these nutrients.

Sodium

There is sodium in most of the foods that we eat—from tiny amounts in some plant foods to higher amounts in some animal foods. But the real culprits are processed foods, which typically have many different forms of sodium added to them. We also get sodium from salt. Small changes can help a lot.

For some people, too much sodium can raise blood pressure. This can lead to heart disease, stroke, and kidney failure. Cutting back on sodium can help lower blood pressure, and prevent hypertension (high blood pressure).

It is easy to get enough sodium to meet our bodies' needs. Thus, most of us get way too much. We need only about 500 milligrams (mg) a day (this is the amount of sodium in less than a fifth of a teaspoon of table salt). Yet most people eat 8–12 times that much. Adults should limit sodium intake to less than 2,300 milligrams a day, which is about the amount in 1 teaspoon of table salt. People who have high blood pressure, kidney disease, or diabetes, may need to limit sodium even more. Middle-aged or older adults and African-American people may need to limit their sodium intake more. Check with your doctor about your situation.

For example, Juanita's care partner, Mo, was having trouble with fluid retention in her legs and her blood pressure was high. Juanita found that cutting back on the sodium at meals by eating fewer high sodium takeout foods, both she and her care partner felt better.

Our love of sodium is learned. It is not something we are born with. Cutting down your sodium intake takes some getting used to, but over time you will learn to enjoy the natural flavors of food. Here are some tips to help you keep your sodium intake in check:

- Always taste your food before salting it; many times, it is good as is.
- Don't add salt to food when cooking; season with spices, herbs, pepper, garlic, onion, or lemon.
- Use fresh or frozen minimally processed poultry, fish, and lean meat, instead of canned, breaded, takeout, or prepared packaged food.
- Choose foods labeled "low sodium" or those with 140 milligrams or less per serving. (Check out the Nutrition Facts food label for this information.) You will find more about food labels on pages 184–185.
- Save high-sodium food for special occasions. Serve bacon, luncheon or deli meats, frozen dinners, packaged mixes, salted nuts, bottled salad dressings, and high-sodium canned soups on rare special occasions, not as everyday fare.
- In restaurants, ask that your food not be salted during preparation.

Potassium

Potassium is a mineral that helps regulate our heartbeat, among other important jobs it does in the body. In contrast to sodium, which raises blood pressure, potassium can help lower blood pressure. When you follow the guidelines for healthy eating on page 182, it is easy to get enough potassium. Many vegetables are good sources, including broccoli, peas, lima beans, tomatoes, potatoes, sweet potatoes, and winter squash. Other sources include nuts and fruits, such as citrus fruits, cantaloupe, bananas, kiwifruit, prunes, and apricots. Meat, poultry, some fish (salmon, cod, flounder, and sardines), milk, buttermilk, and yogurt also contain some potassium.

Calcium

You probably know that calcium helps build bones, but did you know that it is also needed for blood clotting and also helps regulate blood pressure? Calcium may also help protect against colon cancer, kidney stones, and breast cancer. Unfortunately, most people, especially women and young children, do not get enough calcium. Most women under 60 should get the amount of calcium found in 3 cups of milk every day. In addition to milk, other good sources of calcium are yogurt and kefir (a beverage similar to yogurt); calcium-fortified soy, rice, and almond milks and orange juice; seaweed; and leafy greens (bok choy, kale, Brussels sprouts, broccoli, kohlrabi, collards, and some other leafy greens). But note that our bodies cannot use the calcium in spinach, Swiss chard, and rhubarb, so these are not good sources. Most fruits are low in calcium, except for dried figs (there's not

Guidelines for Healthy Eating

Here are some guidelines for daily healthy eating for people eating 2,000 calories a day. You notice we refer to cup equivalents. Within a food group, foods can come in many forms and are not created *equal* in terms of what counts as a *cup* or an ounce. Some foods are more concentrated, and some are airier or contain more water. *Cup-* and ounce-*equivalents* identify the amounts of foods from each food group with similar nutritional content. We have not given equivalents below. A good place to find these is https://health.gov/dietaryguidelines/2015/guidelines/appendix-4/. We offer the following to get started. If you want more information, please talk to your health provider or a registered dietitian.

Vegetables: 2½ cups equivalents per day
Each **week** this can be broken down into:

- **Dark green vegetables:** 1½ cups equivalent
- **Red and orange vegetables:** 5½ cups equivalent
- **Beans and peas:** 1½ cups equivalent
- **Starchy vegetables:** 5 cups equivalent
- **Other vegetables:** 4 cups equivalent

Fruit: 2½ cups equivalent per day

Grains: 6 ounces equivalents per day with as much of this as possible being whole grains

Dairy: 2 cups or the equivalent per day

Protein: 6½ ounce equivalent per day
Each **week** this can be broken down into:

- Seafood: 15 ounces equivalent
- Meat, poultry, eggs: 26 ounces equivalent
- Nuts, seed, soy products: 5 ounces equivalent

Oils: a little less than an ounce equivalent per day (an ounce of oil equals two tablespoons)

Limit calories from other foods such as cookies, ice cream, and chips to 260 calories **per day**. You can find the calories on food labels which are discussed in the box "The Nutrition Facts Label" on pages 184–185.

much in fig cookies, though!) and the tropical cherimoya (custard apple).

Water

Water is the most important nutrient. Like the air you breathe, you cannot live without water. More than half of your body is made up of water, and each cell is bathed in it. Water helps keep our kidneys working, helps prevent constipation, and helps us eat less by making us feel full. It also helps prevent some medication side effects.

Although most people can last weeks without food, you cannot typically live longer than a week or so without water. Most adults lose about 10 cups of water a day. However, most people usually have no problem getting the six to eight glasses each day many experts recommend. This is especially true when you consider that most liquids and foods we eat contain some water so you get water from what you eat as well as what you drink. Even the driest cracker has a tiny bit of water.

To see if you are drinking enough, check your urine. If it is light-colored, you are fine. When you get thirsty, you need more water. Milk, juice, and many fruits and vegetables are good sources of water. Beware, though: Coffee, tea, and other drinks with caffeine or alcohol can cause you to lose water. Do not depend on these drinks for your majority of water.

If you have kidney disease or congestive heart failure or are taking special medications, your needs for water could be different. Talk to a registered dietitian or your health care provider.

Eating for Specific Long-Term Conditions*

The guidelines for healthy eating (on page 182) can be used to create a general plan designed to work for most of us. However, some people have different needs and likes. Our needs and likes depend on age, sex, body size, activity level, health, and even availability and affordability of food. In the following sections, we present some eating information and guidelines for selected long-term health issues.

Diabetes

When you eat a meal, the body breaks down the carbohydrates into glucose, the basic fuel for the body's cells. Glucose is then absorbed into the bloodstream. Protein and fat usually contribute little to the body's blood sugar. The hormone insulin takes the glucose (blood sugar) into the cells. In people with diabetes, cells do not absorb or use glucose very well. Glucose therefore builds up in the bloodstream and can lead to other serious health problems. Managing blood sugar levels is one of the prime goals in diabetes care and involves many different things. These include taking medication, exercising, and keeping a careful eye on diet.

In the past, people with diabetes were told that they could not eat sweets and that they could only eat certain types of carbohydrates. We now know that what a person with diabetes eats should meet their individual needs. There is no perfect diet, but everyone with diabetes needs to watch what and how much they eat. This is especially true for carbohydrates. The American Diabetes Association (ADA) recommends that all people with diabetes eat fewer foods that are high in sugar and foods made with white flour or white rice. They should instead focus on carbohydrates from vegetables, beans, fruits, milk, yogurt and foods made with whole grains. Drinking sugar-sweetened beverages, such as soft drinks (soda pop), and other drinks, such as energy drinks and many juice products, and eating foods with high amounts of processed grains and added sugar, such as breads, pastry and some cereals, is strongly discouraged. Also, because people with diabetes are at higher risk of heart disease, the type of fat they eat is especially important; emphasis should be on the good fats and avoiding the trans fats.

*Please note that while this section is written for you the caregiver, it also applies to your care partner.

The Nutrition Facts Label: "What's in That Package of Food?"

Food labels tell us what is in the packaged foods we eat. The Nutrition Facts panel and the ingredients list are two important parts of food labels. They tell you what is in the food you will be eating, which can help you make more informed and better choices. This can be whether you need to cut back or to increase what you need to eat certain foods or nutrients. Reading and understanding the information on food labels can be overwhelming. Here we focus on helping you understand the key parts of the label.

Serving Size

This is the first thing to look at; all the other information on the label is based on one serving, and many packages contain more than one serving. If the serving size on the package is not the amount you usually eat, you must consider that when you read the rest of the label and change all the amounts accordingly. For example, a serving of rice of 1/2 cup and if you eat a whole cup, you will have eaten two servings.

Calories Are a Measure of Energy

The calories are given for one serving. So, if you eat more or less than one serving, you will have to do a little arithmetic. For example, a serving of corn is 1/2 cup or one ear, and has 80 calories. If you eat two ears of corn you have eaten two servings and 160 calories.

Total Fat and Cholesterol

The Total Fat number lists the amount of all fats in grams (a unit of weight; 30 g = about 1 oz.) in one serving. The bad fats (saturated and trans fats) are specifically listed because of their impact on our health and because many people consume more of these fats than is healthy. The dietary guidelines suggest eating no more than 20 grams of saturated fat a day (based on a 2,000-calorie intake) and as little as possible of trans fats. Although this information is not required to be listed on the label, you might see the good fats, polyunsaturated and monounsaturated fats, also listed. Remember our warning about trans fats! Be aware that food companies can list food as having no trans fats even if they have up to half a gram of trans fats per serving. Thus, you may still be eating trans fats especially if you eat more than one serving. If the ingredients list includes the words *partially hydrogenated* or *hydrogenated,* then the product contains trans fat (even if the amount of trans fats per serving in the Nutrition Facts panel is 0 grams). Trans fats can add up! Trans fats can raise your blood cholesterol level more than the cholesterol from food, increasing your risk of heart disease.

The Cholesterol line tells you the amount of cholesterol by serving size. Because cholesterol is found only in animal foods, this line will show 0 grams for foods that don't contain any animal products. However, if you are watching the amount of cholesterol you eat, you still need to be careful because even if a food does not have any cholesterol, it could have bad or trans fat, particularly if it is a processed food. These foods could cause your body to make cholesterol.

To determine if the fat or cholesterol is high or low, look at the "% Daily Value" column. Any value that is 5% or less is low and 20% or more is high. Note that percent values are not available for trans fats and protein, as there are no recommended daily values.

Nutrition Facts

8 Servings Per Container

Serving size	**2/3 cup (55 g)**
Amount per serving	
Calories	**230**
	% Daily Value*
Total Fat 8 g	**10%**
Saturated Fat 1 g	**5%**
Trans Fat 0 g	
Cholesterol 0 mg	**0%**
Sodium 160 mg	**7%**
Total Carbohydrate 37 g	**13%**
Dietary Fiber 4 g	**14%**
Total sugars 12 g	
Includes 10 g Added Sugars	**20%**
Protein 3 g	
Vitamin D 2 mcg	10%
Calcium 260 mg	10%
Iron 8 mg	10%
Potassium 235 mg	10%

*The % Daily Value (DV) tells you how much a nutrient in a serving of food contributes to a daily diet. 2,000 calories a day is used for general nutrition advice.

Sodium

Surprising to some, most of the sodium in our diet comes from processed foods, not from the salt we add to foods. The dietary recommendations for adults is to consume less than 2,300 milligrams of sodium per day. In the Nutrition Facts label example, that product contains 7% of the recommended daily amount.

Total Carbohydrate, Dietary Fiber, Total Sugars, and Added Sugars

This section of the label breaks out values for carbohydrates, dietary fiber and sugars. It is important for people who want or need to watch or count their carbohydrates. This section of the label also helps you to see if a food is high or low in fiber. Most of us should be eating more fiber.

The Total Sugars row includes the sugars naturally found in food such as those found in fruit or milk as well as those which are added during preparation or packaging. There are many kinds of added sugars in foods, including high fructose corn syrup, honey, malt syrup, molasses, and corn sweetener. The recommendation is to eat less than 10% of daily calories from added sweeteners, which are found in foods such as soda, sport and energy drinks, baked goods, sweet snacks, dairy desserts, candy, and jams. This is important because it is difficult to meet your nutrient needs and calorie limit if 10% or more of your daily calories come from added sugar.

In addition to the Nutrition Facts labels, foods with more than one ingredient must have an ingredient list. This list tells you what is in the food with the ingredient adding the most weight coming first, and going down to the ingredient weighing the least. If you see sugar or added sugars (high fructose corn syrup, honey, malt syrup, molasses, and corn sweetener) listed as the first ingredients, then that food likely contains more sugar than anything else.

You will see that vitamin D and the mineral potassium are also listed. They play significant roles in bone and heart health, respectively, and because many people do not get enough of these two nutrients it is helpful to know how much you are getting (or not getting).

If you have diabetes, please also read the section on heart disease on page 187. Unfortunately, heart disease is the number one complication of diabetes so people with diabetes should follow the recommendations for both diabetes and heart disease.

The American Diabetes Association also encourages the use of the Create Your Plate to plan meals (Figure 10.2). This is the idea of dividing your plate (recommending a 9½ diameter plate) in half. Then take one of those halves and divide it in half again. You should now have three sections. Use the following guidelines to add food to your plate to create a healthy and balanced meal:

- Half of your plate should be non-starchy vegetables, such as spinach, greens, carrots, lettuce, cabbage, bok choy, broccoli, green beans, tomatoes, cauliflower, salsa, cucumber, okra, peppers, mushrooms, beets, or turnips.
- In one of the small sections, choose starchy foods with emphasis on whole grains, such as whole grain bread, cereal, brown rice, pasta, corn tortillas, dal, oatmeal, hominy grits, cooked beans or peas, potatoes, corn, lima beans, green peas, or sweet potatoes,
- In the remaining small section, choose meat or meat substitute, such as chicken or turkey (without the skin), fish, lean cuts of beef or pork, eggs, low-fat cheese, or tofu.
- Add one 8-ounce glass of non- or low-fat milk, or 6 ounces of light yogurt, and a small piece of fruit or a 1/2 cup of fruit salad.

The following are some general suggestions for healthy eating if you or your care partner have diabetes:

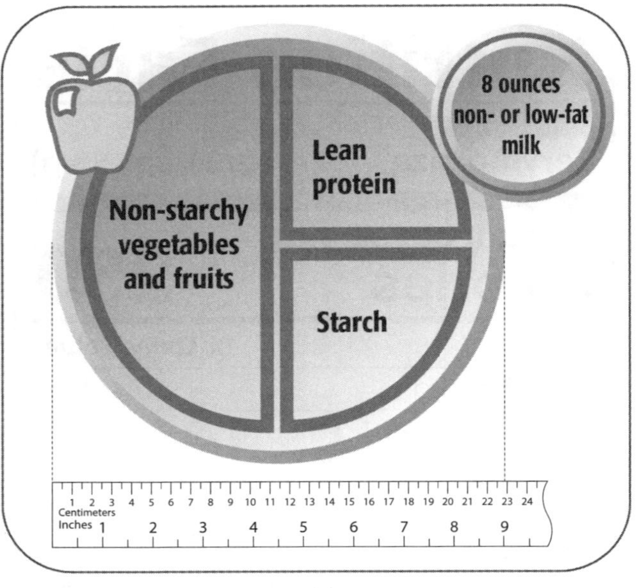

Figure 10.2 **Create Your Plate from the American Diabetes Association (ADA)**

- Use the Create Your Plate (see Figure 10.2) plan for your meals.
- Start each day with something to eat. Eating something in the morning is truly "breaking the fast." It helps fuel the body after a long night of foodless resting; it gives us energy to start the day's activities.
- Regularly space your meals and snacks over the day; don't skip meals. Eating regularly spaced meals at predictable planned times gives your body the chance to produce and use its insulin and time for your medication to work to keep up your energy level. The number of meals you eat and the time between your meals will vary depending on your personal health and lifestyle. You might eat three meals a day, but some people prefer or need to eat smaller meals more frequently.
- Eat the same amount of food at each meal, including snacks. This helps you maintain an even energy flow and blood sugar level

throughout the day. Skipping meals or alternating large meals with small meals can throw off your energy level. It can also lead to overeating or making poorer, less healthy food choices. This can, in turn, cause swings in your blood sugar and result in symptoms such as irritability, shakiness, poor sleep, mood swings, or pain or difficulties breathing due to stomach bloating, heartburn, and indigestion.

Because people with diabetes are at increased risk for heart disease and stroke, they should eat fewer bad fats (saturated and trans fats; see pages 177–179). Replace the bad fats (but don't add to your overall fat intake) with the good fats, such as olive and canola oils. In addition, eat more plant foods and consume less sodium by eating fewer processed, takeout, and prepared foods. Use the salt shaker sparingly, if at all. If you are carrying some extra pounds, the ADA recommends losing 5–7% of your weight. For example, if you weigh 150 pounds work on losing 8–10 pounds, this can help lower your blood sugar. (See "Tips for Choosing Healthier Carbohydrates and Increasing Fiber" on page 178 and "Tips for Choosing Good Fats and Healthier Fats" on page 179.)

Heart Disease and Stroke

Healthy eating for people with heart disease or those who have had a stroke usually means making choices that keep the arteries from hardening or getting clogged. High blood cholesterol levels are a major risk factor for heart disease. Most of the fat you and your care partner eat should come from the good fats (unsaturated fats) and very little from the bad (saturated) fats. You should eat little to no trans fat. Also, increase the amount of fiber you eat. Fiber, especially from oats, barley, dried beans and peas, lentils, apples, citrus fruits, carrots, and psyllium seed, can be helpful in managing blood cholesterol. Eating less salt and sodium can also help prevent or control high blood pressure. Try to limit the daily total amount of sodium you get to no more than that found in one teaspoon of table salt (about 2,300 milligrams). Use herbs, spices, lemon, and vinegar for flavor. Another thing that can affect heart health and diabetes is triglycerides. Triglycerides are a type of fat found in your blood and in food. The amount of this fat in your blood is also made worse by consuming bad fats and a high-carbohydrate diet, especially one containing refined and added sugars, such as honey, other sweeteners, sodas and sugary drinks, and anything made with white flour, such as breads and pastries. To help keep triglycerides in check, eat less of these foods. Exercising, not smoking, maintaining a healthy weight, and avoiding alcohol can also help. If you are overweight losing 5–7% of your weight will help. For example, if you weigh 150 pounds work toward losing 8–10 pounds (See "Tips for Choosing Healthier Carbohydrates and Increasing Fiber" on page 178 and "Tips for Choosing Good Fats and Healthier Fats" on page 179.)

Lung Disease

If you or your care partner have lung disease, especially emphysema, it is sometimes recommended that you increase the amount of protein you eat. This helps increase energy, strength, and the ability to fight lung infections. When it is hard for you to eat enough food, as when you have little or no appetite, try eating higher-calorie foods—fruit nectars instead of juice, dried fruit instead of fresh fruit, sweet potato instead of white potato—or try nibbling on a small handful of nuts over the course of the day.

If you have specific concerns about what to eat, talk to a registered dietitian. These professionals can tell you what's best for you as well as help you fit our general recommendations to your unique health needs.

Osteoporosis

Osteoporosis damages bones so that they are brittle and easily broken. It has been called a silent disease because its first symptom can be a bone fracture, especially in the spine, hip, or wrist. However, it is never too late to help slow its progress. You can do so by getting enough calcium and vitamin D, regularly doing muscle-strengthening and weight-bearing exercise (e.g., walking; see Chapter 9, Exercising for Health and Wellness), and following your health care professional's recommendations, such as taking prescribed medications for bone loss. Osteoporosis is technically not a calcium-deficiency disease, and after bone has been lost, getting more calcium will not fix it. But getting vitamin D along with enough calcium can help the body absorb the calcium.

Everybody needs to eat some calcium every day. The best sources are milk and foods made from milk. Some people avoid milk products because they don't like them, do not eat animal products, or have problems digesting milk sugar (lactose intolerance). You can still get enough calcium from your diet even if you have problems with milk sugar. Many people can enjoy milk products if they eat them in small amounts or eat other foods at the same time (e.g., cereal with milk); if they use lactase tablets to help digest the lactose; or if they can eat calcium-rich foods other than milk, such as kefir or yogurt. There are also some fruits and vegetables that are high in calcium, including kale, collard greens, bok choy, and broccoli. Other sources include calcium-treated tofu; cooked dried beans; and foods with added calcium, such as soymilk, juices, cereals, and pasta. If you think you may not be getting enough calcium, talk to your healthcare provider or a registered dietitian about your diet and whether calcium supplements are needed to meet your calcium needs.

Overcoming Challenges and Making Healthy Food Choices

In this section, we list some common challenges caregivers and care partners face as they try to make better food choices. After each challenge is a strategy for addressing it.

> *"Healthy food doesn't taste the same as food I am used to. When I eat, I want something with substance, like meat and potatoes or a piece of apple pie! The healthy stuff just doesn't fill me up!"*

Making healthier food choices does not mean that you can never eat something you want or crave. It means trading off to occasionally fit in favorite foods while making healthy choices most of the time. And healthy food doesn't have to be unappetizing or dull. There

Being Mindful about What, Why, and When You Eat

Do you eat when you're bored, down in the dumps or sad, or feeling lonely? Many people find comfort in food or just eating as something to do when they need to take their minds off something or have nothing else to do. Some eat when they are feeling angry, anxious, or depressed. At these times, it is easy to lose track of what and how much you eat. Unfortunately, these are often also the times when celery sticks, apples, or popcorn just won't do. Here are some ways to help control these urges:

- Keep a food-mood diary. Every day, list what, how much, and when you eat. Note how you are feeling when you have the urge to eat. Try to spot patterns so you can anticipate when you will want to eat without being overly hungry.
- If you catch yourself feeling bored and are thinking about eating, ask yourself, "Am I really hungry?" If the answer is no, make yourself do something else for 2–3 minutes—go for a short walk around the house or around the block, brush your teeth, work on a jigsaw puzzle, read one article in the news, or play a computer game.
- Keep your mind and hands busy. Getting your hands dirty is helpful (as with gardening).
- Write down action plans for when these situations arise. Sometimes it is easier to refer to the written word than to remember what you said you would do.

Antoine was having a difficult time keeping his weight down after he quit his job to take care of his care partner, Millie. He felt he was hungry most of the time and snacking whenever he went into the kitchen. After meeting with his dietitian, keeping a food diary, and writing down his mood when he was hungry, he was surprised to learn that he was snacking because he was bored. Antoine found that being mindful or aware when going into the kitchen helped him to eat less. He also tried to be mindful when eating out or socializing where tempting foods were present. He learned that he could do other things instead of eating to occupy his free time. For him, distractions, such as playing a computer game, checking out his vegetable garden, or calling a friend, helped him to snack less. He also found that when he waited to snack until he was hungry and not just bored, he enjoyed his snack more.

are many excellent cookbooks with healthy recipes, as well as internet sites with good, healthful recipe ideas.

"But I love to cook!"

If you love to cook, you are in luck. Take a new cooking class, begin watching one on television, buy a new cookbook on healthy cooking, or find an internet site with healthy recipes. If you have odds and ends, even leftovers, in your kitchen, do a computer search to find healthy recipes that include those ingredients. Play around with ways to modify your favorite recipes, making them lower in fat, sugar, and sodium.

"Food doesn't taste as good as before."

Many things can affect how food tastes. Having surgery, taking certain medications, being on oxygen, and even the common cold can make food taste off, bad, or funny. When this happens, you tend to eat less. Many people automatically add extra salt to their food to try to make it taste better. Unfortunately, this can cause you to retain water or feel bloated, which can increase blood pressure.

The following suggestions can make foods taste better:

- Use herbs (basil, dill, oregano, tarragon) and spices (cinnamon, cumin, curry, ginger, nutmeg) while cooking or sprinkle them on top of finished dishes.
- Squirt fresh lemon juice on foods.
- Use a small amount of vinegar in or on top of hot or cold foods. There are dozens of different kinds, from balsamic and fruit-flavored varieties; experiment with new flavors.
- Add healthy ingredients to the foods you usually eat (e.g., carrots or barley to soup, or dried fruits and nuts to salads) to give them more texture and make them tastier.
- Chew your food slowly and well. This will allow the food to remain in your mouth longer and release more flavor.

If the lack of taste is keeping you or your care partner from eating enough, you might need to add more calories to your meals or snacks.

"It takes so long to prepare meals and I do not have any time. By the time I'm done, I'm too tired to eat."

This is a common issue, especially for caregivers who have so many responsibilities and may not have much energy. This situation calls for planning to make sure that you do eat. Here are some hints to help:

- When you do have some energy, cook enough for two, three, or even more servings or meals, especially if it is something you like. Freeze the extra in single sized portions.
- Do a meal exchange with friends or family, and freeze food in single-serving sizes for times when you are tired.
- Break your food preparation into steps, resting in between.
- Ask for help. This is an important caregiver skill. When people ask what they can do to help, suggest they bring you and your care partner a meal once a week or once a month.

Janela finds that on some days, by the time dinner rolls around she is too tired to prepare a meal. She discovered a way to handle that problem that was truly enjoyable. She asks her granddaughter to come over once a week or once every two weeks. Together they prepare food for several meals, such as whole-grain lasagna with her care partner's favorite mushroom sauce, vegetarian chili, and baked chicken breasts. They then put together one-serving packages that fit in her small freezer. Now, when she is tired, she can reheat two packages and not only enjoy her meal but also remember the fun time she had preparing it with her granddaughter.

Thanks to the internet and food delivery services, you can now have food delivered quickly from almost any restaurant. There are also services that deliver the ingredients for an entire healthy meal with instructions about how to cook it. If you do not know how to do this, ask a tech savvy person. If you cannot afford this, call your Area Agency on Aging and ask about Meals on Wheels.

"Sometimes eating causes discomfort."

"I'm afraid I'll become short of breath while I'm eating."

"I really have no appetite."

People who experience shortness of breath or who find it difficult and physically uncomfortable to eat meals tend to eat less. For some, eating a large meal causes stomach problems such as indigestion, discomfort, or nausea. Indigestion, along with a full stomach, reduces the space for your breathing muscles to expand and contract.

If these are challenges you or your care partner sometimes face, try the following:

- Eat four to six small meals a day, rather than the usual three large meals. You will be using less energy for each meal.
- Avoid foods that produce gas or make you feel bloated. Many foods can produce gas, although foods affect people differently. Among the more common foods that can cause discomfort are cabbage, broccoli, brussels sprouts, onions, beans, and certain fruits, including bananas, apples, melons, and avocados.
- Eat slowly, take small bites, and chew your food well. You should also pause occasionally during a meal. Eating quickly to avoid an episode of shortness of breath can cause shortness of breath. Slowing down and breathing evenly reduces the amount of air you swallow while eating.
- Do a relaxation exercise about half an hour before mealtime, or take time out for a few deep breaths during the meal.
- Choose food that is easy to eat, such as yogurt or pudding, or to drink, like a shake, a smoothie or fruit nectar.

"I love to eat out, so how do I know if I'm eating well?"

Whether it is because you don't have time, you hate to cook, or you just don't have the energy to shop for groceries or fix meals, eating out may suit your needs. This is not necessarily bad if you know how to make the best choices possible.

- Select restaurants that have a variety of menu items prepared in healthy ways (e.g., grilled or steamed dishes in addition to or instead of fried foods).
- Order small plates or appetizers rather than an entire meal.
- Ask for a takeout box as soon as the server comes to take your order and put half of the food on your plate in the box before you take a bite.
- Request salad dressing on the side and dip your fork into the dressing before spearing each mouthful.

"I or my care partner snack while doing other things—watching TV, working on the computer, or reading."

If mindless snacking is a problem, plan ahead by keeping a list of healthier snacks to grab. Here are some examples:

- Rather than snack crackers, chips, and cookies, munch on fresh fruit, raw vegetables, or fat-free or plain popcorn.
- Measure out your snack in a single-portion size and put one portion in a separate small bag or container so you won't be tempted to eat more.

- Put healthy snacks at eye level in the refrigerator and cabinet. Put less healthy food out of sight.
- Make specific places at home and work "eating areas," and don't eat anywhere else.
- If weight is a problem for you or your care partner, healthy eating is important whether you want to lose weight and keep it off, maintain your weight, or gain weight.

Healthy eating is about the food choices you make most of the time. It is not about never being able to eat certain foods. There is no such thing as a perfect food or a bad food. Healthy eating means enjoying a moderate amount of a wide variety of minimally processed foods in the proper amounts for your body while allowing for occasional treats. Eating this way can help you maintain your and your care partner's health, help prevent future health problems, and help you manage any disease symptoms.

Eating healthy for you and your care partner might mean making some changes to what you are doing now. These changes could include making more food choices that are higher in good fats and fiber and fewer food choices that are high in bad and trans fats, sugar, and sodium. If you choose to make some of the changes suggested in this chapter, think of this as doing something positive and wonderful for yourself, not as punishment. As a self-manager, it's up to you to find the changes that are best for you. And if you experience setbacks, identify the problems and work at resolving them. You can do it!

Suggested Further Reading

Capron, Mary Ellen, and Elana D. Zucker. *The Ultimate Cooking Companion for At-Home Caregivers*. Upper Saddle River, NJ: Prentice Hall, 2003.

Designed to assist homemaker/home health aides as they plan and cook meals. http://amzn.to/2GrKjeL

Gaines, Fabiola Demps, and Roniece Weaver. *The New Soul Food Cookbook for People with Diabetes*. Alexandria, VA: American Diabetes Association, 2006.

Katz, Rebecca, and Mat Edelson. *The Cancer-Fighting Kitchen: Nourishing, Big-Flavor Recipes for Cancer Treatment and Recovery*. Berkeley, CA: Ten Speed Press, 2017.Features science-based, nutrient-rich recipes that are easy to prepare. http://amzn.to/2C7JGZH

Tarbox, Jonathan, and Taira Lanagan Bermudez. *Treating Feeding Challenges in Autism: Turning the Tables on Mealtime*. London: Elsevier/Academic Press, 2017.

Focuses on the few but highly effective feeding treatment procedures. http://amzn.to/2BDrxlx

Wilson, J. Randy. *I-Can't-Chew Cookbook: Delicious Soft-Diet Recipes for People with Chewing, Swallowing, or Dry-Mouth Disorders*. Alameda, CA: Hunter House Publishers, 2003. Offers new and creative ways to prepare food for the person on a soft-food diet. http://amzn.to/2HsGyaf

Woodruff, Sandra, and Leah Gilbert-Henderson. *Soft Foods for Easier Eating Cookbook: Easy-to-Follow Recipes for People Who Have Chewing and Swallowing Problems.* Garden City Park, NY: Square One, 2010.

Other Resources

Academy of Nutrition and Dietetics. http://www.eatright.org

AgingCare com provides healthy diet tips, nutrition information and benefits of physical activity. https://www.agingcare.com/nutrition-exercise

American Cancer Society. http://www.cancer.org

American Diabetes Association. http://www.diabetes.org

American Diabetes Association Create Your Plate. http://www.diabetes.org/food-and-fitness/food/planning-meals/create-your-plate/?referrer=https://www.google.com

American Heart Association. http://www.heart.org/nutrition

Center for Science in the Public Interest. https://www.cspinet.org

Center for Science in the Public Interest Nutrition Action Healthletter. http://www.cspinet.org

ChooseMyPlate.gov is a U.S. Food and Drug Administration tool to help estimate portions. https://www.choosemyplate.gov

Environmental Nutrition newsletter. http://www.environmentalnutrition.com

Food and Nutrition Information Center. http://www.nal.usda.gov/fnic

Harvard School of Public Health. http://www.hsph.harvard.edu

International Food Information Council Foundation. https://www.foodinsight.org

Mayo Clinic: "Nutrition and Healthy Eating." http://www.mayoclinic.com/health/nutrition-and-healthy-eating/MY00431

SuperTracker looks up the nutrition facts for foods that do not contain a label, such as fruits and vegetables. https://www.supertracker.usda.gov

Tufts University Health & Nutrition. http://www.healthletter.tufts.edu

U.S. Department of Health and Human Services, "Heart Healthy Home Cooking, African American Style." http://www.nhlbi.nih.gov/health/public/heart/other/chdblack/cooking.pdf

There are many online tools available to help you estimate portions, including the USDA tool SuperTracker (https://www.supertracker.usda.gov), where you can look up the nutrition facts for foods that do not contain a label, such as fruits and vegetables.

Chapter 11

Understanding Your Care Partner's Brain

In this chapter, we discuss some common conditions that can cause people to need a caregiver. We know that there are many reasons a person needs care. You may be caring for someone with a mental health disorder, such as schizophrenia, or maybe your care partner has a spinal cord injury, ALS, or some other condition. Unfortunately, we cannot outline every condition. For those of you who wish to find information about a condition not covered in this chapter, we suggest that you look for an organization serving that population. And even if your care partner's problem is not mentioned specifically in this chapter, there is still information in the rest of this book that can be useful to you as you provide assistance to your care partner.

Understanding Dementia

Dementia is a group of brain diseases. Early signs of dementia include memory problems, personality changes, or difficulty in understanding or remembering words. People can also have problems with activities such as driving, using the phone, handling their finances, and shopping. Over time, dementia gets worse. The course of the disease can take a year or two or up to 15 or 20 years. In the later stages of dementia, people can have hallucinations (seeing or hearing things that are not real) or paranoia (thinking that people are listening to or watching them). They can also have problems with bathing, dressing, toileting, transferring, and eating. At these later stages, people usually need care 24 hours a day.

Most people with dementia also have other chronic conditions such as high blood pressure, diabetes, or heart disease. Poor control of these conditions can cause the dementia to worsen more quickly. Thus, it is important to treat the whole person, not just the dementia. As a caregiver, your job is to understand all your partner's medical conditions and determine the best course of care. Your health care provider can help you in determining what lifestyle strategies and medications can be helpful. Organizations, such as the Alzheimer's Association and Parkinson Disease Foundation, can also help you learn about your partner's specific disease and, more importantly, connect you to people like you who are living the caregiving experience. There is also a list of resources at the end of this chapter. You do not have to do this by yourself. People with dementia may or may not be able to participate in their own care. There are at least two possible issues that can interfere with a person who has dementia from making their own decisions about care. The person might deny there is problem or they might not be capable of understanding or remembering what they need to do to care for themselves. As a caregiver, your job is to create a structured means of helping your care partner. It might help to remember that what you see as very difficult behavior is not your care partner's fault. It is the fault of the disease.

Unfortunately, all dementias get worse over time. As we write, there are no cures. As you will find in the rest of this book, there are many things that you can do to make your life less stressful and your care partner's life easier. These are very similar, no matter what the cause of dementia. For example, hearing loss and poor eyesight can contribute to worsening any dementia, so hearing aids or eyeglasses can help with both your and your care partner's lives easier. In the following content, we discuss the major types of dementia.

Alzheimer's Dementia

Greta had always been very involved. As she got older she did lots of volunteer work, played cards with her friends, and still managed to cook for her husband and babysit with her grandchildren from time to time. Her daughter first became concerned one day after Greta had been babysitting. When Greta's daughter returned home after work, her children were very hungry and out of sorts. That had never happened before. When her daughter investigated, she found out that Greta had given the children lunch at 9:30 and then taken them to the park for the rest of

Common Symptoms of Alzheimer's Dementia

Here are some common symptoms of the three Alzheimer's stages: mild, moderate, and severe:

Symptoms of Mild Alzheimer's Dementia

Problems remembering the right word, names, or things they have read

Problems with common tasks in work or social situations

Losing things

Problems with planning and organizing

Personality changes

Symptoms of Moderate Alzheimer's Dementia

Forgetfulness about events or history

Inability to remember address, phone number, or day of the week

Mood changes

Being withdrawn in social situations

Trouble controlling bladder or bowels

Changes in sleep, especially restlessness

Personality changes—repetitive behaviors, suspicion, or paranoia (thinking things are happening that are not real)

Symptoms of Severe Alzheimer's Dementia

Little or no awareness of recent experiences or where they are

Problems walking, sitting, and sometimes swallowing

Inability to recognize or remember people

Usually need 24-hour care

More likely to get infections, especially pneumonia

the day. Greta's daughter talked with her father who said that lately Greta seemed to be confused when driving, even when going to places that they had gone to for the last 20 years. Greta's daughter and husband both decided to watch her more closely and noticed that she was often angry—a very new and unusual development—and sometimes was forgetting words. They urged her to see a doctor. Greta was eventually diagnosed with early Alzheimer's dementia.

For older adults, Alzheimer's dementia is the most common source of dementia. In Alzheimer's dementia, the brain develops abnormal clumps of cells named amyloid plagues and tangled bundles of fibers called neurofibrillary or tau tangles. The medical community believes that these changes take place 10 years before there are any changes in behavior or memory. Unfortunately, there is no way to test for these changes. They can only be seen after death once an autopsy is conducted.

Lewy Body Dementia (LBD)

Lewy body dementia (LBD) is the second most common type of dementia after Alzheimer's. LBD affects 1.4 million Americans. The symptoms of Lewy body disease are similar to those of Alzheimer's but may also include symptoms such as ridged muscles, slow movements, and tremors. Often individuals with Lewy body disease have complex visual hallucinations that are well formed and detailed. They might also have fixed beliefs about events happening that have not been seen or reported by others.

Lewy body disease is caused by deposits of proteins (Lewy bodies) in the parts of the brain that control memory and movement. This is the same part of the brain that produces dopamine, a chemical that affects physical movement. The changes in dopamine production in individuals with LBD causes the symptoms that are similar to Parkinson's disease, such a slowness, muscle rigidity, and tremors. Medications for Parkinson's disease are often prescribed to treat these symptoms for individuals with this disease, but these drugs can cause significant side effects such as hallucinations, confusion, and delusions. If these medications are attempted, they should be used in small doses initially to assess if disease symptoms worsen from the treatment.

It might take a few years to obtain the right diagnosis, but doing so is key as LBD is often treated with specific drugs that are not effective for Alzheimer's. These drugs help improve your care partner's quality of life. Some medications should not be used for LBD as your care partner may be extremely sensitive or have a bad reaction. (See page 199 for a discussion of dementia medications.)

HIV-Associated Dementia or AIDs Dementia

Because Human Immunodeficiency Virus (HIV) can cross into the central nervous system, it can also cause dementia. This usually occurs in cases of advanced HIV disease. The virus can damage the ability to think, impairing memory and the ability to function. HIV-associated dementia can usually be prevented with early diagnosis and treatment of HIV disease.

Frontemporal Dementia (FTD)

Frontemporal dementia (FTD) has a wide range of symptoms and a slow onset and, thus, it is often misdiagnosed as a psychiatric disorder or another form of dementia. Often times, a full specialized neurological evaluation, called a neuropsychological test, is done in order to rule out psychiatric disease. FTD first causes progressive damage to the frontal and/or temporal lobes of the brain. FTD frequently starts as a gradual decline in behavior and language with no memory loss. As the disease continues, the individual loses the ability to plan or organize activities, behave appropriately, interact with others, and care for oneself. FTD often occurs in people in their 50s and 60s, but it can occur in people who are younger and to people up into their 80s.

Mixed Dementia

Many dementias could be a combination of two types of dementia. For example, vascular dementia (dementia that results when the brain does not get enough blood, which might happen with a stroke) may also be accompanied by Alzheimer's dementia This is not uncommon and a definite diagnosis often cannot be made. However, many kinds of dementia and their treatments are similar to Alzheimer's.

Dementia Treatment

All of these types of dementia have three stages (mild, moderate, and severe) similar to the stages of Alzheimer's. Treatment for all dementias is aimed at improving your care partner's quality of life and making your life as a caregiver easier.

Rena and Morris were both aware that Morris was becoming more forgetful. After much discussion, Morris went to the doctor and allowed Rena to come along. The diagnosis of dementia was devastating. The doctor suggested that they go home and come back in a week with questions and concerns. During the week, Rena and Morris talked about the diagnosis. Morris said he wanted to remain active and helpful to others if he could. He was also very clear that he did not want Rena to be a full-time caregiver. Morris was especially concerned about driving. A week later, when they talked with the doctor, it was suggested that Morris start on medications and that both he and Rena attend a group at the Alzheimer's Association. The doctor thought it best for Morris to consider giving up driving and suggested a driving evaluation be done at the local hospital to access Morris's ability. He also told Morris about a transportation program provided by the local senior center. Both Morris and Rena found support in their community, and Morris has become a speaker for the Alzheimer's Association. They both know that the disease will get worse, but working with their doctor and others have helped them make realistic plans to address different things that might happen.

With all dementias and brain disorders, you must work with your care partner's primary care provider and utilize community resources to help you and your partner manage the challenges of the disease. (Please see the resources at the end of this chapter as well as the information in Chapter 7, Getting Help.)

Dementia Medications

Medications used in the treatment of any of these dementias do not keep the disease from getting worse. Instead, they are used to help improve your partner's function and quality of life. For someone already taking many drugs to treat other conditions, the decision to add additional medications has to be made on what combination will give the best quality of life.

Two main classes of medications are prescribed to treat dementia. The first class consists of cholinesterase inhibitors and the second class is the N-methyl-D-aspartate (NMDA) receptor antagonists. The following is a discussion of common drugs used for dementias.

Cholinesterase Inhibitors and Dementia

Cholinesterase inhibitors compensate for the lack of an important brain biochemical called acetylcholine. These medications reduce the breakdown of acetylcholine. The three medications in this class are donepezil, rivastigmine, and galantamine. In general, these medications might provide small symptomatic improvements for some patients in the mild and moderate stages of Alzheimer's dementia. Side effects vary among the three medications but can include stomach upset, diarrhea, weight loss, tiredness, and dizziness. Severe side effects can include low heart rate, which can cause fainting.

The use of cholinesterase inhibitors for other forms of dementia has been studied and the impact has been quite limited. There is some evidence that cholinesterase inhibitors may improve cognition, behavior, and function for those with vascular dementia or mixed dementia. For people with Lewy body dementia, cholinesterase inhibitors may improve cognitive function as well as decrease hallucinations and other behavioral problems. In patients who have dementia associated with Parkinson's disease, the use of cholinesterase inhibitors might have some modest benefit in function. In addition, cholinesterase inhibitors could lessen some of the visual hallucinations.

Due to the limited impact of cholinesterase inhibitors, many practitioners give these medications for a two- to three-month trial and then reassess to see if there is improvement based on the patient's condition or caregivers' observations or on testing. If there is no improvement, often these medications are stopped. Occasionally, people will become worse after the medications are stopped. In this case, the medication could be restarted to see if behavior or function improve or if the new problems are simply due to the disease getting worse.

N-methyl-D-aspartate (NMDA) Receptor Antagonists and Dementia

Memantine is the most common N-methyl-D-aspartate (NMDA) receptor antagonist medication. Memantine works very differently than cholinesterase inhibitors. There is some evidence that memantine may impact Alzheimer's dementia's progress even though this is not seen in improved functioning. Memantine is used to treat people with moderate to severe Alzheimer's dementia. People with mild Alzheimer's dementia have not been shown to benefit. Dizziness is memantine's most common side effect, but confusion as well as agitation and delusions might also occur. Memantine appears to have fewer side effects than the cholinesterase inhibitors. Some medical providers use memantine in combination with a cholinesterase inhibitor for patients with advanced Alzheimer's. A combination capsule is available. Since it may be disease-modifying, a physician could continue memantine even when there is no improvement in symptoms.

Other Medications for Dementia

Antioxidants, such as vitamin E, have been studied for use in patients with Alzheimer's dementia. There is some suggestion that at doses of 2000 IU per day, vitamin E may slow functional loss for people with mild to moderate Alzheimer's. There are no findings of brain function improvement in general; therefore, vitamin E is not used in the care of people with Alzheimer's dementia as the impact is modest at best.

Many other potential dementia medications have been studied and shown not to be effective. These include estrogen replacement; non-steroidal anti-inflammatory medications (or NSAIDs) such as ibuprofen, naproxen, and aspirin; ginkgo biloba; cholesterol-lowering medications such as statins; and dietary supplements such as B vitamins and omega-3 fatty acids. Most medications have side effects. Because your care partner may not be aware of these, you need to be on the lookout and report anything you think might be a medication side effect to your care partner's provider. (See Chapter 12, Managing Medications.)

Antipsychotic Medications and Dementia

Antipsychotic medications are used to treat dementia-related agitation or psychosis that cannot be improved by behavioral techniques. The American Psychiatric Association has outlined how to best use these medications, weighing the risks versus benefits. These medications are often used for a limited time and attempts are made to decrease and/or stop the medications several months after behaviors are no longer present. As a caregiver, you play a central role in how these medications are used and on reporting how these medications impact your care partner. It is important to understand the goals of these medications and to learn how to assess if they are working.

Understanding Stroke

Strokes (also called CVAs or cerebrovascular accidents) are brain injuries caused when the flow of blood to the brain is stopped, which causes brain cell death. There are two main types of stroke: ischemic and hemorrhagic. The less common type of stroke is a hemorrhagic stroke. During a hemorrhagic stroke, a blood vessel in the brain bleeds and damages the surrounding brain tissue. Eighty percent of strokes are ischemic stokes. During an ischemic stroke, an artery in the brain is blocked and the area of the brain served by that artery is damaged. There are two kinds of ischemic strokes: embolic and thrombotic. An embolic stroke occurs when a blood clot travels from another part of the body through the blood stream and lodges in the brain. The lodged clot stops blood flow, causing damage to the brain. One of the most common causes of this type of stroke is atrial fibrillation (an irregular heart beat). Thrombotic strokes result from a fatty deposit (plaque) lining the blood vessel. These can break off and clog the blood vessel or get larger and block the artery.

The Effects of Strokes

The symptoms of a stroke could begin suddenly or slowly over hours to days. Strokes can cause long-term disability and sometimes death. The location of the stroke in the brain determines which part of the body is affected. The location also determines stroke patients' ability to speak, understand, or express themselves. It should also be noted that strokes can cause damage to the part of the brain that controls emotions. A person who has had a stroke may anger or cry very easily. This is not a character flaw and is not the fault of you, the caregiver. The changes in emotions are a result of the stroke.

The injury from a stroke might be temporary or permanent and the outcome depends on how much and which part of the brain is affected, how fast one gets treatment, and the treatment one receives after the stroke. Unfortunately, many stroke survivors are left with physical and/or cognitive (thinking) disabilities and might need supervision for the rest of their lives. This supervision may include medication management as well as lifestyle management, such as help with eating, exercise, hygiene, and emotions as well as social support. Depending on the damage caused by the stroke, this supervision and help may be minimal or might be very demanding. Treatment for strokes includes rehabilitation and medication. Rehabilitation could include physical, occupational, and/or speech therapy depending on your care partner's needs. It is usually best to start rehabilitation as soon as possible after the stroke, although benefit may continue for a year or more. Some communities have community stroke rehabilitation programs. Be sure to ask your health care provider about these.

Stroke Treatment and Medications

The medications that are prescribed post-stroke depend on the type of stroke as well as the type of damage that was done. For ischemic strokes caused by thrombosis or blood clots, medicines are prescribed to prevent blood clots from reforming. Clots can cause another stroke. The types of medicines used to prevent and treat ischemic strokes include medications that thin the blood to help prevent blood clots, antihypertensive medications that lower blood pressure to help stop the damage high blood pressure causes to blood vessel, and cholesterol-lowering medications. Cholesterol can damage or block arteries.

Antiplatelet Medications (Platelet Inhibition Medications)

Antiplatelet medications keep platelets (a part of your blood that helps it to clot) from sticking together and causing an unwanted blood clot. Examples of these medications include aspirin, clopidogrel (brand name Plavix), and dipyridamole (brand name Aggrenox).

Anticoagulant Medications

Anticoagulant medications (like antiplatelet medications) also can prevent blood clots from forming or help break up clots if they exist. Anticoagulants include warfarin (brand name Coumadin), rivaroxaban (brand name Xarelto), dabigatran (brand name Pradaxa), and apixaban (brand name Eliquis). For anyone who has a heart condition that affects the rhythm of the heart, there is a danger of clots forming. People with these conditions may need to take an anticoagulant permanently.

While antiplatelet and anticoagulant medications help prevent a future stroke, they also can cause bleeding. There is a fine line between enough medication to be helpful and too much which can be harmful. Therefore, all of these medications must be carefully monitored. These medications can also interact with other medications. An adjustment in dosage for all medications might be necessary whenever a new medication is started or an old medication stopped. This is usually done with blood tests. Finally, it is important to avoid falls, bumps, and accidents as any of these can cause bleeding. See Chapter 8, Preventing Injuries. As a caregiver, you need to be alert to changes, bleeding, and bruising. Do not hesitate to call your health care provider if you think that there could be a problem.

High Blood Pressure (Hypertension) Treatments and Medications

High blood pressure is a leading cause of stroke. High blood pressure damages the wall of blood vessels and can lead to smaller blood vessels becoming blocked by clots. This is why keeping blood pressure under control is so vital. A low-sodium (salt is our largest source of sodium) and low-cholesterol diet helps prevent further damage and future strokes. While lifestyle choices such as exercising, eating a healthy, balanced diet, and not smoking can help, people with high blood pressure usually also need to take medications. Medications to lower blood pressure include angiotensin-converting enzyme inhibitors such as angiotensin II, receptor blockers, diuretics, calcium channel blockers, such as diltiazem or amlodipine, and beta blockers, such as metoprolol or atenolol. There are many medications for high blood pressure, and sometimes people take more than one. Again, care must be monitored closely and make sure the right medications and the right doses are being taken.

Statins

Statins are medications that help prevent and shrink the plaque (the fatty deposit lining the blood vessels) that cause ischemic stroke. They work by lowering cholesterol, which causes plaque formation. Statin medications include

Taking Medications

Medications cannot help if they are not taken. People who have had strokes or wish to prevent strokes often have to take several medications. Sometimes, people do not want to take medication but do not tell their doctor. What follows is a story of three people. All three go to the doctor with the exact same high blood pressure. In each case, the doctor asks if they have been taking their medication. Each patient answers, "Yes." Lourdes has been taking the medication but has seen little change in her blood pressure. The doctor orders a second medication to be added to the first. Her blood pressure goes down. Henrik has been taking the medication and his blood pressure has been going down but is not quite low enough yet. The doctor notes this and increases the dose of his current medication. His blood pressure goes down. Bonnie has not been taking her medication regularly but is embarrassed to say so. The doctor prescribes a second medication, which the patient also does not take. She eventually has a stroke. The moral of this story is that you have to be honest and work with a doctor to get good treatment. Doctors cannot read minds.

atorvastatin, lovastatin, pravastatin, rosuvastatin, and simvastatin.

Antidepressant Medications

Depression is common one to six months after a stroke. Be aware of this and seek treatment if needed. Antidepressant medications can be helpful, but they can also interfere with some of the other medications taken post-stroke. Again, careful observation, monitoring, and working with health care providers is important.

Understanding Parkinson's Disease

Parkinson's Disease (PD) is a chronic movement disorder that continues to worsen over time. Unfortunately, we do not know the cause or cure of Parkinson's disease. We do know that the symptoms result from a loss of brain cells in a part of the brain called the substantia nigra. This is where dopamine, a chemical our bodies produce that affects movement, is made. The loss of these brain cells decreases the amount of dopamine available. This in turn affects movement and coordination.

The Effects of Parkinson's Disease

People with Parkinson's Disease are unable to control their movements. This could involve the hands, legs, arms, jaw, and feet. Symptoms can include tremors, rigidity, slowness of movement (bradykinesia), and impaired balance. There might also be changes in the voice, especially softening and decreased volume. Other symptoms of Parkinson's disease may include psychosis, hallucinations, daytime sleepiness, pain, fatigue, depression, and dementia. As a caregiver, you need to be aware of these symptoms and report changes when they occur as they may signal a need to change treatment.

Correct diagnosis is important as other diseases might present like Parkinson's disease but progress differently and may or may not respond to PD treatments. These other diseases are known as "Parkinson's Plus Syndrome" and feature classic symptoms of Parkinson's disease as well as additional symptoms that are distinguished from common Parkinson's.

Parkinson's Disease Treatment and Medications

Parkinson's disease treatments include medications and deep brain implantable stimulators. Deep brain implantable stimulation is used for some patients who no longer respond to medications. Drug treatments for Parkinson's disease, like treatments for dementia, do not slow or reverse the natural history and progression of the disease. However, some medications can be very helpful for some symptoms.

Parkinson's disease medications can interact with certain foods, other medications, vitamins, herbal supplements, over-the-counter (OTC) cold medications, and other remedies. The doctor and pharmacist must know all the medications your care partner is taking, including, but not limited to, OTC drugs, vitamins, and supplements. Both you and your care partner must know exactly how these medications should be taken and what foods or other medications should be avoided when taking these medications. For example, alcohol can change the action of some of these medications. Other medication must be taken on an empty stomach to ensure that they are fully absorbed and have maximum effect.

Levodopa and Carbidopa and Parkinson's Disease

Levodopa is the single most effective drug in Parkinson's disease management. As we noted earlier in this section, when a person has Parkinson's, less dopamine is produced; this drug helps replace the missing dopamine. Levodopa is usually given in combination with the drug carbidopa, which helps prevents the nausea caused by levodopa and enhances the action of levodopa. Levodopa is available in immediate-release and long-acting forms. Although levodopa might improve the function and decrease the symptoms, it does not decrease the progression of the disease.

Monoamine Oxidase B (MAO-B) Inhibitors and Parkinson's Disease

Selegiline, a MAO-B inhibitor, is used to help control Parkinson's disease symptoms. People taking this drug often also take levodopa and carbidopa. Selegiline works by increasing the amount of dopamine in the brain. It could help people with Parkinson's disease by decreasing the amount of levodopa/carbidopa needed to control symptoms. Selegiline also helps lengthen the time that the levodopa/carbidopa combination is effective. This drug should not be stopped without talking with a doctor. If the doctor advises that a patient stop taking selegiline, the patient needs to wait at least 14 days before beginning to take certain other medicines.

Dopamine Agonists and Parkinson's Disease

Dopamine agonist medications help improve utilization of existing dopamine in the brain. Dopamine agonists can be used effectively as a single drug in early stages of Parkinson's disease or in combination with carbidopa/levodopa after the disease has progressed. The two primary dopamine agonists are pramipexole and ropinirole. These medications are helpful and play a significant role in reducing tremors, allowing people with Parkinson's disease to carry out the activities of daily living, such as transferring, toileting, bathing, and walking.

Amantadine and Parkinson's Disease

Amantadine was initially developed as a flu treatment and was noted to have benefit for people with Parkinson's disease. It is often used in the early stages of Parkinson's disease with levodopa to treat prominent tremors or abnormality or impairment of voluntary movement.

Catechol-O-Methyl Transerase (COMT) Inhibitors and Parkinson's Disease

COMT inhibitor drugs are only used with levodopa. When a person takes levodopa, an enzyme in the body called catechol-O-methyl transerase (COMT) converts a portion of the levodopa into a form that is useless. These drugs block the COMT enzyme from doing this, which makes more levodopa available in the body for reducing Parkinson's disease symptoms. There are two COMT inhibitors: entacapone and tolcapone. Stalevo is a combination of carbidopa, levodopa, and entacapone. When people are taking stavelo, their liver enzymes might need to be monitored at the beginning of treatment and every six months.

Parkinson's Disease Medications and Psychosis

As noted earlier, psychosis (visual hallucinations and delusions) are common for people with Parkinson's disease. They could also have paranoia. These symptoms are most common as the disease progresses but can also be triggered by hospitalization. Management of these symptoms is dependent on identifying and treating the causes. Medications used for the treatment of Parkinson's disease are the most common cause. Sedatives, anxiolytics, and antidepressants are all medications that can cause psychosis. Be aware of this and if you see changes in your care partner's behavior, contact the doctor. Some of the medications might need changing. Do not try to adjust doses or medications yourself. If these symptoms continue despite attempts at dose adjustments, treatment options include low doses of atypical antipsychotic medications such as quetiapine and clozapine. As mentioned in the previous section on dementia (see page 199), people with Parkinson's disease and dementia may also benefit from cholinesterase inhibitors. These are not helpful in managing psychotic symptoms.

Understanding Traumatic Brain Injury

Traumatic brain injury (TBI) occurs when an individual suffers a jolt or a blow to the head and the brain is damaged and injured. Depending on the extent of the trauma, this can be a mild or severe injury. No two TBIs are alike and every traumatic brain injury patient is different. Traumatic brain injury is very common, and each year an estimated 2.5 million people in the United States suffer TBIs. Men are more than twice as likely to suffer from traumatic brain injury as women. Most people with traumatic brain injury seen in emergency rooms are the very young, but the highest hospitalization rates are for those over age 65. Many different types of injuries can lead to traumatic brain injury. Falls are the leading cause of TBI in older patients, followed by unintentional blunt trauma resulting from auto or bicycle accidents. Risk factors include lower socioeconomic status, alcohol and drug use, and underlying mental health and cognitive disorders. TBI, unfortunately, also is seen too often in young people in the military from combat injuries or from sports injuries.

The Effects of Traumatic Brain Injury

Concussions are the most common traumatic brain injuries and are usually considered a mild form of brain injury. If concussions are not recognized and treated early, there can be major complications. Concussions can be challenging for caregivers. The good news is that if they are treated, they usually improve in days to weeks.

More challenging are moderate and severe traumatic brain injuries. People who have experienced moderate and severe traumatic brain injury often have significant neurological (brain) damage. Depending on the part of the brain damaged, moderate to severe TBIs can interfere with daily function. If your care partner has experienced a moderate to severe TBI, your care partner might lose the ability to be independent (for example, to drive, bank, shop, and clean) and perhaps the ability to carry our activities of daily living, such as dressing, bathing, transferring, eating, and toileting. Depending on the extent of the injury, these changes can be permanent. Because TBIs happen suddenly, sometimes family members become caregivers without warning.

Based on the cause of the traumatic brain injury, there are different treatments. These are all aimed at dealing with the trauma (injury) and getting the best possible outcome. Once this care and treatment plan is started, the challenges for caregivers begins. Caregivers have to deal with and manage the challenges of caring for someone with a TBI, such as giving pills or using special equipment, as well as managing the functions and emotions of care partners. Like other brain diseases and conditions, traumatic brain injury impacts the entire family and is stressful to all those involved in the care of the person with TBI. Understanding how stressful this condition can be for the entire family is critical in developing care plans that are effective and can help all everyone adapt to the new "normal."

Individuals suffering from traumatic brain injury typically face a lot of personal concerns and issues. They may feel they are a burden to the family. In addition, they are likely to develop depression, anxiety, post-traumatic stress disorder (PTSD), or anger about their TBI. Management of these mental health issues is important. Plan for this and talk over what is happening or might happen with your care partner's health care providers. Remaining socially engaged is a key part of treatment. This is where friends, family, and support groups become very important. As a caregiver, you need to understand that care will be long term. Begin early to seek help and make plans. Caring for someone with TBI is like a running a marathon, it requiring requires slow, steady, and persistent effort. As a caregiver, you should not try to do this alone. Get some in-home assistance such as personal care attendants or home health aides. (See Chapter 7, Getting Help.) This will give you a chance to relax and do some of the things you want and need to do. Seek out short-term counseling and longer-term support from brain injury support groups. In addition, having a family and friend support network is important. (See the discussion about family meetings on pages 94–96.)

Traumatic Brain Injury Treatment and Medications

Treatment of traumatic brain injuries involves managing medical and behavioral issues.

Anticonvulsant Medications and TBI

Trauma to the brain can cause areas of the brain to be hyperactive (overly active). This can cause the nerve cells in the brain to cause a seizure. Anticonvulsant medications prevent these seizures by suppressing this activity. Anticonvulsant drugs include gabapentin, sodium valproate, topiramate, and carbamazepine. Common side effects of anticonvulsant medications include confusion, hair loss, lethargy, poor coordination, loss of appetite, nausea, vomiting, tremors, and weight gain. Sometimes the doctor will experiment to find out which drug is best for your care partner. Caregivers play a key role in observing and reporting changes.

Antidepressant Medications and TBI

Antidepressant medications treat anxiety, depression, insomnia, headaches, and pain. All of these symptoms can result from traumatic brain injuries. It might seem strange that antidepressants can treat so many things. In the case of TBIs, many symptoms have very similar origins in the brain. Examples of antidepressants include citalopram, amitriptyline, paroxetine, and sertraline. Side effects of these medications can include dry mouth, dizziness, confusion, constipation, drowsiness, skin rash, seizures, tremors, and urinary retention (that is, problems urinating). Observe care partners who are taking these medicines and report changes to the doctor.

Antipsychotic Medications and TBI

Antipsychotic medications are prescribed to treat some people with traumatic brain injuries who have severe mental or emotional issues or lose contact with reality (psychosis). In addition, antipsychotic medications are sometimes prescribed for severe sleep disturbances and aggressive or agitated behaviors. Antipsychotic medications include risperidone, quetiapine, and olanzapine. Common side effects of these drugs include blurred vision, dizziness, dry mouth, headache, low blood pressure, abnormal movements of the body, tremors, weight gain, and urinary retention (that is, problems urinating). If your care partner is taking antipsychotic medications, it is especially important that you observe and report changes as your care partner might not be an accurate reporter.

Understanding Post-Traumatic Stress Disorder

Post-traumatic stress disorder (PTSD) is a mental health disorder that develops after a person experiences or witnesses trauma. That trauma could be a life-threatening event, such as a natural disaster; an assault; military combat, some other violent experience; or involvement in an accident. PTSD is often long-term and severely disabling. People with PTSD may have nightmares, flashbacks (sudden and disturbing vivid memories of events in the past), or sleep disorders and may be on edge. In addition, they often are unable to take part in social, work, or family relationships. Another common symptom is blaming their problems on someone other than themselves.

Diagnosing Post-Traumatic Stress Disorder

PTSD is diagnosed after symptoms continue for at least four weeks after the traumatic event. Unfortunately, it sometimes takes years to diagnose PTSD because health care professionals, family, and friends fail to recognize the symptoms and connect them with a traumatic event. Early identification and treatment of this condition might help PTSD from becoming long-term. As a caregiver, you have a central role. You may know your care partner better than anyone else, and so it is up to you to report changes, tell health professionals about any trauma, and help your care partner find treatment. In many instances, people with post-traumatic stress disorder are unaware for a long time that they have this condition. We know of one case of a World War II officer with PTSD who returned home and had a successful career and was not diagnosed until fifty years after the trauma occurred. If your care partner is violent, or if you experienced the same trauma as your care partner, you might also suffer from PTSD. If you think this might be possible, ask your doctor for an assessment. We have said this before, but we will say it again: Being a caregiver should never expose you to physical harm. See Chapter 3, Dealing with Stress and Difficult Care Partner Behavior, to read more about this topic.

Post-Traumatic Stress Disorder Treatment

The first step to PTSD recovery is for the people who experience the trauma to recognize that they have been exposed to experiences that have altered their world views. This is often difficult, as people with PTSD are typically distrustful of others and unwilling to accept a "diagnosis" which brings with it an accompanying suggestion of weakness or mental instability. The most important step for people with PTSD is that they form trusting relationships with someone who can be impartial and an advocate for the individual in need. Your care partner must find a person to talk to who neither disbelieves nor judges your care partner's history in any way. Once individuals with PTSD have established trusting relationships, they are more open to observations and opinions.

People with PTSD typically are able to establish only one or two such trusting relationships and often disregard opinions of people whom they see as lacking traumatic life experiences. This could include you, the caregiver. Remember that this lack of trust comes from the condition, not the individual. Care partners might relate better to others who have experienced similar trauma than they do to their caregivers. In fact, your care partner may find your opinions, no matter how well intentioned, uninformed at best and patronizing at worst. Traumatized individuals are typically rigid in their thinking and easy to anger. Your care partner might see the world in black and white with very few shades of gray (in other words, either good or bad with nothing in between). If you or anyone else suggest that you know how they feel, you will be rejected. To combat this, listen to the story without adding your own ideas or assumptions. Just listen!

Many people with PTSD also abuse drugs and/or alcohol. They use these as coping mechanisms. This means that drug or alcohol use must be treated at the same time as one is trying to come to terms with a PTSD diagnosis. The continued use of illicit drugs or alcohol gets in the way of PTSD treatment and recovery. This is difficult, as traumatic events often encourage isolation, depression, distrust, and alienation. All of these can lead to drug or alcohol abuse. If you do not believe this, just think how often have you heard someone say, "I have had a really hard day. I need a drink." Unfortunately, alcohol and drugs are a common but not successful attempt to deal with stress. PTSD treatment aims at getting rid or decreasing the troubling symptoms as well as getting people to become aware of the triggers and what active steps they can take in preventing or getting rid of symptoms.

One of the common treatments for PTSD is cognitive behavioral therapy (CBT). Cognitive behavioral therapy can take place in individual therapy sessions or in groups and has been effective in treating people with a variety of mental health issues. CBT helps people develop personal coping strategies. In CBT treatment, patients learn to develop action plans and new ways of dealing with problems. CBT is often recommended when medications for PTSD are prescribed. We discuss PTSD medications in the following section.

Post-Traumatic Stress Disorder Medications

Before we talk about specific medications, it is important to review a few things. Not everyone responds to every medication. Therefore, it may take several trials of medications until the right one is found. Of course, medications will never work if they are not taken. Unfortunately, many people with PTSD do not believe they need medications and thus do not ever begin taking their medications, take less or more than was prescribed, or stop taking their medications altogether. For this reason, medications are often prescribed as part of a treatment plan that includes therapy, such as CBT, so the patient can be regularly encouraged by a therapist to take their medications. It is also very important that people with PTSD trust the health care providers who prescribe medications.

Sometimes, people do not respond to medications. Medications are typically more effective in treating mood disorders, agitation, anger, anxiety, and depression and less effective in managing flashbacks and behavioral issues. The medical community knows less about PTSD in older people than about military-related PTSD in younger people.

Antidepressants and PTSD

Selective serotonin reuptake inhibitors (SSRIs) include paroxetine or sertraline. SSRI antidepressants have been widely studied for people with PTSD. The amount of medication (the dose) is low at first and is slowly increased until symptoms decrease. If nothing happens within two months, then the dose is tapered off and another medication is tried. Patients should not stop these medications suddenly without their doctor's approval. Serotonin-norepinephrine reuptake inhibitors (SNRIs) are similar to the SSRIs and include venlafaxine extended release. Some older antidepressant medications, such as tricyclic antidepressants, and atypical antidepressants, such as mirtazapine, have not been shown to be effective for PTSD.

Second-Generation Antipsychotics (SGAs) and PTSD

If antidepressants and cognitive behavioral therapy are not working after multiple tries, second-generation antipsychotics (SGAs) may be prescribed for PTSD. Often, the individual with PTSD has agitation and psychotic symptoms combined with depression that require the use of these. Unfortunately, these medications do not have a strong evidence base to support their use. In particular, use of either risperidone or quetiapine is often tried.

Other Medications and PTSD

Alpha-adrenergic receptor blockers have been used to reduce nightmares and improve sleep for PTSD patients. The alpha-adrenergic receptor drug most often used is Prazosin, which is also used in the treatment of high blood pressure. It is used with SSRI medications and is usually given at a very low dose and then increased.

Sometimes people with PTSD are hypervigilant. This means that they are constantly searching for any sign of threat and are aware of sights, sounds, and smells that many of us take for granted such as cars backfiring, children shouting at play, or planes flying overhead. They are very anxious and this leads to mental and physical exhaustion. Although benzodiazepines are often used to treat these symptoms, they have a down side as they are easily abused. Thus, benzodiazepines should be avoided if possible. If prescribed, a medication contract and close monitoring is necessary. As a caregiver, you might be asked to monitor your care partner.

Suggested Further Reading

Agronin, Marc E. *The Dementia Caregiver: A Guide to Caring for Someone with Alzheimer's Disease and Other Neurocognitive Disorders*. Lanham, MD: Rowman & Littlefield, 2016. Guides readers through a better understanding of the changes their loved ones may be going through and helps them tap into the various resources available to them. http://amzn.to/2o7tRJS

Ali, Naheed. *Understanding Parkinson's Disease: An Introduction for Patients and Caregivers*. Lanham, MD: Rowman & Littlefield Publishers, Inc., 2015. An introduction to essential information on the risk factors associated with Parkinson's, the signs and symptoms, the different stages of the disease, the various treatments, as well as how the disease develops. http://amzn.to/2EOc2Jj

Barrick. Ann Louise, Joanne Rader, Beverly Hoeffer, Philip D. Sloane, and Stacey Biddle. *Bathing without a Battle: Person-Directed Care of Individuals with Dementia*. 2nd ed. New York: Springer Publishing, 2008. (Also available as a training DVD.)

Cassidy, John W. *Mindstorms: The Complete Guide for Families Living with Traumatic Brain Injury*. Cambridge, MA: Da Capo Press, 2009.

Explains the different types of brain injury; common myths surrounding it; and demonstrates the ways in which TBI may affect memory, behavior, and social interaction. http://amzn.to/2EMUWf1

Friedman Joseph H. *Making the Connection between Brain and Behavior: Coping with Parkinson's Disease*. New York: Demos Medical Publishing, 2013.

Gitlin, Laura N. and Catherine Verrier Piersol. *A Caregiver's Guide to Dementia: Using Activities and Other Strategies to Prevent, Reduce, and Manage Behavioral Symptoms*. Philadelphia: Camino Books Inc., 2014.

Hart, John. *The Brain Book: Understanding How the Brain Works and How to Improve Brain Performance*. Chatswood, Australia: New Holland Publishers, 2016. Provides the medical background to effective brain performance, but also offers an easy to follow, step-by-step guide to caring for your brain in an ever-changing world. http://amzn.to/2FcSOLc

Owen, Adrian. *Into the Gray Zone: A Neuroscientist Explores the Mysteries of the Brain and the Border between Life and Death*. New York: Scribner, 2018.Helps readers understand the so-called "gray zone" between full consciousness and brain death experienced by people who have sustained traumatic brain injuries or are the victims of stroke or degenerative diseases. http://amzn.to/2BCNi4W

Radin, Gary, Lisa Radin, eds. *What If It's Not Alzheimer's? A Caregiver's Guide to Dementia*. 3rd ed. New York: Prometheus Books, 2013.

Rao, Vani, Sandeep Vaishnavi, and Peter V. Rabins. *The Traumatized Brain: A Family Guide to Understanding Mood, Memory, and Behavior after Brain Injury*. Baltimore: Johns Hopkins University Press, 2015. Case studies and suggestions for appropriate medications, counseling, other treatments and targeted tips for coping. http://amzn.to/2C53wVe

Spencer, Beth, and Laurie White. *Coping with Behavior Change in Dementia: A Family Caregiver's Guide*. Whisppub.com, 2015.

Wolfelt, Alan. *Reframing PTSD as Traumatic Grief: How Caregivers Can Companion Traumatized Grievers through Gatch-Up Mourning*. Fort Collins, CO: Companion Press, 2014. A guide for counselors and caregivers reframing PTSD as a form of grief. http://amzn.to/2FbtwwN

Other Resources

American Stroke Association Life After Stroke. http://www.strokeassociation.org/STROKEORG/LifeAfterStroke/ForFamilyCaregivers/For-Stroke-Family-Caregivers_UCM_308560_SubHomePage.jsp

Anxiety and Depression Association of America. https://www.adaa.org/understanding-anxiety/posttraumatic-stress-disorder-ptsd

Area Agencies on Aging (AAAs) were established under the Older Americans Act (OAA) in 1973 to respond to the needs of Americans 60 and over in every local community. By providing a range of options that allow older adults to choose the home and community-based services and living arrangements that suit them best, AAAs make it possible for older adults to "age in place" in their homes and communities by providing access to the resources that will allow them to maintain their lives in the community. There is an Area Agency on Aging in every area of the United States. To find the one nearest to you, go to https://www.n4a.org and you can then put in your zip code.

Association for Frontotemporal Dementia. https://www.theaftd.org/understandingftd/ftd-overview

Banner Beacon Newsletters houses seven years of newsletters on specific care issues such as driving, travel, living alone, holidays, weight loss. http://banneralz.org/education-events/the-bai-beacon-newsletter.aspx

Eldercare Locator Nationwide is a service of the federal government that helps caregivers locate local support and resources. 1-800-677-1116. https://eldercare.acl.gov/Public/Index.aspx

On the **Family Caregiver Alliance** site, you can find the Family Care Navigator list of disease-specific organizations. https://www.caregiver.org/state-list-views?field_state_tid=152

National Alzheimer's Association is the leading voluntary health organization in Alzheimer's care, support and research. Connection with local chapters can be found on the website. Their professionally staffed 24/7 Helpline (1-800-272-3900) offers information and advice to more than 300,000 callers each year and provides translation services in more than 200 languages. They host face-to-face support groups and educational sessions in communities nationwide. They provide caregivers and families with comprehensive online resources and information through the Alzheimer's and Dementia Caregiver Center, which features sections on early-stage, middle-stage, and late-stage caregiving. Their free online tool, Alzheimer's Navigator®, helps those facing the disease to determine their needs and develop an action plan, and the online Community Resource Finder is a comprehensive database of programs, housing and care services, and legal experts. http://www.alz.org

National Center for PTSD. https://www.ptsd.va.gov/public/PTSD-overview/basics/what-is-ptsd.asp

National Institute of Neurological Disorders and Stroke (NINDS) conducts and supports research on brain and nervous system disorders. 1-800- 352-9424. https://www.ninds.nih.gov

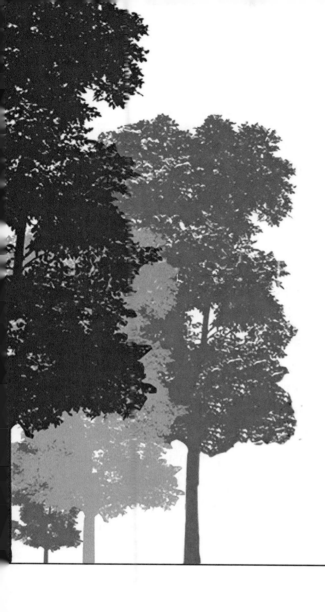

Chapter 12

Managing Medications

WHETHER YOU ARE TAKING MEDICATIONS for yourself or giving them to your care partner, understanding how to manage medications is a critical job. Working closely with your doctor and your care partner's medical team is essential for the safe and effective use of medications. The suggestions offered in this chapter can be useful in managing your medications as well as those you may be giving to your care partner.

Understanding the Purpose of Medications

Few products are more heavily advertised than medications. If we read a magazine, listen to the radio, or watch TV, we see a constant stream of drug ads. These are aimed at convincing us that if we just use this pill, our symptoms will be cured. "Recommended by 90% of the doctors asked," the voiceover may say. But be aware that the drug producer might have asked doctors working for the company or only a handful of doctors. These ads are designed to influence your decisions and they use a number of tactics to do just that. For example, have you noticed that on TV, the ads present the benefits in a slow, upbeat voice, while the side effects are recited very rapidly? Yet many of us have also been taught to avoid excess medications. And we have all heard about, or personally experienced, some of the bad effects of medications. It can be very confusing.

Your body is often its own healer, and, given time, many common symptoms and disorders improve. The prescriptions filled by the body's own "internal pharmacy" are frequently the safest and most effective treatment. There is no rule that says you should rush to fix everything that goes wrong with a pill. Patience, careful self-observation, and monitoring with your doctor are often excellent choices.

It is also true that medications can be a very important part of managing your care partner's or your own illness. These medications do not cure the disease. They generally serve one or more of the following purposes:

- **To relieve symptoms.** For example, an inhaler delivers medications that help expand the bronchial tubes and make it easier to breathe. A nitroglycerin tablet expands the blood vessels, allowing more blood to reach the heart, thus quieting angina. Acetaminophen (Tylenol) can relieve pain.
- **To prevent further problems.** For example, medications that thin the blood help prevent blood clots, which cause strokes and heart and lung problems.
- **To improve or slow the progress of the disease.** For example, nonsteroidal anti-inflammatory drugs (NSAIDs) can help arthritis by quieting the inflammatory process. Likewise, antihypertensive medications can lower blood pressure. The medications for Alzheimer's dementia discussed in Chapter 11, Understanding Your Care Partner's Brain, act in this way.
- **To replace substances that the body is no longer producing adequately.** For example, thyroid hormone for underactive thyroid and insulin for diabetes. This is also how drugs for Alzheimer's dementia work. See Chapter 11, Understanding Your Care Partner's Brain, for more details about medications used for Alzheimer's and other brain diseases.

In other words, the primary purpose of medication is to lessen the consequences of disease or to slow the course of a disease. Sometimes the effects of drugs are hard for us to see. You may not be aware that the medication is doing anything but it might be slowing the course of your care partner's disease—keeping them from getting worse or helping them get worse more slowly. It is important to continue taking medications, even if you cannot see how they are helping. If you have concerns about whether or how a drug is working, ask your doctor.

We pay a price for having such powerful weapons against diseases and their symptoms. Besides being helpful, all medications have undesirable side effects. Some of these effects are predictable and minor, and some are unexpected and life-threatening. Some 5% to 10% of all hospital admissions are due to unwanted drug reactions. At the same time, not taking medications as prescribed is also a major cause of hospitalization. When considering a new medication for yourself or your care partner, it is important to talk with the doctor about the possible benefits and harms of both taking the medication and not taking it.

Enlisting Mind Power: Expect the Best

Medication affects your body in two ways. The first is determined by the chemical nature of the medication. The second is triggered by your beliefs and expectations. Many studies have shown the power of the placebo—the power of mind over body. When people are given a placebo (a pill containing no medication), some of them improve anyway. Placebos can relieve back pain and chronic pain, fatigue, arthritis, headache, allergies, hypertension, insomnia, asthma, irritable bowel syndrome and chronic digestive disorders, depression, anxiety, and pain after surgery. The placebo effect clearly demonstrates that our positive beliefs and expectations can turn on our self-healing mechanisms. Your beliefs and confidence can change your body chemistry and your symptoms. The placebo effect is an example of how closely the mind and body are connected.

You can learn to take advantage of this powerful connection and use your mind to help your body. ***Every time you take a medication, you are swallowing your expectations and beliefs as well as the pill. So. expect the best!***

The following are some ways to do that:

- **Examine your beliefs about the treatment.** If you tell yourself, "I'm not a pill taker" or "medications always give me bad side effects," how do you think your body is likely to respond? If you don't think the prescribed treatment is likely to help your symptoms or condition, your negative beliefs will undermine the ability of the pill to help you. You can change these negative images into more positive ones.
- **Think of your medications the way you think of vitamins.** Many people associate healthful images with vitamins—more so than with medications. Taking a vitamin makes you think that you are doing something positive to prevent disease and promote health. If you regard your medications as health-restoring and health-promoting, like vitamins, you may obtain more powerful benefits.
- **Imagine how the medicine is helping.** Develop a mental image of how the medication is helping your body. For example, if

you are taking thyroid hormone replacement medication, tell yourself it is filling a missing link in your body's chemical chains to help balance and regulate your metabolism. For some people, forming a vivid mental image is helpful. An antibiotic, for example, might be seen as a broom sweeping germs out of the body. Don't worry if your image of what's happening chemically inside of you is not physiologically correct. It's your belief in a clear, positive image that counts.

- **Keep in mind why you are taking or giving the medication.** You are not using the medication just because your doctor told you to. You are taking the medication to help you and your care partner live as full a life as possible. It is therefore important to understand how the medicine is helping. You can use this information to help the medicine do its job. Suppose a woman with cancer is given chemotherapy. She has been told that it will make her feel like she has the flu, she will vomit, and her hair will fall out. So, of course, that is what she thinks about and that is what happens. But suppose she is also told that the symptoms will last only a few days, that hair falling out is a good sign because it means that cells that grow fast (like cancer cells and hair cells) are being destroyed, and that her hair will grow back after chemo. In that case, she might regard her hair loss, flu-like symptoms, and vomiting as signs the drugs are working. She can then take actions to counter these effects and often have an easier time tolerating them. The presence of side effects can sometimes be your proof that the medicine is working.
- **Present the positive.** Your positive (or negative) attitude about medication can be contagious! Even if care partner has major cognitive (thinking) problems feelings about medication influence the way your care partner acts when given medications. If you are positive and calmly persistent, your care partner might be more likely to take the medication.

Taking Multiple Medications

People with multiple problems often take many medications: a medication for dementia, a medication to lower blood pressure, anti-inflammatory drugs for arthritis, a pill for angina, a bronchodilator for asthma, antacids for heartburn, plus a handful of over-the-counter (OTC) remedies and herbs. The more medications (including vitamins and OTC remedies) you and/or your care partner are taking, the greater the risk of unpleasant reactions. Also, not all drugs work well together, and when they are taken together, they sometimes cause problems. Fortunately, it is often possible to take fewer medications and lower the risks. However, you should not do this without the help of your or your care partner's doctor. Most people would not change the ingredients in a complicated cooking recipe or throw out a few parts when fixing something in the car or home. It is not that these things can't be done.

It is just that if you want the best and safest results, you may need expert help.

How you or your care partner respond to any one medication depends on age, metabolism, daily activity, the waxing and waning of symptoms, any particular chronic conditions, genetics, and frame of mind. For you and your care partner to get the most from your medications, your doctor depends on you. Report what effect, if any, the drug has on symptoms and any side effects. You might have to observe your care partner closely to determine these. Based on this critical information, medications could be continued, increased, discontinued, or otherwise changed. In a good doctor–patient partnership, there is a continuing flow of information in both directions (see the following section, Sharing Information with the Doctor.)

The goal of treatment is to maximize the benefits and minimize the risks. This means taking the fewest medications, in the lowest effective doses, for the shortest period. Whether the medications you or your care partner are taking are helpful or harmful often depends on how much you know about your medications and how well you communicate with the doctors.

Sharing Information with the Doctor

Unfortunately, the vital conversation between doctors and patients and caregivers about medication is often shortchanged. Studies indicate that fewer than 5% of patients who are given new prescriptions asked any questions about them. Doctors tend to interpret patient silence as understanding and satisfaction. Problems often occur because patients do not receive enough information about medications or do not understand how to take them. In addition, all too often people do not follow instructions.

Safe, effective drug use depends on your doctor's expertise and equally on your understanding of when and how the drug should be taken. You must ask questions. Some people are afraid to ask their doctors questions. They are afraid that they will seem foolish or stupid or that they might be perceived as challenging the doctor's authority. But asking questions is a necessary part of a healthy doctor–patient relationship. As a caregiver, it is especially important to ask questions because your care partner might not be able to do so.

Even if your doctor doesn't ask, there is certain vital information about medications you should report during every consultation. Ask yourself these questions before each appointment and share your answers with your health care providers.

Are you or your care partner taking any other medications?

Report to your physician or you care partner's physician and dentist all prescription and nonprescription medications including birth control pills, vitamins, aspirin, antacids, laxatives, alcohol, and herbal remedies. An easy way to do this is to carry a list of all medications along with the amount you take (dosage). Keep one list for you and one for your care partner. Or bring all medications to the doctor visit, and make sure to check that your electronic medical record is up-to-date. Saying that your care partner is taking "the little green pills" isn't very helpful.

This is particularly key if you or your care partner are seeing more than one physician. Each doctor may not know what the others have prescribed, particularly if they are in different medical groups that don't share their electronic medical records. Keeping a detailed record of all your and your care partner's medications and supplements, and sharing that record with all your doctors, is essential for correct diagnosis and treatment. For example, if you have symptoms such as nausea or diarrhea, sleeplessness or drowsiness, dizziness or memory loss, impotence or fatigue, they might be caused by a drug side effect rather than a disease. If your doctors do not know all your medications, they cannot protect you from drug interactions.

Have you or your care partner had allergic or unusual reactions to any medications?

Describe any symptoms or unusual reactions that you suspect could be caused by medications. Be specific: Which medication and exactly what type of reaction? A rash, fever, or wheezing that develops after taking a medication is often a true allergic reaction. If any of these develop, call your doctor immediately. Nausea, diarrhea, ringing in the ears, light-headedness, sleeplessness, and frequent urination are likely to be side effects rather than true drug allergies.

What chronic diseases and other medical conditions do you or your care partner have?

Many diseases can interfere with the action of a drug or increase the risk of using certain medications. Diseases involving the kidneys or liver are critical to mention because these diseases can slow the metabolism of many drugs and increase toxic effects. The doctor may also avoid certain medications if you or your care partner now or in the past have had such diseases as high blood pressure, peptic ulcer disease, asthma, heart disease, diabetes, or prostate problems. Be sure to let your doctor know if you are possibly pregnant or are breastfeeding. Many drugs cannot be safely used in those situations. What medications were tried in the past to treat this condition or disease?

It is a good idea to keep your own records and, a record for your care partner. What medications were used in the past and what were the effects? Knowing what has been tried and how you or your care partner reacted will help guide the doctor's recommendation of any new medications. However, the fact that a medication did not work in the past does not necessarily mean that it can't be tried again. Diseases change, and the same medication might work the second time.

Asking the Doctor Questions about Medication

There is important information that you need to know about all medications that you and your care partner take. Be sure to ask the following questions.

Is this medication really needed?

Some doctors prescribe medications not because they are really necessary but because they think patients want and expect drugs. Doctors often feel pressure to do something for the patient, so they prescribe a new drug. Don't pressure a doctor for medications. Many new medications are heavily advertised and promoted by their manufacturers. Quite a few medications that were heavily marketed were later found to be not helpful or so hazardous that they were withdrawn from the market.

Be cautious about requesting the newest medications. All reactions or effectiveness cannot always be accurately learned just from the clinical trial of the medication; things may change over time as more people take them. If the doctor doesn't prescribe a medication during a visit, consider that good news. Ask about nondrug alternatives. In some cases, lifestyle changes, such as exercise, diet, and stress management, should be considered first. When any treatment is recommended, ask what is likely to happen if treatment is postponed. Sometimes the best medicine is none at all, and sometimes it is taking a powerful medication early to avoid permanent damage or complications.

What is the name of the medication, dosage, and when it should be taken?

Keep a record of each medication prescribed by your doctor. Note its brand name, if any; the generic (chemical) name; and the dosage prescribed. If the label on the medication you get from the pharmacy doesn't match this information, ask the pharmacist to explain the difference. Your pharmacist and this precaution are your and your care partner's best protection against medication mix-ups.

What is the medication supposed to do?

The doctor should tell you why the medication is being prescribed and how it might help. Is the medication intended to prolong life, completely or partially relieve symptoms, or improve the ability to function? For example, if your care partner is given a medicine for high blood pressure, the medication is given primarily to prevent later complications (such as stroke or heart disease) rather than to stop a headache. On the other hand, if you are told to take a pain reliever such as acetaminophen (Tylenol), the purpose is to help ease the headache. You should also ask how soon you can expect results from the medication. Drugs that treat infections or inflammation may take several days to a week to show improvement. Antidepressant medications and some dementia drugs can sometimes take several weeks to start providing relief.

How and when should the medicine be taken, and for how long?

If medications are going to work they must be taken when they are supposed to be taken in the correct dosage (amount) for as long as they are supposed to be taken. This is crucial to their safe and effective use. Does "every 6 hours" mean every 6 hours just during the day time or every 6 hours around the clock? Should the medication be taken before meals, with meals, or between meals? What should you do if you accidentally miss a dose? Should you skip it, take a double dose next time, or take it as soon as you remember? Should you refill and continue taking the medication until you or your care partner have fewer symptoms or until the current prescription is finished? Some medications are prescribed on an as-needed ("prn") basis, so you need to know when to begin and end treatment and how much medication to take. Work out a plan with the doctor to suit your or your care partner's individual needs.

Taking medication properly is vital. Yet nearly 40% of people report that their doctors fail to tell them how to take the medication or how much to take. If you are not sure about your prescription, contact your doctor or pharmacist.

What foods, drinks, other medications, or activities should I or my care partner avoid while taking this medication?

Having food in your stomach may help protect the stomach from irritation when taking some medications but make other drugs ineffective. For example, milk products or antacids block the absorption of the antibiotic tetracycline. This drug is best taken on an empty stomach. Some medications might make you more sensitive to the sun, putting you at increased risk for sunburn. Ask whether the medication prescribed will interfere with driving safely. Other drugs, even over-the-counter drugs and alcohol, can amplify or lessen the effects of the prescribed medication. Taking aspirin along with an anticoagulant medication can result in possible bleeding. The more medications being taken, the greater the chance of an undesirable drug interaction. Tell the physician or pharmacist about all the medications you or your care partner take and ask about possible drug–drug and drug–food interactions.

What are the most common side effects, and what should I do if they occur?

All medications have side effects. Your doctor may have to try several medications before hitting on the one that is best for you or your care partner. You need to know what symptoms to look for and what action to take if they develop. Should you seek immediate medical care, discontinue the medication, or call the doctor? While you cannot expect the doctor to tell you every possible adverse reaction, the most common and most important ones should be discussed. Unfortunately, a recent survey showed that 70% of people starting a new medication did not recall being told by their physicians or pharmacists about precautions and possible side effects. So, it could be up to you to ask.

Are there any tests necessary to monitor the use of this medication?

Most medications are monitored by the improvement or worsening of symptoms. However, some medications can disrupt body chemistry before any symptoms develop. Sometimes these adverse reactions can be detected by laboratory tests such as blood counts or liver function tests. In addition, the levels of some medications in the blood need to be measured on a regular basis to make sure you or your care partner are getting the right amounts. Ask the doctor if the medication being prescribed has any of these special requirements.

Can a less expensive alternative or generic medication be prescribed?

Every drug has at least two names, a generic name and a brand name. The generic name is the name used to refer to the medication in the scientific literature. The brand name is the unique name given to the drug by its developer. When a drug company develops a new drug in the United States, it is granted exclusive rights to produce that drug for 17 years. After this

17-year period, other companies may market chemical equivalents of that drug. These generic medications are generally considered as safe and effective as the original brand-name drug but often cost much less. In some cases, a physician might have a good reason for preferring a particular brand. Even so, if cost is a concern, ask the doctor if a less expensive but equally effective medication is available.

You may also be able to save money by knowing how to best use your insurance. For example, your co-payment might be less if you obtain your medications from a company designated by your insurer. Mail order pharmacies will often offer a lower co-payment if you fill a prescription for 90 days' supply instead of 30 days. Also, many national pharmacies have discount programs for seniors and individuals with incomes below a certain level. It pays to ask and then ask again. And it is wise to shop around. Even in the same town, different stores sell the same medication at different prices.

Is there any written information about the medication?

Your doctor may not have time to answer all of your questions. You many not remember everything you heard. Fortunately, there are many other good sources of information, including pharmacists, nurses, package inserts, pamphlets, books, and websites. Several useful sources are listed at the end of this chapter.

Reading the Prescription Label

A valuable source of information about medications is the prescription label. The following illustration will help you learn how to read the labels on your prescriptions.

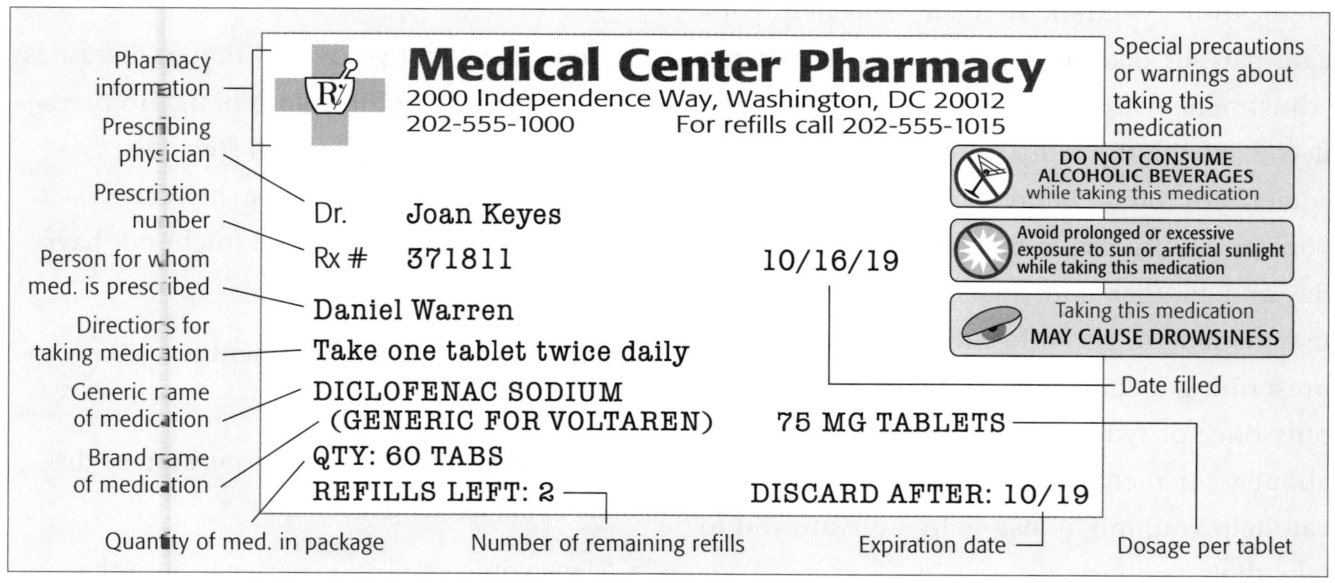

A Special Word about Pharmacists

Pharmacists are an underutilized resource. Pharmacists go to school for many years to learn about medications, how they act in your body, and how they interact with each other. Your pharmacist is an expert on medications and can readily answer questions face to face, over the phone, or even via email. In addition, many hospitals, medical schools, and schools of pharmacy have medication information services that you can call to ask questions. As a caregiver, don't forget pharmacists. They are valuable and helpful consultants.

Taking Your Medications

Medications don't work if they are not taken. Nearly half of all medicines are not taken as prescribed. There are many reasons why people don't take their prescribed medication: forgetfulness, lack of clear instructions, complicated dosing schedules, bothersome side effects, cost of the medications, and so on. Whatever the reason, if you are having trouble taking your medications or giving your care partner their medications, discuss this with your doctor. (In the next section, Remembering to Take Medications, we talk about how to help your care partner take medications.) Often simple adjustments can make it easier. For example, if you are taking many different medications, sometimes one or more can be eliminated. If you are taking one medication three times a day and another four times a day, your doctor may be able to simplify the regimen, perhaps prescribing medications that you need to take only once or twice a day. Understanding more about your medications, including how they can help you, might also help motivate you to take them regularly.

If you are having trouble taking your medications, or giving them to your care partner, ask yourself the following questions and discuss the answers with your doctor or pharmacist:

- Do you tend to be forgetful?
- Are you confused about the instructions for how and when to use the medications?
- Is the schedule for taking your medications too complicated?
- Do your medications have bothersome side effects?
- Is your medicine too expensive?
- Do you feel that your condition or disease is not serious or bothersome enough to need regular medications? (With some diseases such as high blood pressure, high cholesterol, or early diabetes, you might not have any symptoms.)
- Do you feel that the treatment is unlikely to help?
- Are you in denial about a condition or disease that needs treatment?
- Have you had a bad experience with the medicine you are supposed to be taking or another medication?

- Do you know someone who had a bad experience with the medication, and are you afraid that something similar will happen with you?
- Are you afraid of becoming addicted to the medication?
- Are you embarrassed about taking the medication, view it as a sign of weakness or failure, or fear you'll be judged negatively if people know about it?
- Do you need further information about the benefits you might get if you take the medication as prescribed?

Remembering to Take Medications

If forgetting to take your medications or give medications to your partner is a problem, here are some suggestions:

- **Make it obvious.** Place the medication or a reminder next to your toothbrush, on the breakfast table, in your lunch box, or in some other place where you're likely to "stumble over" it. (But be careful where you put the medication if children are around.) Or you might put a reminder note on the bathroom mirror, the refrigerator door, the coffee maker, the television, or some other conspicuous place. If you connect taking the medication or giving medication to your partner with some well-established habit such as meal times or watching a favorite television program, you'll be more likely to remember.
- **Use a checklist or an organizer.** Make a medication chart listing each medication you and your partner are taking and the time when it needs to be taken. Or check off each medication on a calendar as you or your care partner takes it. You might also buy a medication organizer for each of you at the drugstore. This container separates pills by the time of day they should be taken. You can fill the organizer once a week so that all your pills and your care partner's pills are ready to take at the proper time. A quick glance at the organizers lets you know if anyone has missed any doses and prevents double dosing. There are also websites that allow you to print out charts to help you track medications; PictureRx (https://mypicturerx.com) is one, but it requires a subscription.
- **Use a color-coded system.** You and your care partner should have clearly labeled organizers that are different colors so that there is less chance of mixing them up.
- **Use an electronic reminder.** Get a watch or cell phone that can be set to beep at pill-taking time. There are also "high-tech" medication containers that beep at a preset time to remind you about medication. If you have a smartphone, you can also download apps that can track and remind you to when you need to take medication or give it to your care partner.
- **Get prepackaged medications.** Some pharmacies are beginning to offer personalized prepackaged doses of medications to help patients who need to take multiple medications several times a day. Each packet has the date, time, and description of the

medications and nutritional supplements. Ask your pharmacist.

- **Have others remind you.** Ask members of your household to remind you to take your medications at the appropriate times.
- **Don't run out.** Don't let yourself run out of your medicines. When you get a new prescription, mark on your calendar the date a week before your medications will run out. This will serve as a reminder to order and get your next refill. Don't wait until the last pill. Some mail-order pharmacies offer automatic refills, so your medications arrive when you need them.

Getting Your Care Partner to Take Medications

Sometimes it is difficult to get care partners to take their medications. Here are some tips:

- Your care partner might resist taking the medication because of side effects such as nausea. Your care partner may not be able to tell you this so look for signs of side effects.
- Your care partner might need to take more control. Put the pill and glass of water near your partner but let them take their own medication. Help only as needed.
- If pills are hard for your care partner to swallow, ask about liquid medication or if pills can be crushed. Not all pills are crushable and some may be dangerous if you do crush them. Sometimes pills and liquid medications can be "hidden" or combined with foods or beverages.
- Ask the doctor if the medication is really necessary.
- Be a good role model and take your pills at the same time as your care partner.
- Use short sentences. Do not explain or reason. Stay calm and try again in 15 or 20 minutes.
- Find the best time of day (as long as medications do not have to be given at certain times). Care partners with Alzheimer's often are more cooperative in the morning than in the afternoon or evening.
- Try to stick to a daily routine, but be flexible if needed.
- Reward good behavior. Try giving a treat once the medications are taken.

Self-Medicating

In every two-week period, nearly 70% of people will take a nonprescription over-the-counter (OTC) drug. Many OTC drugs are highly effective and may be recommended by your doctor. But if you self-medicate, or are giving an OTC to your care partner, you should know what you are taking, why you are taking it, how it works, and how to use the medication wisely.

More than 200,000 nonprescription drug products are offered for sale to the American public, representing about 500 active ingredients. Nearly 75% of the public receives its education on over-the-counter (OTC) drugs solely from TV, radio, newspaper, and magazine advertising. This advertising is aimed at you.

The main message of drug advertising is that there is a pharmaceutical solution for every symptom, every ache and pain, and every problem. While many OTC products are effective, many are simply a waste of your money. They might also keep you from using better ways to manage your illness or may interfere or interact badly with your prescription medications.

Whether you are taking prescribed medications or using over-the-counter medications or herbs, here are some helpful suggestions:

- **If you or your care partner are pregnant or nursing, have a chronic disease, or are already taking multiple medications, consult your doctor before self-medicating.**
- **Always read drug labels and follow directions carefully.** Reading the label and reviewing the individual ingredients, could prevent you from taking medications that have caused problems for you in the past. If you don't understand the information on the label, ask a pharmacist or doctor before buying it.
- **Do not exceed the recommended dosage or length of treatment** unless you have discussed the change with your doctor.
- **Use caution with over-the-counter (OTC) medications if you or your care partner are taking other drugs.** Over-the-counter and prescription drugs can interact, either canceling or exaggerating the effects of the medications. If you have questions about drug interactions, ask your doctor or pharmacist before mixing medicines.
- **Try to select OTC medications with a single active ingredient rather than combination ("all-in-one") products.** A product with multiple ingredients is likely to include drugs for symptoms you don't even have, so why risk the side effects of unneeded medications? Single-ingredient products also allow you to adjust the dosage of each medication separately for optimal symptom relief with minimal side effects.
- **When choosing OTC medications, learn the ingredient names and then look for generic alternatives.** Generics contain the same active ingredient as the brand-name product, usually at a lower cost.
- **Never take or give a drug from an unlabeled container or a container whose label you cannot read.** Keep your medications in their original labeled containers or transfer them to a labeled medication organizer or pill dispenser. Do not make the mistake of mixing different medications in the same bottle.
- **Do not take medications that were prescribed for someone else**, even if you have similar symptoms.
- **Drink at least a half glass of liquid with pills**, and remain standing or sitting upright for a short while after swallowing. This can prevent the pills from getting stuck in the esophagus.
- **Store medications where children or young adults cannot find them.** Poisoning from medications is a common and preventable

A Special Word about Alcohol and Recreational Drugs

The use of alcohol and recreational drugs (illegal or prescription medications used for nonmedicinal purposes) has been increasing in recent years, particularly among people over the age of 60. These drugs, whether legal or illegal, can cause problems. They can interact with prescription medications, making them less effective or even causing harm. They can fog judgment and cause problems with balance. This can, in turn, cause accidents and injure both you and others. In some cases, alcohol or recreational drugs can make existing long-term conditions worse. Alcohol use is associated with increased risk of hypertension, diabetes, gastrointestinal bleeding, sleep disorders, depression, erectile dysfunction, breast and other cancers, and injury.

Limiting alcohol use to no more than two drinks per day is advised. "At risk" alcohol use for women is drinking more than seven drinks per week or more than three drinks per day and for men more than 14 drinks per week or more than four drinks in a day. This means that women of any age and anyone over age 65 should average no more than one drink per day and men under 65 should have no more than two drinks per day on average.

Please consider these two pieces of advice:

- If you are at the "at risk" level for alcohol or are regularly using recreational drugs, seriously consider cutting down or stopping their use.
- Talk to your doctor about your use of these drugs. Doctors are often hesitant to raise the issue because they don't want to embarrass you, so it is up to you to bring up the subject. Doctors will be very willing to talk about it once you raise the subject. They have heard it all, and they will not think less of you. An honest conversation might save your life.

problem among the young. And the primary sources of recreational drugs used by teens and young adults are prescription medications of relatives or the relatives of friends. Some people, regardless of age, with cognitive problems might take extra medication, believing they have missed a dose. Take precautions to prevent this. Despite its name, the bathroom medicine cabinet is not usually an appropriate place to store medications. A kitchen cabinet or tool box with a lock is far safer.

Medications can help or harm. What often makes the difference is the care you exercise and the partnership you develop with your doctor.

You will find more about the specific medications used for people with cognitive impairment (thinking problems) in Chapter 11, Understanding Your Care Partner's Brain.

We have all heard of opioid pain medications and many of us have been prescribed opioids or know an opioid user. (Please note that we did not say abuser). Like all prescription medications, this class of drugs is useful and it can also cause many problems. Many people who take opioids legally would like to use less or to not use opioids at all but are afraid of pain, withdrawal, or even letting health professionals know their wishes. There is probably no group of drugs that is less understood, either by the

A Special Word about Opioids

Today, the overuse of prescription opioids is a problem in many countries. These drugs are used both legally by people who have prescriptions, and illegally by people who steal or purchase these drugs "on the street." Because their use is so widespread, there are many myths and half-truths about them. This information is for anyone who is using prescription opioids or knows someone who is using them.

public or health professionals. This content is written to try to put the use of prescription opioids into perspective.

Opioids are the most commonly used prescription pain medications. In the United States, medical use of opioids requires a prescription and you cannot buy opioids over-the-counter without a prescription. Examples of prescription opioids include:

- acetaminophen/hydrocodone (Vicodin, Norco)
- acetaminophen/oxycodone (Percocet)
- oxycodone (Oxycontin, Roxicodone)
- oxymorphone (Opana)
- fentanyl (Duragesic, Abstral)
- hydromorphone (Dilaudid, Exalgo)

There are many resources that exist to help you learn more about opioids and their use and abuse. As a starter see the book by Beth Darnell cited below.

Suggested Further Reading

Castleman, Michael. *The New Healing Herbs: The Essential Guide to More Than 130 of Nature's Most Potent Herbal Remedies*. 3rd ed. New York: Rodale, 2017.

Darnall, Beth. *Less Pain, Fewer Pills: Avoid the dangers of prescription opioids and gain control over chronic pain*. Boulder: Bull Publishing, 2014

Griffith, H. Winter, and Stephen W. Moore. *Complete Guide to Prescription and Nonprescription Drugs, 2018–2019*. New York: TarcherPerigee Books, 2017.

Leonard, Peggy C. *Quick and Easy Medical Terminology*. St. Louis, MO: Elsevier, 2017. Clearly and concisely covers disorders, diagnosis, and treatment with a strong focus on anatomy for self-study. http://amzn.to/2Fce5o7

Lippincott Drug Guide for Nurses 2018. Philadelphia: Lippincott Williams & Wilkins, 2017. A handy pocket guide with essential information on over 2,000 medications in an easy-access A-to-Z format. http://amzn.to/2oaDEyN

Physicians Desk Reference. *The PDR Pocket Guide to Prescription Drugs*. 10th ed. New York: Pocket Books, 2013.

Silverman, Harold M. *The Pill Book*, 14th ed. New York: Bantam Books, 2018.

Other Resources

AgingCare provides information on medication interactions, awareness and assistance. https://www.agingcare.com/medications

ConsumerLab. http://www.consumerlab.com

MedlinePlus: Drugs, Herbs, and Supplements is a service of the U.S. National Library of Medicine and National Institutes of Health. http://www.nlm.nih.gov/medlineplus/druginformation.html

National Center for Complementary and Integrated Health (NCCIH). http://nccih.nih.gov

National Institutes of Health: Rethinking Drinking: Alcohol and Your Health. http://rethinkingdrinking.niaaa.nih.gov

Natural Medicines Comprehensive Database. http://naturaldatabaseconsumer.therapeuticresearch.com/home.aspx

PictureRx. https://mypicturerx.com

PubMed Heath. https://www.ncbi.nlm.nih.gov/pubmedhealth

WebMD. Drugs and Medications A–Z. http://www.webmd.com/drugs

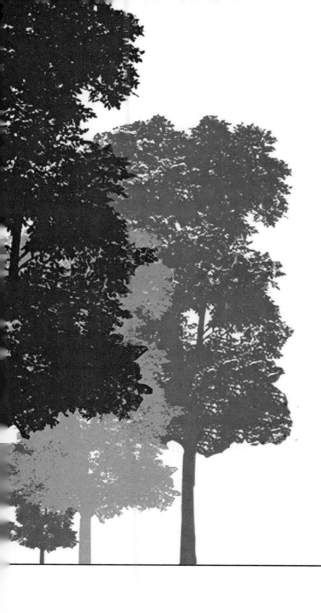

Chapter 13

Making Treatment Decisions

We hear about new treatments, new drugs, nutritional supplements, and alternative treatments all the time. Hardly a week goes by without a new treatment of some kind being reported in the news. Drug companies and nutritional supplement companies run commercials during the television news and place large ads in newspapers, magazines, and social media sites. Our email boxes are filled with promises of treatments or cures from spammers. We are bombarded in the market or pharmacy with signs for over-the-counter alternative treatments. Not only that, our health care providers may recommend new procedures, medications, or other treatments that we don't know much about.

What can we believe? How can we decide what might be worth a try?

Asking Questions about New Treatments

A significant part of managing our own care and that of our care partner is being able to evaluate these claims or recommendations and make informed decisions about trying something new. There are some key questions that you should ask yourself when making decisions about any treatment, whether it is a mainstream medical treatment or a complementary or alternative treatment.

Where did I learn about this?

Was it reported in a scientific journal, a supermarket tabloid, a print or TV ad, a website, or a flyer you picked up somewhere? Did your doctor suggest it?

The source of the information is important. Results that are reported in a respected scientific journal are more likely to be true than those you see in a supermarket tabloid or on social media. Results reported in scientific journals, such as the *New England Journal of Medicine, Lancet,* or *Science,* are usually from research studies. These studies are carefully reviewed for scientific integrity by scientists, who are very methodical in their review and cautious about what they approve for publication.

When you hear about a cure or treatment that is not based on scientific research that was reported in a scientific journal, you need to be extra careful and critical about analyzing what you read or hear. Everyone now has access to at least the abstracts (written summaries of studies) from scientific journals. Before the internet, medical scientific literature was generally hard to find. This is no longer true. You can read the abstract of the most up-to-date articles by going to Google Scholar or PubMed. Like any search, the more specific you can be the better. Sometimes these searches are more than you want to undertake or you are afraid you might not understand what you find. If this is the case, connect with a health library, run by a hospital or other health organizations. Health libraries have professionals and volunteers to help you. Usually, you can connect with them by phone or via email. To find a health library, just type "health library near me" into a search engine on your computer or smartphone. Even if there is not a library nearby, you can visit the online site of a major health care facility, such as Stanford, and connect with their health library. It does not matter where you live.

Were the people who got better like me?

In the past, many research studies were done with easy-to-get people, so older studies were often done on college students, nurses, or white men. This has changed, but it is still important to find out if the people that got better were like you. Were they from the same age group? Did they have similar lifestyles? Did they have the same health problems? Were they the same sex and race? If the people aren't like you or your care partner, the results may not be the same.

Could anything else have caused the positive changes reported by users of the treatment?

A woman returns from a two-week stay at a spa in the tropics and reports that her arthritis improved dramatically thanks to the special diet and supplements she received. But is it appropriate to attribute her improvement to the treatment when the warm weather, relaxation, and pampering might have had even more to do with her improvement?

It is important to look at everything that has changed since starting a treatment. It is common to take up a generally healthier lifestyle when starting a new treatment—could that be playing a part in the improvement? Did the people whose health improved start another medication or treatment at the same time? Has the weather improved? Can you think of anything else that could have affected the change?

Does treatment suggest stopping other medications or treatments?

Does it require stopping another basic medication because of dangerous interactions? If the basic medication is important (and even if it isn't), discuss the new treatment with your health care provider before making any changes.

Does treatment involve not eating a well-balanced diet?

Does it eliminate any necessary nutrients or stress only a few nutrients that could be harmful? Maintaining a balanced diet is important for overall health. Be sure that you're not sacrificing needed nutrients or make certain that you're getting them from another source. Also, be sure to avoid putting excessive stress on your organs by concentrating on only a few nutrients to the exclusion of others.

Can I think of any possible dangers or harm?

Some treatments take a toll on the body. All treatments have side effects and possible risks. Discuss these matters thoroughly with your health care provider. Only you can decide if the potential problems are worth the possible benefit, but you must have all the information to make that decision.

Many people think that if something is natural, it must be good for you. This may not be true. "Natural" isn't necessarily better. Something isn't mild or gentle just because it comes from a plant or animal. For example, the powerful heart medication digitalis, which comes from the foxglove plant, is "natural," but the dosage must be exact or it could be dangerous. Hemlock comes from a plant, but it is a deadly poison. Some treatments could be safe in small doses but dangerous in larger doses. Be careful.

In most countries, governments do not monitor and control non-pharmaceutical treatments. Except in Germany and Canada, no regulatory agency is responsible for verifying that what is listed on the label of a nutritional supplement is what's in the bottle, or that it is safe. Supplements don't have the same safeguards as medications. Do some research about the company selling the product before you try it. *Consumer Reports*, for example, often writes about alternative treatments.

Can I afford it?

Do you have the money to give this treatment the time it needs to produce an improvement? Is your health or your care partner's health strong enough to maintain this new regimen? Will you be able to handle it emotionally? Will this put a strain on your relationships at home or at work?

Am I willing to go to the trouble or expense?

Do I have the necessary support in place?

If you ask yourself these questions and decide to try a new treatment, it is very important to inform your or your care partner's health care professional. Only in this way can you get the best help and the best advice.

Finding Reliable Resources

The internet can provide information about new treatments very quickly and is therefore a resource for up-to-date information about these treatments. But be cautious. Some information on the internet is incorrect or unsafe. Seek out the most reliable sources by noting the author or sponsor of the site and the URL (internet address). Internet addresses ending in .edu, .org, and .gov are generally more objective and reliable; they originate from universities, nonprofit organizations, and governmental agencies, respectively. Some .com sites can also be good, but because they are maintained by commercial or for-profit organizations or are accepting commercial advertising, their information may be biased in favor of their own products and advertisers. The National Institutes of Health has a center for Complementary and Integrative Health. They maintain the following excellent website for researching these treatments: https://nccih.nih.gov/health/atoz.htm.

Sometimes it is wise to say no to conventional medical treatments as well. For example, various medical specialty organizations, after reviewing the medical evidence, have recommended that nearly 50 common treatments and procedures should *not* be done. See www.choosingwisely.org.

In the end, you make the choices for yourself and your care partner. Our hope is that this discussion will help you with your decisions.

Suggested Further Reading

Hogan, Paul, and Lori Hogan. *Stages of Senior Care: Your Step-by-Step Guide to Making the Best Decisions*. New York: McGraw-Hill, 2010. A guide through a comprehensive range of things to consider, step by step, so you can make better informed decisions and ensure the senior in your life is receiving the best care possible. http://amzn.to/2oeSvHG

Kind, Viki. *Caregivers Path to Compassionate Decision Making: Making the Choices for Those Who Can't*. Austin, TX: Greenleaf, 2010. Offers tools and techniques that will limit your frustration and fears and help you make informed, respectful decisions. http://amzn.to/2FcDv5d

Levy, David. *The Family Caregivers Manual: A Practical Planning Guide to Managing the Care of Your Loved One*. Las Vegas: Central Recovery Press, 2016. How to evaluate priorities, understand options, and face legal, financial, emotional, and social issues, so caregivers can make wise and informed decisions. http://amzn.to/2EnDZUL

McCullough, Dennis M. *My Mother, Your Mother: Embracing "Slow Medicine," the Compassionate Approach to Caring for Your Aging Loved Ones*. New York: HarperCollins, 2009. A new approach advocating for careful anticipatory "attending" to an elder's changing needs rather than waiting for crises that force medical interventions. http://amzn.to/2sDxkEK

Rubinstein, Nataly. *Alzheimer's Disease and Other Dementias: The Caregiver's Complete Survival Guide*. Minneapolis, MN: Two Harbors Press, 2011. A resource to make informed decisions regarding the best possible care for you and your loved one. http://amzn.to/2HpjtFm

Siles, Madonna. *Brain, Heal Thyself: A Caregiver's New Approach to Recovery from Stroke, Aneurysm, and Traumatic Brain Injuries*. Charlottesville, VA: Hampton Roads Publishing, 2006. A guidebook for individuals who have to make life and death decisions for those they love. http://amzn.to/2Gp9pdZ

Zarit, Steven H., and Judy M. Zarit. *Mental Disorders in Older Adults Fundamentals of Assessment and Treatment*. New York: Guilford Press, 2011. Demonstrates how to evaluate and treat frequently encountered clinical problems including dementias, mood and anxiety disorders, and paranoid symptoms. http://amzn.to/2EAecsI

Other Resources

American Board of Internal Medicine Foundation's Choosing Wisely. http://www.choosingwisely.org

Better Health Channel provides information on making healthcare decisions for someone else. https://www.betterhealth.vic.gov.au/health/servicesandsupport/making-healthcare-decisions-for-someone-else

The Caregiver Network webinar on decision-making. https://thecaregivernetwork.ca/event/decision-making-caregivers

CaringInfo on decision making and advance care planning. http://www.caringinfo.org/i4a/pages/index.cfm?pageid=3325

Google Scholar. https://scholar.google.com/

National Caregivers Library on making caregiving decisions. http://www.caregiverslibrary.org/caregivers-resources/making-caregiving-decisions.aspx

Chapter 14

Planning for the Future: Fears and Reality

Caregivers often worry about what will happen next. In fact, they have double worries. What will happen to their care partners over time and what will happen if they can no longer be caregivers? One way people can deal with fears of the future is to take control and plan. We may never need to put our plans into effect, but there is reassurance in knowing that we have some plans in place if the events we fear come to pass. Because of the special relationship between caregivers and care partners, you might be responsible for both planning for your own future and your care partner's future at the same time. Although these can be difficult events and topics to discuss and plan for, you are in a unique position and are likely best suited to help your care partner better prepare for the future. In this chapter, we examine the most common concerns people have about the future and offer some suggestions.

What if I Can't Take Care of Myself or My Care Partner Anymore?

Regardless of how healthy we are, most of us fear becoming helpless and dependent. This fear is even greater among caregivers and has physical as well as financial, social, and emotional aspects.

Problem Solving about Physical Day-to-Day Living Needs

As your own health condition changes, you may need to consider changing how and where you and your care partner live. This could involve hiring someone to help you in your home or moving to a place where more help is provided. How you make this decision depends on your needs and how they can best be met. Most people think only of the physical needs, but we all have social and emotional needs, too. All these aspects must be considered.

Start by evaluating what you can do yourself and for your care partner. Remember that we are most concerned in this book about you and your health. What caretaking tasks are a problem and affecting your own health? Which of your own activities of daily living (ADLs) will require help? ADLs are everyday tasks, such as getting out of bed, bathing, dressing, preparing and eating meals, cleaning house, shopping, and paying bills. Most people can do these things, even though they may have to do them slowly, with some modification, or with some help from gadgets. However, when you are responsible for doing these things for your care partner as well as yourself, you need to evaluate which of these tasks that you can continue to do and which are becoming more difficult for you.

Some people eventually find one or more of these tasks is no longer possible without help from somebody else. For example, you might still be able to fix meals but are no longer able to do the shopping. Or if you have problems with fainting or sudden bouts of unconsciousness, you might need to always have somebody present and available to help. You may also find that some things that you enjoyed in the past, such as gardening, are no longer pleasurable. Use the problem-solving steps discussed in Chapter 2, Becoming a Better Caregiver: The Basics, analyze and make a list of what the potential problems might be. Once you have this list, solve the problems one at a time, first writing down every possible solution you can think of.

The following is an example of a problem list and possible solutions:

Can't go shopping

- Find a volunteer shopping service.
- Shop at a store that delivers.
- Ask another family member to shop for me.
- Ask a neighbor to shop for me.
- Use the internet.
- Get home-delivered meals or meal kits.

Can't be by myself or can't leave my care partner alone

- Hire in-home care.
- Move in with a relative.
- Get a Lifeline Emergency Response system.
- Move to a skilled-nursing or assisted-living facility.

When you have listed your problem and the possible solutions to the problem, choose one problem-solving method or solution to try that seems the most workable, acceptable, and within your financial means (step 3 of problem-solving).

Getting Help with Decision Making

It might help to discuss your wishes, abilities, and limitations with a trusted friend, relative, or social worker. Sometimes another person can spot things we ourselves overlook or would like to ignore. Making use of other resources is step 6 in the problem-solving steps in Chapter 2, Becoming a Better Caregiver: The Basics.

If possible, make changes in your life slowly, one step at a time. You don't need to change your whole life to solve one problem. Remember that you can always change your mind. Don't burn your bridges behind you. If you think that moving out of your own place to another living arrangement (relatives', assisted-living home, or elsewhere) is the thing to do, don't give up your present home until you and your care partner are settled in your new home(s) and are sure you want to stay there. Here, we would like to note that the solution might not be the same for you and your care partner. For example, it may be that you go to live with a relative and your care partner goes to live in a nearby skilled-nursing facility, assisted-living facility, or board-and-care home.

A social worker at your local senior center, center for people with disabilities, or hospital social services department can be very helpful in providing information about resources in your community. This person can also give you ideas about how to deal with your care needs. There are several kinds of professionals who can be of great help. Social workers are good for helping you decide how to solve financial and living arrangement problems and locating appropriate community resources. Some social workers are also trained in counseling the disabled or the elderly in relation to emotional and relationship problems that could be associated with your health problem and/or your care partner's.

An occupational therapist can assess the daily living needs for both you and your care partner, and if needed suggest assistive devices or accommodations in and around your home. You also might get some ideas by looking at Chapter 8, Preventing Injuries.

If you or your care partner end up in a hospital, you can draw on the hospital resources for help. Most hospitals have a discharge planner. These planners, usually a nurse or social worker, will see you or your care partner before you go home and check that you know what to do and how to do it. It is very important that you be honest with this person. If you have concerns about your ability to care for your care partner or yourself, say so. Solutions are usually available, and the discharge planner is a real expert. However, the planner can help only if you share your concerns. Many hospitals also have chaplains that can often be helpful and might know of resources within your own religious or spiritual community.

An attorney specializing in estate planning or elder law should be on your list for helping you set your financial affairs in order—to preserve your assets, to prepare a proper will, and perhaps to execute a durable power of attorney for both health care and financial management. If finances are a concern, ask your local senior center for the names of attorneys who offer free or low-cost services to seniors. Your local bar association chapter can also refer you to a list of attorneys who are competent in this area. These attorneys are generally familiar with the laws applying to younger persons with disabilities as well. Even if you are not a senior, your legal needs are much the same as those of the older person. You will find more information about legal concerns later in this chapter.

Will I Have Enough Money to Pay for Care?

Next to the fear of physical dependence, many people fear not having enough money to pay for their own and their care partner's needs. Being sick often requires expensive care and treatment. If you are not able to work because of illness or because you are caregiving full time, the loss of income, and especially the loss of your health insurance coverage, might present an overwhelming financial problem. You can, however, avoid some of the risks by planning and knowing your resources.

Health insurance and Medicare may meet only a part of the ultimate cost of care. Medicare does not cover everything and most private "Medigap" insurance policies cover only the 20% that Medicare does not cover. Usually, they do not cover any procedure or treatment that isn't also covered by Medicare.

However, supplemental insurance policies offer the kind of coverage that provides for care needs that Medicare and Medigap insurance do not pay for. If you plan to buy such insurance for yourself and/or your care partner, carefully read the sections on limitations and exclusions. Be sure the policy covers nursing home care at a daily rate that is realistic for your community. Make sure you know how long they will pay for care. There is usually a cap of three months or so in a skilled nursing or rehabilitation facility, less if you or your care partner are judged to not be getting better and only need "custodial" care.

Health care reform continues to bring many changes in both Medicare and private insurance, some of which could be difficult to understand. We suggest that you talk to people at your local senior center, Area Agency on Aging, or disability organization to find trustworthy sources of information.

If you are too sick to work—either permanently or for some extended period—you may be entitled to draw Social Security based on your disability. If you have dependent children, they would also receive benefits. If you have been disabled for a specified period (as of this writing, it is two years), you might be entitled to Medicare coverage for your medical treatment needs. Disability payments are based only on disability, not on need. If Social Security benefits are unavailable or insufficient, the Supplemental Security Income (SSI) program is available to individuals who meet the eligibility criteria for Medicaid.

If you have minimal savings and little or no income, the federal Medicaid program may pay for medical treatment and long-term skilled or custodial care. The eligibility rules on assets and income differ from state to state. You should consult your local social services department to see if you are entitled to benefits. An elder care attorney could also be able to help.

The social services department in a hospital where you or your care partner have obtained treatment can advise you about your own situation and the probability of being eligible for these programs. The local agency serving the disabled usually has advisers who can refer you to programs and resources for which you may be eligible Senior centers often have counselors knowledgeable about the ins and outs of health care insurance.

If your or your care partner are a United States military veteran, check with your nearest VA facility or the VA website about services. You may be eligible for a range of services at very low or no cost.

If you or your care partner own a home, you might be able to get a reverse mortgage, whereby the bank pays you a monthly amount based on the value of your home. The nice thing about a reverse mortgage is that no matter how long you live, you can never be thrown out of your home. It is usually better to take out a reverse mortgage than to borrow against the assets you have in your house. Be sure to talk to a good financial planner who is knowledgeable about health- and aging-related issues before making any decisions; there are both risks and benefits to reverse mortgages.

I Need Help but Don't Want Help—Now What?

Let's talk about the emotional aspects of needing help. Every human being emerges from childhood reaching for and cherishing every possible sign of independence—the driver's license, the first job, the first credit card, the first time we go out and don't have to tell anybody where we are going or when we will be back, and so on. In these and many other ways, we demonstrate to ourselves as well as to others that we are "grown up"—in charge of our lives and able to take care of ourselves without any help from parents.

If a time comes when we must face the realization that we can no longer manage our own and our care partner's needs, it may seem like a return to childhood and having to let somebody else oversee our lives. This can be very painful and embarrassing.

Some people in this situation become extremely depressed and can no longer find any joy in life. Others fight off the recognition of their need for help, thus placing themselves and their care partners in possible danger and making life difficult and frustrating for those who would like to be helpful. Still others give up completely and expect others to take total responsibility for their lives, demanding attention and services from their children or other family members. If you are having one or more of these reactions, you can help yourself feel better and develop a more positive response.

The concept of "changing the things I can change, accepting the things I cannot change, and being able to know the difference" is fundamental to being able to stay in charge of our lives. You must be able to evaluate your situation accurately. You must identify the activities that require the help of somebody else (going shopping and cleaning house, for instance) and those that you can still do on your own (getting dressed, paying bills, writing letters). Another way to look at this is to get help from others for the things you least like to do, giving you the time and energy to do the things you would rather or want to do.

This means making decisions, and if you are making the decisions, you are in charge. It is important to decide and act while you are still able to do so, before circumstances intervene and the decision gets made for you and your care partner. That means being realistic and honest with yourself. Decision-making tools can be found on pages 12–14 in Chapter 2, Becoming a Better Caregiver: The Basics.

Some people find that talking with a sympathetic listener, either a professional counselor or a sensible close friend or family member, is comforting and helpful. An objective listener can often point out alternatives and options you may have overlooked or were not aware of. The person can provide information or contribute another point of view or interpretation of a situation that you would not have come upon yourself.

Be very careful, however, in evaluating advice from anyone who has something to sell you. There are many people whose solution to your problem just happens to be whatever it is they are selling—health or burial insurance policies, annuities, special and expensive furniture, "sunshine cruises," special magazines, or health foods with magical curative properties.

When talking with family members or friends who offer to be helpful, be as open and reasonable as you can and, at the same time, try to make them understand that you reserve for yourself the right to decide how much and what kind of help you will accept. They will probably be more cooperative and understanding if you say, "Yes, I do need some help with __________, but I still want to do __________ myself." More tips on asking for help can be found in Chapter 6, Communicating Effectively, and Chapter 7, Getting Help.

Asking for help does not mean giving up your right to choose and decide about issues relating to you and your care partner's lives. Insist on being consulted. Lay the ground rules with your helpers early on. Ask to be presented with choices so that you can decide what is best for you and your care partner as you see it. If you try to objectively weigh the suggestions made to you and not dismiss every option out of hand, people will see that you can make reasonable decisions and will continue to give you the opportunity to do so.

Be appreciative. Recognize the goodwill and efforts of people who want to help you and your care partner. Even though you might be embarrassed, you maintain your dignity by accepting with grace the help that is offered, if you need it. If you are truly convinced that you are being offered help you don't need, decline it with tact and appreciation. For example, you can say, "I appreciate your offer to have Thanksgiving at your house, but I'd like to continue having it here. I could really use some help, though—I will roast the turkey, but could the rest of you bring the other food and clean up after dinner?"

If you reach the point of being unable to come to terms with your increasing dependence on others, you should consult a professional counselor. Find a counselor who has experience with the emotional and social issues of people with disabling health problems and the complexities of caregiving. Your local agency providing services to the caregivers or the disabled can refer you to the right kind of counselor. The local or national organization dedicated to serving people with your care partner's specific health condition (Alzheimer's Association, Parkinson's Association, American Lung Association, American Heart Association, or American Diabetes Association, for example) and Veterans Affairs can also direct you to support groups and classes. You can locate the agency you need through the internet or telephone book Yellow Pages under the listing "social service organizations."

Akin to the fear and embarrassment of becoming physically dependent is the fear of being abandoned by family members who would be expected to provide needed help. Tales of being "dumped" in a nursing home by children who never come to visit haunt many people, who worry that this may happen to them. Your care partner might have these same fears.

We need to be sure that we do reach out to family and friends and ask for the help we need when we recognize that we can't go on alone. It sometimes happens that in expectation of rejection, people fail to ask for help. Some people try to hide their need in fear that their need will cause loved ones to withdraw. Families often complain, "If we'd only known . . . ," when it is revealed that a loved one had needs for help that were unmet. If you cannot turn to close family or friends because they are unable or unwilling to become involved, there are agencies dedicated to providing for such situations. Through your local social services department's "adult protective services" program or Family Services Association, you should be able to locate a case manager who will be able to organize the resources in your community to provide the help you need. The social services department in your local hospital can also put you in touch with the right agency.

Grieving: A Normal Reaction to Bad News

When we experience any kind of a loss—small losses (such as losing one's car keys) or big ones (such as seeing your care partner decline or losing a loved one)—we go through an emotional process of grieving and coming to terms with the loss.

Caregivers experience a variety of losses. These include loss of companionship, loss of confidence, loss of self-esteem, loss of independence, loss of the lifestyle we knew and cherished, and perhaps the most painful of all, loss of a positive self-image. Many caregivers tell us that no matter what they do, they feel they do not do enough and are not good enough.

Elizabeth Kübler-Ross, a psychiatrist who wrote extensively about this process, describes the stages of grief:

- **Shock**, when we feel both a mental and a physical reaction to the initial recognition of the loss

- **Denial**, when we think, "No, it can't be true," and proceed to act for a time as if it were not true
- **Anger**, when we fume "Why me?" and search for someone or something to blame (if the doctor had diagnosed it earlier, it is my care partner's fault because they refused to stop smoking, for example)
- **Bargaining**, when we promise, "I'll never smoke again," or "I'll follow my treatment regimen absolutely to the letter," or "I'll go to church every Sunday, if only I can get over this"
- **Depression**, when awareness sets in, we confront the truth about the situation, and experience deep feelings of sadness and hopelessness
- **Acceptance**, when we recognize that we must deal with what has happened and make up our minds to do what we must do to move forward

We do not necessarily pass through these stages in a linear fashion. We are more apt to flip-flop between them. Don't be discouraged if you find yourself angry or depressed again when you thought you had reached acceptance.

Making End-of-Life Decisions

The feelings around death can be very confusing. Our attitudes about death are shaped by our own central attitudes about life. This is the product of our culture, our family's influences, perhaps our religion, and certainly our life experiences. We might wish that our care partner be released from suffering, feel guilty for having this wish, or fear death. Sometimes we can experience several of these feelings. You are not alone. Many people try to avoid facing the future because they are afraid to think about it.

If you are ready to think about your own and your care partner's future—about the near or distant prospect that your lives will most certainly end at some time—then the ideas that follow will be useful to you. If you are not ready to think about it just yet, put this aside and come back to it later.

As with depression, the most useful way to come to terms with eventual death is to take positive steps to prepare for it. This means you must get your house in order by attending to all the necessary details, large and small. If you continue to avoid dealing with these details, you will create problems for yourself and for those involved with your situation.

It is very important that you decide and then convey to others your wishes about how and where you want your care partner to be during those last days and hours. Do you want the same thing for yourself? Do you want to be in a hospital or at home? When do you want procedures to prolong life stopped? At what point do you want to let nature take its course when it is determined that death is inevitable? Who should be with your care partner (or you)—only the few people who are nearest and dearest or all the people you care about and want to see one last time? What will happen if you can no longer give care? What will happen if your care partner cannot manage their affairs? What do you want to happen at the end of life? Most people have very definite ideas of what they would like.

Planning is hard and sometimes frightening. We do not like thinking about the "what ifs." Nevertheless, such planning is necessary for both you and your care partner. Good planning will help protect both of you.

However, if your plans are not in writing, and more importantly into legal documents, your wishes or your care partner's wishes might not be followed. The following section is a discussion of the legal documents you need to have in place. If you are not sure what you have or do not have any of these, consult a lawyer. This is not something you can do yourself. Many people fear that going to a lawyer will be very expensive. Many lawyers will allow a free meeting where you discuss your needs and the price of each service. The two documents that we discuss in the following section are relatively inexpensive to have prepared and executed.

Legal Planning

Setting out your wishes in legal documents is something you should do now, not later. If your care partner is declining mentally, an attorney will not prepare these documents for them. They are required by law to determine that the person is "of sound mind" and able to make these decisions for themselves. If you wait, you could get caught in this situation.

First, we want to state a disclaimer: **This discussion is not complete. Also, the laws are different for each state and country. For complete details, you will need to seek legal counsel. These are just the basics to prepare you for a deeper discussion.** It should also be noted that both you and your care partner need these documents.

Durable Power of Attorney (DPA)

A Durable Power of Attorney (DPA) is a document in which one person (the care partner) gives another person (the caregiver or someone else), the "attorney in fact," which is the legal authority to act on their behalf when they cannot. The authority can be limited to something specific, such as selling the house or using a specific bank account, or it can be general. The following list helps explain what a DPA is and how it can help you plan:

- A general DPA gives the person designated the power to make all legal decisions, including handling all the money as the designated person sees fit.
- A durable power of attorney is different from a simple power of attorney. A simple power of attorney is valid only if the person signing the documents can understand its meaning. A DPA, on the other hand, continues to be valid even if the person signing no longer can think or act for themselves or understands the document.
- There are two types of DPAs. Both types are valid if people cannot act on their own behalf.
  - One is legal when it is signed and stays legal if the person becomes completely incapacitated.
  - The other type is legal only when the person is incapacitated.
- A DPA can avoid the need for a *conservator.* Conservatorship involves a court hearing

where one person, the "conservatee" (care partner), is found to be unable to handle their own affairs, and another person, the "conservator" (caregiver or some other person), is appointed to handle these affairs. This is expensive and usually means going to court many times.

- A DPA is not usually used for medical care decisions. For this, there is another document—the advance health care directive. We talk about this next.

Advance Directives for Health Care

Although none of us can have absolute control over our own death, death, like the rest of our lives, is something we can help manage. That is, we can have input, make decisions, and probably add a great deal to the quality of our and our care partner's final days. Proper management can lessen the negative impact of death on our family and friends. An advance health care directive can help you manage some of the medical and legal issues concerning death as well as help you plan for both expected and unexpected end-of-life situations. Your care partner, if they are able, needs to have an advance health care directive as early as possible. Without this, your wishes as a caregiver may not be followed unless you have conservatorship.

Advance directives are written instructions that tell your doctor what kind of care you would like to receive when your care partner or you are not able to make medical decisions for yourselves (for example, if you are unconscious, in a coma, or mentally incompetent). Usually, an advance directive describes both the types of treatments you want and those you do not want.

There are different types of advance directives. The most common types are described in the following list:

- **Living will.** A living will is a document that states the kind of medical or life-sustaining treatments you or your care partner would want if you were seriously or terminally ill. A living will, however, does not let you legally appoint someone to make those decisions for you.
- **Durable power of attorney (DPA) for health care.** A durable power of attorney for health care (or more simply a power of attorney for health care) allows you or your care partner to name someone to act for you as your agent but also gives guidelines to your agent about your health care wishes. If you want, you can let your agent make the decisions. Many people, however, prefer to give guidance to their agent. This guidance can indicate almost anything you want done for your care; it may range from the use of aggressive life-sustaining measures to the withholding of these measures. Whereas a living will is good only in the case of a terminal illness, a DPA can be used anytime you are unconscious or unable to make decisions due to any illness, accident, or injury. It is important to understand that a DPA allows you to appoint someone else to act as your agent for only *your health care*. It does not give this person the right to act on your behalf in other ways, such as in handling your financial matters. In general, a DPA is more useful than a living will because it allows you to appoint someone to make decisions for you, and it can be activated at any time when you

are unable to make decisions. The only time a DPA might not be the best choice is if there is no one you trust to act on your behalf. The following section contains more detailed information on preparing a durable power of attorney (DPA) for health care.

- **Do not resuscitate (DNR) order.** A DNR is a request that you not be given cardiopulmonary resuscitation (CPR) if your heart stops or if you stop breathing. A DNR can be included as part of a living will or durable power of attorney for health care; however, you do not need to have either a living will or a DPA to have a DNR order. Your doctor can put a DNR in your medical chart so that it may guide the actions of the hospital and any health care provider. You can also post a DNR on your refrigerator or elsewhere in your home so that emergency personnel will know your wishes. Without a DNR order, hospital or emergency personnel will make every effort to resuscitate you. DNR orders are accepted in all states in the United States.
- **Advance directive for mental health care.** Although advance directives for health care are generally used for end-of-life situations, they may also be prepared to request the type of mental health treatment given in the event a person with dementia or mental illness becomes incapacitated due to that illness. Under U.S. federal law, most states may combine advance directives for health care and mental health care in one document and allow you to appoint an agent to act on your behalf for both health and mental health issues. Some states, however, require separate documents, which also allow you to choose different agents, one for health care and another for mental health care. For more information on mental health advance directives and the specific practices in your state, check the website of the National Resource Center on Psychiatric Advance Directives given at the end of this chapter.
- **Power of attorney (POA).** A general power of attorney is a document that gives someone you appoint the power to make your financial or business decisions. If you are no longer able to make these decisions and you do not have a POA in place and you need to pay for care, your family or friends, or even sometimes the state, must go to court to pay your bills. This can be very expensive. You should talk to your lawyer about the advantages and disadvantages of a POA.

Preparing a Durable Power of Attorney (DPA) for Health Care

Adults (anyone age 18 or older) should prepare a durable power of attorney (DPA) for health care. Unexpected events can happen to anyone at any age. This is a different document from a regular power of attorney. The DPA for health care applies only to health care decisions.

Although each state has different regulations and forms for advance directives, the information presented in the following pages should be useful wherever you live. Check out some of the websites at the end of this chapter for forms you can download. You can also find them at the local health department, Area Agency on Aging, hospitals, VA facilities or the offices of your health care providers.

Note that many states recognize durable powers of attorney for health care that are created in another state. However, this is not always the case. As of now, this is an unclear legal issue. To be on the safe side, if you move or spend a lot of time in another state, it is best to check with a lawyer in that state to see if your document is legally binding there.

Choosing Your Agent

To prepare a DPA, first you must choose your agent. Your agent can be a friend or family member, but it cannot be the physician who is providing your care. This person should probably live in your area. If the agent is not available on short notice to make decisions for you, the agent won't be much help. Just to be safe, you can also name a backup or secondary agent who would act for you if your primary agent were not available.

Be sure that your agent thinks like you or at least would be willing to carry out your wishes. You must be able to trust that this person has your interests at heart and truly understands and will respect your wishes. Your agent should be mature, composed, and comfortable with your wishes, and should be someone you know will be able to carry them out. Sometimes a spouse or child is not the best agent because this person is too close to you emotionally. For example, if you wish not to be resuscitated in the case of a severe heart attack, your agent must be able to tell the doctor not to resuscitate. This could be very difficult or impossible for a family member to decide then and there. Be sure the person you choose as your agent is up to this task and would not say "do everything you can" at this critical time. You want your agent to be someone who will not find this job too much of an emotional burden.

In review, look for the following characteristics in an agent:

- Someone who is likely to be available should they need to act for you
- Someone who understands your wishes and is willing to carry them out
- Someone who is emotionally prepared, able to carry out your wishes, and will not feel burdened by doing so

Finding the right agent is a significant task. This may mean talking to several people. These might be the most important interviews that you will ever conduct. We talk more about discussing your wishes with your family, friends, and doctor later in this chapter.

Expressing Your Choices

Once you have chosen your agent, spend some time thinking about your choices and determine what you want. In other words, what are your directions to your agent? What you want will be guided by your beliefs and values. Some DPA forms give several general statements of desires concerning medical treatment. These can help you decide what you want. The following are some examples of general statements:

- *I do not want my life to be prolonged and I do not want life-sustaining treatment to be provided or continued (1) if I am in an irreversible coma or persistent vegetative state, or (2) if I am terminally ill and the application of life-sustaining procedures would serve only to artificially delay the moment of my death, or (3) under any other circumstances where the burdens of the treatment outweigh the expected benefits. I want my agent to consider the relief of suffering and the quality as well as the extent of the possible extension of my life in making decisions concerning life-sustaining treatment.*

- *I want my life to be prolonged, and I want life-sustaining treatment to be provided unless I am in a coma or vegetative state that my doctor reasonably believes to be irreversible. Once my doctor has reasonably concluded that I will remain unconscious for the rest of my life, I do not want life-sustaining treatment to be provided or continued.*
- *I want my life to be prolonged to the greatest extent possible without regard to my condition, the chances I have for recovery, or the cost of the procedures.*

If you use a form containing such suggested general statements, all you need to do is initial the statement that applies to you.

Other forms make a "general statement of granted authority," in which you give your agent the power to make decisions. However, you do not have to write out the details of what these decisions should be. In this case, you are trusting that your agent will follow your wishes. Since these wishes are not explicitly written, you must discuss them in detail with your agent.

All forms also have a space in which you can write out any specific wishes. You are not required to give specific details but may wish to do so. Knowing what details to write is a little complicated. None of us can predict the future or knows the exact circumstances in which the agent will have to act. You can get some idea by asking your doctor what the most likely developments are for someone with your or your care partner's condition. Then you can direct your agent on how to act. Your directions can include outcomes, specific circumstances, or both. If you specify outcomes, the statement should focus on which types of outcomes would be acceptable and which would not (for example, "resuscitate if I can continue to fully function mentally").

The following are some of the more common specific circumstances encountered with major chronic diseases:

- **You or your care partner have been diagnosed with Alzheimer's dementia and other neurologic problems that may eventually leave you with little or no mental function.** These conditions are not generally life-threatening, at least not for many years. However, things happen if you have one of these conditions that can be life-threatening, such as pneumonia and heart attacks. You need to decide how much treatment you want. For example, do you want antibiotics if you get pneumonia? Do you want to be resuscitated if your heart stops? Do you want a feeding tube if you are unable to feed yourself? Remember, it is your choice as to how you answer each of these questions. You may not want to be resuscitated but may want a feeding tube. If you want aggressive treatment, you might want to use all means possible to sustain life; alternatively, you might not want any special means to be used to sustain life. For example, you may want to be fed but may not want to be placed on life-support equipment.

- **You or your care partner have very bad lung function that will not improve.** Should you become unable to breathe on your own, do you want to be placed in an intensive care unit on a mechanical ventilator (a breathing machine)? Remember, in this case you will not improve. To say that you never want ventilation is very different from saying that you don't want it if it is used to sustain life when no improvement is likely. Obviously, mechanical ventilation can be lifesaving in cases such as a severe asthma attack when it is used for a short time until the body can regain its normal function. Here, the issue is not whether to use mechanical ventilation ever but rather under what circumstances you wish it to be used.
- **You or your care partner have a heart condition that cannot be improved with surgery.** Imagine you are in the cardiac intensive care unit. If your heart stops functioning, do you want to be resuscitated? As with artificial ventilation, the question is not "Do you ever want to be resuscitated?" but rather "Under what conditions do you or do you not want resuscitation?"

From these examples, you can begin to identify some of the directions that you might want to give in your advance directive or durable power of attorney for health care. Again, to understand these better or to make them more personal to your own condition, talk with your physician about what the common problems and decisions are for people with these conditions.

In summary, there are several decisions you need to make in directing your agent on how to act in your behalf:

- Generally, how much treatment do you want? This can range from the very aggressive, that is, doing many things to sustain life—to the very conservative—which is doing almost nothing to sustain life, except to keep you clean and comfortable.
- Given the types of life-threatening events that are likely to happen to people with your condition, what sorts of treatment do you want and under what conditions?
- If you become mentally incapacitated, what sorts of treatment do you want for other illnesses, such as pneumonia?

Remember, although each state has different regulations and forms for advance directives, the information presented here should be useful wherever you live. Check out some of the websites at the end of this chapter for forms you can download.

While we have primarily focused on the kinds of decisions you want yourself, you should also think about the different scenarios that might happen with your care partner. Even if your care partner's wish is recorded on a document, you can prepare yourself emotionally for the time you will need to act on those decisions. Asking your care partner's physician about what is the usual course of your care partner's condition can help you think about how you would react when they happen. You will be better able to effectively direct the health care team when you have prepared yourself emotionally.

Sharing Your Wishes about End-of-Life Issues with Others

Writing down your wishes and having a durable power of attorney is not the end of the job. A good manager must do more than just write a memo. A good manager must see that the memo gets delivered. If you want your wishes carried out, you need to share them fully with your agent, family, and doctor. This is often not an easy task.

Before you can have this conversation, though, everyone involved needs to have copies of your power of attorney for health care. Once you have completed the documents, have them witnessed and signed. In some places, you can have your DPA notarized instead of having it witnessed. Make several copies. You will need copies for your agents, family members, and doctors. Also, it does not hurt to give one to your lawyer if your lawyer did not prepare them for you.

Now you are ready to talk about your wishes. People don't like to discuss their own death or that of a loved one. Therefore, it is not surprising that when you bring up this subject, the response is often, "Oh, don't think about that," or, "That's a long time off," or "Don't be so morbid; you're not that sick." Unfortunately, this is usually enough to end the conversation. Your job is to keep the conversation open. There are several ways to do this. First, plan on how you will have this discussion. Here are some suggestions:

- Prepare your durable power of attorney, and then give copies to the appropriate family members or friends. Ask them to read it and then set a specific time to discuss it. If they give you one of the avoidance responses, explain that you understand that this is a difficult topic but that you must discuss it with them. This is a good time to practice the "I" messages discussed in Chapter 6, Communicating Effectively. For example, say, "I understand that death is a difficult thing to talk about. However, it is very important to me that we have this discussion."
- Another strategy is to get blank copies of the DPA form for all your family members and suggest that you all fill them out and share them. This could even be part of a family get-together. Present this as an important aspect of being mature adults and family members. Making this a family project involving everyone may make it easier to discuss. Besides, it will help clarify everyone's values about death and dying.
- If these two suggestions seem too difficult or for some reason are impossible to carry out, you can write a letter or email or prepare a video that can then be sent to family members. Talk about why you feel your death is an important topic to discuss and that you want them to know your wishes. Then state your wishes, providing reasons for your choices. At the same time, send them a copy of your DPA for health care. Ask that they respond in some way or that you set aside some time to talk in person or on the phone.

Of course, as mentioned previously, when deciding on your agent, it is key that you choose someone with whom you can talk freely and exchange ideas. If your chosen agent is not willing to or is unable to talk to you about your wishes, you have probably chosen the wrong agent. Remember, the fact that someone is very close to you does not mean that that person understands your wishes or would be able to carry them out. This topic should not be left to an unspoken understanding unless you don't mind if your agent decides differently from what you wish. For this reason, choosing someone who is not as close to you emotionally and then talking things out with your agent are essential. This is especially true if you have not written out the details of your wishes. Making these decisions at what is an extremely emotional time can be a burden that you might not want to ask of a family member. If you do choose someone else, make sure your family knows who you have appointed and why.

Talking with Your and Your Care Partner's Doctor about End-of-Life Issues

From our research, we have learned that people often have a more difficult time talking with doctors about their wishes surrounding death than they do with their families. In fact, only a very small percentage of people who have written DPAs for health care or other advance directives ever share these with their physician.

Even though it is difficult, you should talk with both your doctor and your care partner's doctor. You need to be sure that the doctors' values are similar to yours. If you and the doctors do not have the same values, it may be difficult for them to carry out your wishes. Second, the doctors need to know what you want. This allows them to take appropriate actions such as writing orders to resuscitate or not to use mechanical resuscitation. Third, each of your doctors needs to know who your agent is and how to contact this person. If an important decision must be made and your wishes are to be followed, the doctor must talk with your agent. One last thought, your wishes for yourself and what your care partner wants or what you want for your care partner, might not be the same. This is OK, but the doctors giving care for each person must know that person's wishes and have those wishes in writing.

Be sure to give your doctor a copy of your DPA for health care so that it can become a permanent part of your medical record. The same is true for the doctor of your care partner. There is another advance directive form that is becoming more common, called a "POLST" (Physician Orders for Life-Sustaining Treatment Paradigm Form). This form is completed by you and your doctor. Many doctors introduce these forms (which is usually pink) to their patients during an appointment, and it gives both you and your physician an opportunity to discuss what could happen and what you want when it does. A POLST is added to your medical record, but does not appoint someone to act on your behalf, so a power of attorney for health care is still an important document to have.

As surprising as it may seem, many physicians also find it hard to talk to their patients about their end-of-life wishes. After all, doctors are in the business of keeping people alive and well; they don't like to think about their patients dying. On the other hand, most doctors want their patients to have durable powers of attorney for health care (and sometimes a POLST). These documents relieve both you and your doctor from pressure and worry.

If you wish, plan a time with your doctor when you can discuss your wishes. This should not be a side conversation at the end of a regular visit. Rather, start a visit by saying, "I want a few minutes to discuss my wishes in the event of a serious problem or impending death." When put this way, most doctors will make time to talk with you. If the doctor says that there is not enough time to talk, ask when you can make another appointment. This is a situation where you might need to be a little assertive. Sometimes a doctor, like your family members or friends, might say, "Oh, you don't have to worry about that; let me do it," or "We'll worry about that when the time comes." Again, you must take the initiative, using an "I" message to communicate that this is important to you and that you do not want to put off the discussion.

Sometimes doctors do not want to worry you. They think they are doing you a favor by not describing all the unpleasant things that might happen to you or the potential treatments in case of serious problems. You can help your doctor by telling them that having control and making some decisions about your future will ease your mind. Not knowing or not being clear on what will happen is more worrisome than being faced with the facts, unpleasant as they may be, and dealing with them.

Even knowing all that's been said so far, it is still sometimes hard to talk with your doctor. Therefore, it might also be helpful to bring your agent with you when you have this discussion. The agent can facilitate the discussion and at the same time make your doctor's acquaintance. This also gives everyone a chance to clarify any misunderstandings. It opens the lines of communication so that if your agent and physician have to act to carry out your wishes, they can do so with few problems. If you can't talk with your doctor, your doctor should still receive a copy of your DPA for health care for your medical record.

When you go the hospital, be sure the hospital has a copy of your DPA. If you cannot bring it, be sure your agent knows to give a copy to the hospital. This is important, as your doctor may not oversee your care in the hospital. The same is true for care partners. If your care partner goes to the hospital, the hospital must have your care partner's wishes in writing.

Do not put a durable power of attorney in a safe deposit box—no one will be able to get it when it is needed. And remember, you do not need to see a lawyer to draw up a durable power of attorney. You can do this by yourself with no legal assistance. If you are writing a DPA for your care partner, however, you probably need legal advice.

Preparing Yourself and Others

Now that you have done all the important things, the hard work is over. However, remember that you can change your mind at any time. Your agent may no longer be available, or your wishes or your care partner's might change. Be sure to keep your DPA for health care updated. Like most legal documents, it can be revoked or changed at any time. The decisions you make today do not have to be forever.

Making your wishes known about how you want to be treated in case of serious or life-threatening illness is one of the most important tasks of self-management. As we have just stated, the best way to do this is to prepare a durable power of attorney for health care and share this with your family, close friends, and physician.

Here are some other steps to help reduce the emotional burden to your care partner and/or your family:

- **Make a will.** Even if your estate is a small one, you may have definite preferences about who should inherit what. If you have a large estate, the tax implications of a proper will might be significant. A will also ensures that your belongings go where you would like them to go. Without a will, some distant or "long-lost" relative might end up with your estate. You may also want to consider a trust. Your will should include information about what you want done with your digital accounts and give directions as to who can access them and how. Do not put passwords in a will. Talk with your lawyer about these.
- **Plan your funeral and that of your care partner.** Write down your wishes or make arrangements for your funeral and burial. You and/or your grieving family will be very relieved not to have to decide what you would want and how much to spend. Prepaid funeral plans are available, and you can purchase a burial space in the location and of the type you prefer.
- **Organize your papers.** You can purchase (at any well-stocked stationery store) a kit in which you place a copy of your will, your durable powers of attorney, important papers, and information about your financial and personal affairs. Another useful source to help organize this information is "My Life in a Box." which is listed in the reading and resources section at the end of this chapter. There are forms that you fill out about bank and charge accounts, insurance policies, the location of important documents, passwords to you online accounts, your safe deposit box and where the key is kept, and so on. This is a handy, concise way of getting everything together that anyone might need to know about. Some of us keep these documents on our computers. If this is the case, be sure others can find your passwords and accounts.
- **Finish your dealings with the world around you.** Mend your relationships. Pay your debts, both financial and personal. Say what needs to be said to those who need to hear it. Do what needs to be done. Forgive yourself.

Forgive others. (By the way, this is a good idea at any time, not just at end of life.)

- **Talk about your feelings about death.** Most family and close friends are reluctant to initiate such a conversation but will appreciate it if you bring it up. You may find that there is much to say to and to hear from your loved ones. If you find that they are unwilling to listen to you talk about your death and the feelings that you are experiencing, find someone who will be comfortable and empathetic in listening to you. Most hospitals and hospice services have chaplains who hold these conversations daily. You may find one helpful. Your family and friends might be able to listen to you later. Remember, those who love you will also go through the stages of grieving when they think about the prospect of losing you.

A large component in the fear of death is fear of the unknown: "What will it be like?" "Will it be painful?" "What will happen after death?" Most people who die of a disease are ready to die when the time comes. Painkillers and the disease process itself weaken body and mind, and the awareness of self diminishes without the realization that this is happening. Most people just "slip away," with the transition between the state of living and that of no longer living hardly identifiable. Reports from people who have been brought back to life after being in a state of clinical death indicate they experienced a sense of peacefulness and clarity and were not frightened.

A dying person could sometimes feel lonely and abandoned. Regrettably, many people cannot deal with their own emotions when they are around a person they know to be dying and so deliberately avoid a dying person's company, or they may engage in superficial chitchat, broken by long, awkward silences. This is often puzzling and hurtful to those who are dying, and for you, the caregiver, who are seeking companionship and solace from the people they count on.

You can sometimes help by telling your family and friends what you want and need from them—attention, entertainment, comfort, practical help, and so on. Again, a person who has something positive to do is more able to cope with difficult emotions. If you can engage your family and loved ones in specific activities, they can feel needed and can relate to you around the activity. This will give you something to talk about, to occupy time, or at least provide a definition of the situation for them and for you.

Considering Palliative Care and Hospice Care

In most parts of the United States, as well as in many other parts of the world, both palliative care and hospice care are available. The goal of both palliative care and hospice care is to provide comfort. Palliative care can begin at diagnosis and occur at the same time as treatment. Hospice care begins after treatment of the disease is stopped, when it is clear the illness will not be survived. In everyone's life. there comes a time when regular medical care is no longer helpful and we need to prepare for death. Today, we often have several weeks or months, and sometimes years, to make these preparations. This is when hospice care is so very useful. In hospice, medical and other care is aimed at making the patient as comfortable as possible and providing a good quality of life. Recently, we have learned that at least for some diseases, people who receive hospice care live longer than those who receive more aggressive treatment. Most hospices only accept people who are expected to die within six months. This does not mean that you or your care partner will be thrown out if you live longer.

At the same time, they make the patient more comfortable, hospice professionals help both the patient and the family prepare for death with dignity and help the surviving family members. Today, most hospices are "in-home" programs. This means that patients stay in their own homes and the services come to them. In some places, there are also residential hospices where people can go for their last days. Skilled nursing facilities often bring in hospice as well, and they oversee the comfort for the last days, for both the person and for the family. Hospices usually include support services for the family, which can extend after the death of loved ones.

One of the problems with hospice care is that often people wait until the last few days before death to ask for this care. They somehow see asking for hospice care as "giving up." By refusing hospice care, they often put an unnecessary burden on themselves, friends, and family. The reverse is also often true. The caregiver or family might say they can cope without help. This may be true, but you or your care partner's life and dying may be much better if hospice cares for all the medical things so that loved ones are free to give love and support.

It is important to recognize that if your care partner, you, a family member, or a friend is in the end stage of illness, you should find and make use of your local hospice. It is a wonderful final gift. Hospice workers are very special people who are kind, thoughtful, and supportive. An added benefit of hospice care is that many services are paid for that are not covered by regular insurance or Medicare.

In closing, we would like to thank you for choosing to be a caregiver. We have tried to give you some tips and tools to make this easier. We truly believe that all caregivers are doing the best they can. If we have forgotten something, or if there is something you would like to share, please feel free to contact us.

Suggested Further Reading

Atkinson, Jacqueline M. *Advance Directives in Mental Health: Theory, Practice and Ethics.* London: Jessica Kingsley Publishers, 2007.

Cullen, Melanie, and Shae Irving. *Get It Together: Organize Your Records So Your Family Won't Have To.* Berkeley, CA: Nolo, 2016.

Provides a complete system for structuring and organizing your information and documents into a records binder, including helpful content, rich resources, and step-by-step instructions as well as downloadable forms. http://amzn.to/2Hvnfx0

Doukas, David John, and William Reichel. *Planning for Uncertainty: Living Wills and Other Advance Directives for You and Your Family,* 2nd ed. Baltimore: John Hopkins University Press, 2007.

Godkin, M. Dianne. *Living Will, Living Well: Reflections on Preparing an Advance Directive.* Edmonton: University of Alberta Press, 2008.

Kübler-Ross, Elizabeth. *On Death and Dying.* New York: Simon & Schuster, 2011.

Kurz, Gary. *Cold Noses at the Pearly Gates: A Book of Hope for Those Who Have Lost a Pet.* New York: Citadel Press, 2008.

Long, Laurie Ecklund. *My Life in a Box: A Life Organizer: How to Build an Emergency Tool Box,* 4th ed. Fresno, CA: AGL, 2010.

Pettus, Mark C. *The Savvy Patient: The Ultimate Advocate for Quality Health Care.* Sterling, VA: Capital Books, 2004.

Rosen, Harris N. *My Family Record Book: The Easy Way to Organize Personal Information,*

Financial Plans, and Final Wishes for Seniors, Caregivers, Estate Executors, Etc. S.l.: Harris N. Rosen Books, 2015. A complete step-by-step guide that will help you keep track of and organize final wishes and arrangements, computer information and passwords, estate planning documents, employment records, insurance policies, tax records, retirement accounts, government benefits, real estate records, house maintenance, and more. http://amzn.to/2EC10Uh

Saavedra, Mary Jo, Susan Cain McCarty, Theresa Giddings, Lawrence Hansen, Benjamin B.

Hellickson, Joyce Sjoberg, Sara K. Yen, and Ruth Matinko-Wald. *Eldercare 101: A Practical Guide to Later Life Planning, Care, and Well-Being.* Lanham, MD: Rowman & Littlefield, 2016. An easy-to-understand guide for families in need of help as they care for their aging loved ones, organized into "six pillars of aging well-being": legal, financial, living environment, social, medical, and spiritual. http://amzn.to/2sDZTSd

Sitarz, Daniel. *Advance Health Care Directives Simplified.* Carbondale, IL: Nova, 2007.

Stolp, Hans. *When a Loved One Dies: How to Go on After Saying Goodbye.* Hampshire, England: O Books, 2005.

Other Resources

AARP. https://www.aarp.org/caregiving/financial-legal/free-printable-advance-directives

Benefits Check Up. http://www.benefitscheckup.org

Five Wishes (Aging with Dignity). http://www.agingwithdignity.org

Growth House, Improving Care for Dying. http://www.growthhouse.org

Leading Age (homes for the aged). http://www.leadingage.org

My Life in a Box: A Life Organizer. http://mylifeinabox.com

National Council on Aging. http://www.ncoa.org

National Council on Aging Use Your Home to Stay at Home. https://www.ncoa.org/economic-security/home-equity/housing-options/use-your-home-to-stay-at-home

National Hospice and Palliative Care Organization. http://www.caringinfo.org

National POLST Paradigm. http://polst.org

National Resource Center on Psychiatric Advance Directives. http://www.nrc-pad.org

U. S. Department of Housing and Urban Development: "Frequently Asked Questions about HUD's Reverse Mortgages." https://www.hud.gov/program_offices/housing/sfh/hecm/rmtopten

U. S. Department of Veterans Affairs. https://www.va.gov/vso/

Index

Note: Page numbers followed by *f* or *t* indicate a figure or table

Academy of Cognitive Therapy, 34, 37
Academy of Nutrition and Dietetics, 193
Acceptance, 37, 44, 61, 244
Acting out, 29
Action plans
  carrying out, checking results, 20
  elements for success, 19
  My Action Plan, 22
  realistic plans, 17–19
  short-term plans, 16–17
Activities of daily living (ADLs)
  description, 17, 109
  helping care partner with, 109
  mindfulness and, 64
  self-evaluation related to, 238
  traumatic brain injury and, 206
ADA. *See* American Diabetes Association
Adaptive thinking, 39–40
Adult daycare, 104
Adult Protective Services, 33
Advance directives
  DNR order, 247
  DPA for health care, 245–254
  living will, 246, 247
  for mental health care, 247
Aerobic, low-impact exercise, 113
Aggrenox (dipyridamole), 202
AgingCare.com, 142, 167, 193, 230
Agingpro, online directory, 106
AIDS-related dementia, 198
Alcohol
  alcohol abuse, 32–33, 228
  interactions with medications, 204, 222, 228
  prescription labels and, 223
  PTSD and, 209
  traumatic brain injury and, 206
Alcohol abuse, 32–33
Alcoholics Anonymous, 44
Alpha-adrenergic receptor blockers, 210
Alzheimer's Association, 11, 33–34, 39, 45, 99, 106
Alzheimer's dementia
  caregiving in, 3–4
  impaired cognition and, 44
  "sundowning" effect in, 44–45
  symptoms, 196–197
Amantadine, 205

American Association of Retired Persons (AARP), 47, 99, 143, 258
American Cancer Society, 193
American Diabetes Association (ADA), 186*f*, 193
American Heart Association, 99, 193
American Stroke Association, 44, 212
Americans with Disabilities Act (ADA), 136
Amitriptyline, 207
Angiotensin-converting enzyme (ACE) inhibitors, 202
Anticoagulant medications, 202
Anticonvulsant medications, 207
Antidepressant medications
- depression and, 203–204
- Parkinson's related-diseases and, 45, 205
- PTSD and, 210
- TBI and, 207

Antihypertensive medications, 202, 216
Antioxidants, 200
Antiplatelet medications, 202
Antipsychotic medications
- dementia and, 45, 200
- Parkinson's disease, psychosis, and, 205
- PTSD and, 210
- traumatic brain injury and, 207–208

Anxiety and Depression Association of America, 212
Apixaban (Eliquis), 202
Area Agencies on Aging (AAA), 15, 98, 212
Arm and leg exercises, 150–152
Aspirin, 86, 200, 202, 219, 222
Assisted living facilities, 105, 106, 238–239
Association for Frontotemporal Dementia, 212
Association of Cancer Online Resources (ACOR), 106
Atorvastatin, 203

Back exercises, 147–150
Balance exercises, 156–159
Banner Beacon Newsletters, 212
Behavior diary, 32
Behavior of care partners
- causes/triggers of, 4, 17
- frustrations caused by, 3, 14
- stress cycle and, 3, 18, 26

Benefits Check Up, 258
Benson, Herbert, 52–53
Benzodiazepines, 210
Beta blockers, 202
Better Health Channel, 235
Blaming communication, 73, 74, 76, 208
Board and care homes, 106
Body-scan script, 53
Boredom, difficult behavior and, 28–29
Brain, 195–210. *See also* cognitive abilities; traumatic brain injury
- eating, nutrition, and, 170, 173–175, 177
- imagination *vs.* reality, 58
- injuries, 28, 44
- loss of cognitive functions, 37
- scheduling worry time, 65

Brainstorming, 65, 126, 127
Breath/breathing
- body scan script and, 53
- Do Not Resuscitate order and, 247
- exercising and, 149, 152, 155, 160
- guided imagery and, 59, 62
- mindful breathing, 63–64
- nutrition, indigestion, and, 191
- relaxation breathing, 17
- stress and, 3, 26–27, 50
- thoughtful breathing, 26–27

Broken record method, of communication, 43–44

Calcium channel blockers, 202
Carbamazepine, 207
Carbidopa, 204, 205
Caregiver.com, 106
Caregiver Network, 235
Caregiver's Toolbox, 2, 7, 11, 12
CaringBridge, 106
Caring.com, 8
CaringInfo, 8, 235
Catechol-o-methyltransferase (COMT) inhibitors, 205
Catholic Family Services, 15, 99
CBT. *See* cognitive behavioral therapy
Center for Advancing Health, 106
Center for Science in the Public Interest, 193
Centers for Disease Control and Prevention (CDC), 106, 142
Certified aging in place specialist (CAPS), 136
Changes (personal changes)
- of caregivers, 9
- decision-making and, 12
- overcoming obstacles and, 20

priority-setting and, 13
problem-solving and, 15, 18
self-rewards and, 21
studies of, 20
Children, communicating with, 91
Cholesterol
absence of, in plant foods, 180
fiber and, 177
good fats and, 178
healthy eating and, 170, 187
heart disease, stroke, and, 187, 201–202
nutrition label information, 184
statin medications for, 202–203
Cholinesterase inhibitors, 199
ChooseMyPlate.gov, 176, 193
Citalopram, 207
Clopidogrel (Plavix), 202
Cognitive abilities
adaptations for loss of, 138, 139
cause of impairment of, 44
cholinesterase inhibitors and, 199
communication issues and, 73
medication and, 228
mind power and, 50
social skills and, 37
stroke and, 201
traumatic brain injury and, 206
Cognitive behavioral therapy (CBT)
for depression, 36–37
for PTSD, 209
Communication/effective communication, 71–91
asking for information, saying no, 79
asking questions, 80–81
blaming and, 73, 74, 76
body language, 72, 79, 82
broken record tool, 43–44
with care partners, 28, 71–91
conversational styles, 82
frustration and, 71
"I" messages, 75–76, 251
ineffective, consequences of, 71
listening skills, 74, 79–80
minimizing conflict, 76–77
paraphrasing, 81
receiving/giving help, 78–79
stress and, 3, 18, 71
thoughtful communication, 72–74
with young children, 91
Communication with health care team, 82–91
asking, 85
clarifying communication, 90–91
positive feedback, 87
preparing for, 84–85
repeating, 85–86
second opinions, 86
sharing medical decisions, 87
taking action, 86
working within health care system, 87–90
Community resources, 96–102
family meetings, 97
Internet, 100–102
libraries, 99–100
newspapers, 100
organizations, referral services, 98–99
social media, networking, 5, 101–102, 231, 232
voluntary agencies, 99
Complementary and Integrative Health Center (NIH), 234
Conflict, strategies for minimizing, 76–77
ConsumerLab, 230
Continuing care communities (CCRC), 105–106
Control
facing the facts and, 43
in guided imagery, 58
improved health and, 18
letting go of, 44
positive thinking, self-talk, and, 56
stress management and, 49
success and, 6, 18
uncertainty and loss of, 12
Coping with caregiving, 5
Coumadin (warfarin), 202
Council of Churches, 99
Counseling, 16, 20, 207
Create Your Plate eating plan (ADA), 186*f*, 193

Dabigatran (Pradaxa), 202
Daily Strength, online support communities, 106
Dangerous behaviors of care partners, 32–34
support system help for, 33–34
triggers of, 17
Decision-making
assumptions as enemies of, 16
examples/keeping score charts, 13–14
shared decision-making, 104
steps, 12–13

Dementia. *See also* Alzheimer's dementia
adult daycare and, 104
AIDS/HIV-associated, 198
children's understanding of, 91
description, 196
difficult behavior and, 28
frontotemporal dementia, 198
Lewy body dementia, 197–198
medications/treatments, 199–200
memory and, 196
mixed dementia, 198
NMDA receptor antagonists, 200
NMDA receptor antagonists, 200
Parkinson-related, 45
sundowning in, 45
Depression
in caregivers, 36
challenges created by, 36
in Parkinson's related dementia, 45
stress compared with, 36
treatment approaches, 36–37
Diabetes
absence of symptoms, 224
breakfast and, 174
Create Your Plate plan, 176, 186
dementia and, 196
healthful eating and, 170–171, 183, 186–187
risk factors with, 187
Difficult behaviors, strategies for managing, 27–32
causes/triggers of, 27–29
changing reactions to, 30–31
eliminating triggers, 30, 32
identifying steps leading to, 29–30, 32
naming of, 27–28
self-evaluation of progress, 31–32
Difficult emotions, of caregivers, 38–44
adaptive thinking strategy, 39–40
dealing with peer pressure, 43–44
establishing priorities, 40–42
facing the facts, 42–43
giving up control, 44
identifying/management of, 38–39
Difficult emotions of care partners, 44–46
Dipyridamole (Aggrenox), 202
Discussion groups, on the Internet, 102
Distraction techniques, 54–55
Diuretics, 202
Do Not Resuscitate (DNR) order, 247
Doomsayers, 43
Dopamine agonists, 205
DPA. *See* Durable Power of Attorney
Drug abuse, 32–33, 209, 229
Durable Power of Attorney (DPA), 245–254

Eating. *See also* healthful eating; nutrients; overeating
action planning and, 18
activities of daily living and, 17, 109
avoiding overeating, 17
avoiding spills, 135
avoiding spoiled foods, 139
care partner demands and, 126
food labels, 184
long-term conditions and, 183–188
mindful eating, 64, 175, 189
personal preferences, 169
speech therapy and, 139–140
tools related to, 135
Eldercare Locator, 106
Eldercare Locator Nationwide, 212
Electronic support groups, 5
Eliquis (apixaban), 202
Embarrassment
of caregivers, 37, 67
of care partners, 243
Emotions. *See also* difficult emotions
attitudes/thoughts, links with, 49–50
of difficult care partners, 44–46
"I" messages and, 75
stress's impact on, 66
End-of-life issues and decisions, 244–250
DPA for health care, 245–254
forgiveness of self, others, 254–255
funeral planning, 254
hospice care, 8, 63, 255–256
legal planning, 245–247
palliative care, 255–256
sharing wishes with others, 251–253
talking about feelings about death, 255
talking with doctors, care partners, 253–254
will preparation, 254
Endurance exercises, 159–163
stationary bicycling, 162–163
swimming, 162
walking, 160–162
Evidence-Based Leadership Council, 142

Exercise/exercise programs, 145–166
in adult day care centers, 104
aerobic, low-impact, 113
for arms and legs, 150–152
for balance, 156–159
benefits of, 146–147
for better posture, 152–153
for body pain reduction, 140
with care partners, 163–164
developing/sticking with, 165–166
for endurance, 159–163
for falling prevention, 112*t*, 113, 115, 140
for flexibility, 147–152
inactivity consequences *vs.*, 112
for leg strength, 154–156
for low back pain, 112–113
national senior programs, 115
for neck and back, 147–150
overcoming barriers to, 164–165
positive impact of, 111
for reducing injury risks, 111–115
relaxation exercises, 15, 17–18, 52
types of classes, 163

Facebook, 5, 101–102
FaceTime, 5
Falling/fall risk reduction, 42, 110, 113–115, 128, 132*t*, 134*t*, 137, 139, 140, 141
Family Caregiver Alliance, 8, 107, 142, 212
Family meetings, 5, 94–96
Flexibility exercises
arm and leg, 150–152
neck and back, 147–150
whole-body stretcher, 147
Food. *See also* eating; healthful eating; nutrients
action planning and, 18
as behavior trigger, 29
depression and, 36
mindfulness and, 64
overeating, 17, 18, 38
spills, 135
spoiled foods, 139
Frontotemporal dementia (FTD), 198
Future planning, 237–256
end-of-life issues, decisions, 244–256
physical day-to-day living needs, 238–239

Gabapentin, 207
Goals and goal setting, 14–21. *See also* action plans
evaluating successes, 19
exploring options, 15–16
midcourse corrections, 20
self-rewards, 20–21
tools for, 6, 11
Google+, 101
Grab bars, in bathrooms, 136
Guided imagery
description, 58–59
for fatigue, 60–61
for pain, depression, 61
for tension, stress, 60
Walk in the Country script, 59
Walk on the Beach script, 62
Guilty feelings (of caregivers), 5, 36

Harvard School of Public Health, 193
HealthCentral, 107
Healthful eating, 169–193. *See also* eating; nutrients
amount/portion control, 174–176
benefits/importance of, 146, 170
breakfasts, 174
challenges and choices, 188–192
Choose My Plate guidelines, 176
description, 170–171
diabetes and, 183, 186–187
guidelines, 182
heart disease and, 187
lung disease and, 187–188
nutrients, 176–183
nutrition facts labels, 184
osteoporosis and, 188
principles, 172–174
stroke and, 187
vitamins and minerals, 180–183
Heart disease
dementia and, 196
diabetes and, 183, 186, 187
fats, cholesterol, and, 178, 184
healthful eating and, 170, 187
sodium and, 180
strokes and, 187
Help, seeking and getting
action planning and, 16–19
adaptive thinking and, 39–40
adult daycare, 104
asking for and accepting, 78–79

Help, seeking and getting (*continued*)
community resources, 96–102
for dangerous care partners, 32–34
decision-making and, 12, 13–14
emotions/feelings and, 38
family meetings, 94–96
friends/family, challenges of, 5
getting, 78, 79, 93–106
giving, 78, 79
in-home care, 102–104
letting go and, 44
peer pressure and, 43
receiving and giving, 78–79
resources for, 8, 10
seeking, 10–11, 15, 30, 36, 93–106
self-help groups, 20
stress management and, 50–52, 54, 60–63
thoughtful communication and, 72–73
HIV-associated dementia, 198
Hormones
regulatory functions of, 179, 183, 216, 218
thoughts as triggers of, 49–50
Hospice care, 8, 63, 255–256
Hypertension (high blood pressure)
alcohol use and, 228
medications/treatments for, 202
placebos and, 217
sodium and, 180

"I" messages, 75–76, 251
In-home care, 102–104
Injury prevention, 109–144
adaptive devices for, 128, 135–139, 135*f*
bathroom grab bars, 136
body mechanics, 115–117, 118
communication and, 124, 125
environment cues for, 138
exercise, physical activity, and, 111–115
fall risk reduction, 42, 110, 113–115, 128, 132*t*, 134*t*, 137, 139, 140, 141
getting into bed, 119–120
getting out of bed, 120–212
getting up from floor, 122–123
health professional guidance for, 139–140
low back pain, 112–113
mindful movement practice, 127–128
mobility aids, prevention tips, 128, 129*t*–131*t*
music, nature, and, 126
reducing injury risks, 111–117
risk assessment exercise, 112
risk factors for injury, 109–110
self-care needs, priorities, 125–126
sharing activities, 127
sitting posture, 117*f*
sitting to standing, 119
special equipment, 132*t*–134*t*
standing posture, 116*f*
swinging away wheelchair leg rests, 123
teamwork for, 124–127
transfer (changing positions) postures, 117–118, 121, 123
unintentional injury cycle, 110–111
Instagram, 5, 101
International Food Information Council Foundation, 193
Internet, 10–11, 100–102
Ischemic strokes, 201, 202–203
Isolation
failure to communicate and, 71
help in overcoming, 2, 5
inactivity as cause of, 156
trauma, PTSD, and, 209

Jewish Family Services, 15, 99
Journaling, 39

Legal planning, end-of-life
Do Not Resuscitate order, 247
DPA for health care, 245–254
living will, 246, 247
Leg strengthening exercises, 154–156
Levodopa, 204, 205
Lewy body dementia (LBD), 197–198
Libraries, 100
Live-in care, 103
Lovastatin, 203
Lung disease
exercise and, 160
healthful eating and, 187–188

A Matter of Balance, fall prevention program, 115, 142
Mayo Clinic, 107
Meals on Wheels, 98

Medical alert systems, 143
Medications. *See also* specific medications
alcohol's interactions with, 204, 222, 228
allergic reactions, 220
alternative/generic versions, 222–223
communication with doctors, 219–223
for dementia, 199–200
for depression, 36, 203–204
dosages/length of time, 221
effects/purposes of, 217–218
getting care partners to take, 226
for hypertension, 202
multiple medication issues, 218–219
opioids, 228–229
OTC (over-the-counter), 204, 218, 226–227
for Parkinson's-related diseases, 45, 204–205
pharmacists as resources, 224
placebos, 217, 221
positive expectation toward, 217–218
for posttraumatic stress disorder, 209–210
for PTSD, 210
reading prescription labels, 223
remembering to take, 224–226
self-medicating, 226–229
side effects of, 216–217, 222
source reliability, 234
for strokes, 201–203, 202
for traumatic brain injury, 207
treatment decisions, 232–233
types of, 218
Medline Plus, 107
Memantine, 200
Memorial Sloan-Kettering Cancer Center, 107
Memory. *See also* cognitive abilities; dementia
Alzheimer's disease and, 4, 197
gratitude and, 66
HIV/AIDS and, 198
impaired cognition and, 44
Lewy body disease and, 197–198
medication side effects and, 220
mindfulness practices and, 63
music's effect on, 126
nature walks and, 126
responses triggered by, 50
Midcourse corrections, 20
Mind
body, stress, and, 49–51
distraction techniques, 54–55
positive thinking, self-talk, 56–57
stress management and, 49–68
Mindfulness
application to ADLs, 64
defined, 64
mindful eating, 64, 175, 189
mindful movement, 127–128
Monoamine oxidase B (MAO-B) inhibitors, 204
Moving Easy and Exercise for Chronic Conditions, CDs, 167
MyPlate website (USDA), 176

National Alzheimer's Association, 212–213
National Association of Area Agencies on Aging, 142
National Cancer Institute, 107
National Caregivers Library, 235
National Center for Complementary and Integrated Health (NCCIH), 230
National Center for PTSD, 213
National Council on Aging, 143, 258
National Hospice and Palliative Care Organization, 8, 258
National Institute of Neurological Disorders and Stroke (NINDS), 213
National Institutes of Health (NIH), 107, 230, 233
National Library of Medicine, 107
National POLST Paradigm, 258
National Resource Center on Psychiatric Advance Directives, 247, 258
National Volunteer Caregiving Network (NVCN), 8
Natural Medicines Comprehensive Database, 230
Nature therapy, 64
Neck and back exercises, 147–150
Newsletters for caregivers, 5
Newspapers, 100
N-methyl-D-aspartate (NMDA) receptor antagonists, 200
Numbing, defined, 45
Nursing homes, 105
Nutrients, 176–183. *See also* eating; healthful eating
calcium, 173, 176, 180, 181–182, 188, 202
carbohydrates, 177, 178, 179, 183, 185
fiber, 146, 172, 177, 178, 180, 185, 187, 192
nutrition facts labels, 184
oils, solid fats, 177–178, 179

Nutrients (*continued*)
potassium, 180, 181, 185
protein, 146, 176, 179–180, 182, 183, 184
sodium, 171, 180–181, 185, 187, 189, 192
vitamins, minerals, 180–183
water, 182–183

Olanzapine, 207
Online support groups, 4, 5, 8, 102, 106
Opioids, 228–229
Organizations, referral services, 98–99
Osteoporosis, 173, 188
Otago Exercise Program, 142
Overeating
depression and, 36
management of, 174–175, 178, 186–187
stress and, 17, 18
Over-the-counter (OTC) medications, 204, 218, 226–227

Palliative care, 255–256
Parkinson's disease
effects of, 203–204
impaired cognition and, 44
Lewy body dementia comparison, 198
medications/treatments, 204–205
psychosis and, 205
Parkinson's Foundation, 99, 107
Parkinson's-related dementia, 45
Paroxetine, 207, 210
Partnership for Healthy Aging, 143
PatientsLikeMe, 107
Peer pressure, 43–44
Personal care assistant, 103
Physical therapy, 124–125, 139, 140
Physician Order for Life-Sustaining Treatment Paradigm Form (POLST), 252–253
PictureRX, 230
Pinterest, 101
Plavix (clopidogrel), 202
Positive thinking, 4, 56–57
Posttraumatic stress disorder (PTSD)
diagnosis, 208
emotional difficulties in, 45
impaired cognition and, 44
medications, 209–210
treatments, 208–209
Posture-related exercises, 152–153
Pradaxa (dabigatran), 202
Pramipexole, 205
Pravastatin, 203
Prayer
health and, 61, 63
serenity prayer, 44
Prazosin, 210
Prescription labels, medication, 223
Problem-solving
action plan and, 19
assumptions as enemies of, 16
midcourse corrections, 20
seeking help with, 15, 98
speech therapy and, 140
steps, 10–12, 27, 238–239
Psych Central, 107
Psychotherapy
for depression, 36
for PTSD, 45
PTSD. *See* posttraumatic stress disorder
PubMed Health, 230

QuackWatch, 107
Quetiapine, 207
Quieting reflex technique, 64

Reddit, 101
Registries (referral services), 103–104
Relapses, 20
Relaxation response, 52–53
Relaxation techniques. *See also* mindfulness
body scan, 52, 53
quick/easy methods, 51–52
relaxation response, 52, 54
Respite care, 103
Risperidone, 207
Rivaroxaban (Xarelto), 202
Ropinirole, 205
Rosuvastatin, 203

Second generation antipsychotics (SGAs), 210
Selective serotonin reuptake inhibitors (SSRIs), 210
Selegiline, 204
Self-confidence, 20
Self-help groups, 20
Self-rewarding, 20–21
Self-talk, 56–57
Senior List, 8
Senior living communities, 104–106
Serenity prayer, 44

Serotonin-norepinephrine reuptake inhibitors (SNRIs), 210
Sertraline, 207, 210
Silver Sneakers program, 167
Simvastatin 203
Sit and Be Fit classes, 167
Skilled nursing homes, 105, 238
Skype, 5
Smart Patients, online group, 102
Snapchat, 101
Social media, 5, 231, 232
Social networking sites, 101–102. *See also* specific social networking sites
Sodium valproate, 207
Spirituality, 61, 63
Statins, 202–203
Stay Active and Independent for Life (SAIL) program, 115, 142
Stepping On, fall prevention program, 115, 142
Steps in problem-solving, 10–12
Strength exercise
  for better posture, 152–153
  for legs, 154–156
Strengths inventory, 66
Stress
  caregiving and, 3–4
  causes of, 50
  consequences of, 25
  depression comparison, 36
  emotional reactions to, 3, 66
  identification of, 26
  ineffective communication and, 71
  management strategies, 4, 17, 18, 27
  mind, body, and, 49–51
  overeating and, 17, 18
  Selye's definition of, 3
  uncertainty and, 12
Stress cycle, 3, 27
Stress management
  action plans, 17–19
  body-scan script, 53
  change of perspective, 65
  distraction techniques, 54–55
  gratitude practices, 65–66
  guided imagery, 58–59
  key principles, 50–51
  kindness practice, 66
  mind and, 49–68
  mindfulness, 63–64
  nature therapy, 64
  positive thinking, self-talk, 56–57
  prayer/spirituality, 61, 63
  "quieting reflex" technique, 64
  relaxation techniques, 51–54
  strengths inventory, 66
  support groups, 4
  thoughtful breathing, 27
  worry time technique, 64–65
  writing away stress, 66–68
Stroebel, Charles, 64
Strokes (CVAs, cerebrovascular events)
  cognitive impact of, 44
  dementia and, 198
  description/effects of, 201
  diabetes and, 187
  emotional swings in, 45
  health eating and, 187
  healthful eating and, 187
  impaired cognition and, 44
  ischemic strokes, 201, 202–203
  medications/treatments, 201–203
  mobility aids/injury prevention tips, 130*t*
  mobility-related aids, 130*t*
  sodium and, 180
Substance abuse
  alcohol, 32–33, 228
  drugs, 32–33, 209, 229
Success strategies, 5–6
"Sundowning" effect, 44–45
Support groups
  online groups, 4, 5, 69, 106, 107
  for stress management, 4
  for TBI sufferers, 207

Tai Chi for Arthritis program, 115, 142
Tai Ji Quan: Moving for Better Balance program, 115, 142
TBI. *See* traumatic brain injury
Thoughtful breathing, 27
Thoughtful communication, 72–74
Thoughts, as trigger of hormones, 49–50
Time management, 5
Today's Caregiver, 8
Topiramate, 207
Traumatic brain injury (TBI)
  caregiving for care partners with, 45–46

Traumatic brain injury (TBI) (*continued*)
  description, 206
  effects of, 206–207
  emotional difficulties in, 45–46
  impaired cognition and, 44
  medications/treatments, 207–208
Treatment decisions, 231–235
Triggers
  identification of, 27
  in PTSD, 209
  strategies for dealing with, 30–32, 45, 46
  sundowning and, 45
  types of, 29, 50, 58, 205, 217
Tumblr, 101
Twitter, 101

Uncertainty
  body language and, 82
  doomsayers and, 43
  living with, 11, 12
Ups and downs, 6
U.S. Administration on Aging, 106
U.S. Department of Agriculture, 176
U.S. Department of Veterans Affairs, 258
U.S. Department on Housing and Urban Development, 258

VA Caregiver Support, 142
Vascular dementia, 198
Veterans Administration (VA), 34, 99
Video chatting, 5
Violence in the home, 10
Visualization, 60
Vitamins and minerals, 180–182

Warfarin (Coumadin), 202
WebMD, 107, 230
Well Spouse Association, 8
Whole-body stretcher (exercise), 147
Worry time technique, 64–65
Writing away stress, 66–68

Xarelto (rivaroxaban), 202